CONSTRUCTING DEAFNESS

Edited by Susan Gregory and Gillian M. Hartley

at The Open University

PINTER PUBLISHERS IN ASSOCIATION WITH THE OPEN UNIVERSITY

Open University 'Issues in Deafness' Course Team

Lorna Allsop, Juliet Bishop, Laraine Callow, Tim Dant, Anne Darby, Mary Fielder, Vic Finkelstein, Susan Gregory, Gerald Hales, Fiona Harris, Gillian Hartley, Lynne Hawcroft, Yvonne Holmes, Linda Janes, Mary John, Jim Kyle, Paddy Ladd, Carlo Laurenzi, Clive Mason, Rukhsana Meherali, Dorothy Miles, Bob Peckford, Christine Player, Sharon Ridgeway, Janice Silo, George Taylor

This Reader forms part of the Open University course *Issues in Deafness (D251)*. For further information about this course, please write to the Student Enquiries Office, The Open University, PO Box 71, Milton Keynes MK7 6AG.

Published in Great Britain by
Pinter Publishers Limited
25 Floral Street, London WC2E 9DS
in association with
The Open University
Walton Hall
Milton Keynes MK7 6AB

British Library Cataloguing in Publication Data

Constructing deafness.
1. Man. Deafness – Sociological perspectives
I. Gregory, Susan, *1945– Jan. 18–* II. Hartley, Gillian M.
III. Open University
305.908162

ISBN 0–86187–057–3
ISBN 0–86187–056–5 pbk

Grateful acknowledgement is made to Trevor Landell for permission to use his painting on the cover of this book.

This reader is one part of an Open University course and the selection is therefore related to other material available to students. Opinions expressed in it are not necessarily those of the course team or of the University.

Typeset by Medcalf Type, Bicester
Printed in Great Britain by Redwood Books, Trowbridge, Wiltshire

Contents

Preface

This book is about deafness as it affects prelingually profoundly deaf people in the United Kingdom. It is not about partially hearing people or about hearing loss that develops later in life. It is a book edited by hearing people and the discourses with which we are concerned belong to the public domain of the hearing world. We believe that a truly deaf construction of deafness would be possible only in the language of deaf people. Deaf authors have written on a number of the issues addressed in this book and we have included extracts from their work. The deaf authors have, however, been constrained by the language they have been forced to adopt. In attempting to influence dominant ideologies of deafness, they have been compelled to operate within already established conceptual frameworks. The political situation of deaf people in hearing society at present means that hearing perspectives of deafness impinge on many areas of their lives. Thus Jacobs (1974) writes, 'I felt more handicapped from the treatment I received at the hands of hearing people than from my deafness' (p. 99).

Our aim within this book has been to indicate the perspectives within which discourses defining deafness have arisen, and to illustrate how the very definitions of deafness, and what it is to be deaf, have been socially constructed. The book illustrates current debates and those of the recent historical past by bringing together previously published material from disparate sources, and specially commissioned articles. An underlying theme is the power of different definitions of deafness, either explicit or implicit, in constraining the scope of particular debates and in influencing participants' views. It suggests how recent challenges to established ideologies are leading to shifts in the debates.

We were faced with the problem of whether to include a small number of complete papers and extracts, or whether to include a large number of papers more severely cut and edited. We chose the latter option in order to present as wide ranging a view of differing, but influential, models of deafness as possible. The result inevitably fails to do full justice to some areas and some authors. The section on audiology and technology, for example, makes no mention of speech audiometry or the measurement of functional hearing loss. Nor does it mention the controversial but extremely influential debates surrounding cochlear implants. We have chosen an introduction to objective measurement of hearing to represent a powerful scientific paradigm which has had, and continues to have, an enduring impact on models of deafness.

The longest sections of the book, on education, linguistics and social welfare, are concerned with those areas which have had most impact on deaf people's lives: education and social welfare since they represent powerful institutions of deafness within society, and linguistics because of its crucial role in developing the cultural minority model of deafness which is changing current ideologies. We were guided further in our selection of papers by our concern with constructions of deafness specifically in the United Kingdom. The articles by American and other European authors have been included because of their role in establishing or influencing debates in this country. Extracts from work which has been published previously have been reproduced in their original form unless otherwise indicated; they may, therefore, include language which would now be considered sexist or disablist.

Constructing Deafness is one of two Readers which form part of the Open University course *D251 Issues in Deafness*. This course as a whole aims to question and explain commonly held conceptions about deafness and deaf people—conceptions which define deaf people as 'victims' and deafness as a problem requiring intervention by social agencies. Thus, whilst this book is free-standing and independent of the course, the readings it contains also reflect its integration with other course materials. If you are interested in enquiring about the availability of any of the other course components, please write to: Open University Educational Enterprises Ltd, 12 Cofferidge Close, Stony Stratford, Milton Keynes MK11 1BY, UK.

We would like to acknowledge the lively discussion, active encouragement and honest criticism we have received from members of the Open University course team for *Issues in Deafness* in the preparation of this book. We are also grateful for constructive suggestions from Rob Baker, Mary Brennan and Jim Kyle. We would particularly like to thank Fiona Harris for her considered and careful editorial support. We are further indebted to Yvonne Holmes for her invaluable secretarial assistance which has made the preparation of this book possible.

Susan Gregory
Gillian M. Hartley

Reference

Jacobs, L. (1974) *A Deaf Adult Speaks Out*, Washington, DC, Gallaudet College Press.

Acknowledgements

Grateful acknowledgement is made to the following sources for permission to reproduce extracts in this Reader:
C. Padden and T. Humphries (1988) *Deaf in America: Voices from a Culture*, Harvard University Press, Cambridge, Mass, copyright © 1988 by the President and Fellows of Harvard College, reprinted by permission of the publishers; N.E. Groce (1985) *Everyone Here Spoke Sign Language: Hereditary Deafness on Martha's Vineyard*, Harvard University Press, Cambridge, Mass, copyright © 1985 by Nora Ellen Groce; P. Higgins (1980) *Outsiders in a Hearing World: A Sociology of Deafness*, Sage Publications Inc.; L. Lawson (1981) 'The role of sign and the structure of the deaf community', in B. Woll, J. Kyle and M. Deuchar (eds) *Perspectives in British Sign Language and Deafness*, Croom Helm; P. Ladd (1988) 'The modern deaf community', in D. Miles (ed.) *British Sign Language*, BBC Enterprises Ltd; C. Padden (1980) 'The deaf community and the culture of deaf people', in C. Baker and R. Battison (eds) *Sign Language and the Deaf Community: Essays in Honour of William Stokoe*, National Association of the Deaf, USA; D. Brien (1981) *Paper from the Study Weekend, Loughborough*, National Council of Social Workers with the Deaf; S. Quigley and P. Paul (1984) *Language and Deafness*, Croom Helm; J. Kyle (1983) 'Looking for meaning in sign language sentences', in J. Kyle and B. Woll (eds) *Language in Sign*, Croom Helm; T. Basilier (1964) 'Surdophrenia', *Acta Psychiatrica Scandinavica Supplementium*, 40, copyright © 1964 Munksgaard International Publishers Ltd, Copenhagen, Denmark; H. Lane (1988) 'Is there a "Psychology of the Deaf?"', *Exceptional Children*, vol. 55, no. 1, 1988, pp. 7–19, copyright © 1988 by The Council for Exceptional Children (USA), reprinted with permission; B. McCormick (1983) *Screening for Hearing Impairment in Young Children*, Croom Helm; W. Noble (1978) *Assessment of Impaired Hearing: A Critique and a New Method*, copyright © 1978 by Academic Press, Inc.; I. Tucker and M. Nolan (1984) *Educational Audiology*, Croom Helm; R. Baker 'Information technology: a breakthrough for deaf people?', in J. Kyle (ed.) *Adjustment to Acquired Hearing Loss*, The Centre for Deaf Studies; BATOD (1981, amended 1985) 'Audiological descriptors', British Association of Teachers of the Deaf; A. Markides (1983) *The Speech of Hearing Impaired Children*, Manchester University Press; H. Lane (1984) 'Why the deaf are angry', *Address to the National Union of the Deaf (Manchester)*, September 15, copyright © Professor Harlan Lane; R. Conrad (1979) *The Deaf School Child, Language and Cognitive Function*, Harper and Row Ltd; W. Lynas, A. Huntington and I. Tucker (1988) *A Critical Examination of the Different Approaches to Communication in the Education of Deaf Children*, Ewing Foundation; L. Evans (1982) *Total Communication Structure and Strategy*, Gallaudet University Press; M. Llwellyn-Jones (1988) 'Bi-lingualism and the education of the deaf child', *Educating the Deaf Child: Proceedings of a Conference Held in Derby*, October 1987, copyright © Miranda Pickersgill (née Llwellyn-Jones); D. Wood, H. Wood, A. Griffiths and I. Howarth (1986) *Talking and Teaching with Deaf Children*, copyright © 1986 John Wiley and Sons Ltd, reproduced by permission of John Wiley and Sons Ltd; W. Lynas (1986) *Integrating the Handicapped into Ordinary Schools*, Croom Helm; T. Booth (1988) 'Challenging conceptions of integration', in L. Barton (ed.) *The Politics of Special Educational Needs*, Falmer Press Ltd; S. Gregory and J. Bishop (1989) 'The mainstreaming of primary age deaf school children in the United Kingdom', in H. Hartmann and K. Hartmann (eds) *Hard of Hearing Pupils in Regular Schools*, Bundesgemeinschaft der Eltern und Freunde schwerhoriger Kinder e.v.; B. Woll (1987) 'Historical and comparative aspects of BSL', in J. Kyle (ed.) *Sign and School: Multilingual Matters*, Centre for Deaf Studies, University of Bristol; A. Van Uden (1986) *Sign Languages of Deaf People and Psycholinguists: A Critical Evaluation*, SWETS Publishing Service; W. Stokoe (1987) 'Tell me where is grammar bred?: "Critical evaluation" or another chorus of "Come back to Milano"?', *Sign Language Studies*, vol. 54, spring, Linstok Press Inc.; V. Volterra (1986) 'What sign language research can teach us about language acquisition', in B. Tervoort (ed.) *Signs of Life: Proceedings of the Second European Congress on Sign Language Research*, 50, The Institute of General Linguistics of the University of Amsterdam; K. Lysons (1979) 'The development of local voluntary societies for adult deaf persons in England', *British Deaf News*, British Deaf News; G. Taylor (1986) 'Deaf people, ethnic minorities and social policy', *The Journal of the National Council of Social Workers with Deaf People*, vol. 2, no. 2, National Council of Social Workers with Deaf People/British Deaf Association; D. Parratt and B. Tipping (1986) 'The state, social work and deafness', *The Journal of the National Council of Social Workers with Deaf People*, vol. 2, no. 4, National Council of Social Workers with Deaf People/British Deaf Association; J. Kyle (1986) 'Deaf people and minority groups in the UK', in B. Tervoort (ed.) *Signs of Life: Proceedings of the Second European Congress on Sign Language Research*, 50, The Institute of General Linguistics of the University of Amsterdam; J. Schuchman (1988) *Hollywood Speaks: Deafness and the Film Industry*, University of Illinois Press, copyright © 1988 University of Illinois Press.

Introduction

This book is concerned with the meaning of the term deafness. Constructing deafness is an active process. We have attempted to put that process into historical context and to show how debates within a range of discourses both construct and are constructed by implicit or explicit definitions of deafness.

The first section of the book considers examples of the emergence of the construction of deafness. It illustrates how deafness may be taken for granted until the values of the hearing world impinge and difference is constructed. In the extract about Martha's Vineyard, it is the non-deaf author who creates deafness as a topic. The very idea of defining deafness may itself, therefore, be seen as a social construction.

Further sections of the book focus on areas within which professionals have had a major impact on deaf people's lives and perceptions, and on developing ideologies of deafness. These include psychology, audiology, education, linguistics and social welfare. Two views of deaf people have either implicitly or explicitly informed the work of hearing professionals: the view of deaf people either as subjects of enquiry or clients of proffered services, and the alternative view of deaf people as active participants whose own constructions of deafness are of paramount importance.

Historically, notions of deafness in professional discourse have been dominated by non-deaf people. Section 2 presents early attempts to articulate the foundation of a deaf construction of deafness by addressing the issues of who belongs to the Deaf community and whether there is a Deaf culture.[1]

Lay notions of deafness, being more diffuse, appear less tangible than those of academic or professional discourse. Nevertheless, they exert an important influence since they inform everyday interactions between deaf and hearing people in a non-deaf world. Section 8 is concerned with conceptions of deafness portrayed in certain areas of popular culture. It indicates some of the ways in which public constructions of deafness reflect and are reflected in film and fiction.

Models of deafness within both professional and lay discourses may be categorized in a number of ways. A major distinction may be made between the relative emphasis placed on audiological or social factors. Perhaps the most widespread lay notion of deafness is that of sensory impairment. Section 3 suggests how the view of deafness as physical deficit has also dominated psychological discourse. Basilier's paper on surdophrenia illustrates how, within an area of clinical psychology, deafness has been seen as a defining characteristic of a deaf person in a way that hearing would be unlikely to be used in defining a hearing person. It is as if deafness, viewed as pathology, accounts for concomitant pathologies.

Similarly, the definition which has dominated medical models of deafness is of deafness as a pathological condition. Deafness is viewed as deviation from the normal, healthy state and emphasis is placed, therefore, on remediation and normalization—on overcoming hearing loss to restore 'normal' functioning. We have chosen an area of audiology to illustrate this construction of deafness. Objective measurement of hearing loss is seen as providing information about degree of deafness. The extract by Noble in Section 4 has been included to suggest that the foundation of the objective measurement of hearing, audiometric zero, is itself a social construction relying for its validity on the consensus of audiologists and the criteria used in selecting the samples for the original development of an audiometric scale.

The influence of the audiological construction of deafness in education is illustrated in Section 5 by the paper from the British Association of Teachers of the Deaf. Within education, deaf children are often categorized according to audiological criteria and the resultant labelling of children has important implications for the educational expectations held by educationalists for particular deaf children. The audiological model of deafness has important social implications. By focusing on one aspect of deafness—lack of hearing—it suggests notions of pathology, deficit, impairment and disability, with an attendant emphasis on normalization and amplification to overcome a sensory deficit.

Few professional ideologies of deafness are based wholly on audiological considerations, most take at least some account of social factors. An important consideration in evaluating the significance of these factors is whether they are viewed from the perspective of hearing or deaf people. From the point of view of the majority of hearing people in society, deaf people have been perceived as disabled. Educationalists who have adopted a disability model have focused primarily on the area of communication. The emphasis has been on deaf people acquiring the language which is the vehicle of socialization and participation in society: hence the development of an oral approach (see Markides, and also Lynas, Huntington and Tucker, in Section 5). Historically, within social welfare an ideology of disability has led to a focus on inadequacy and has generated a caring paternalistic model as discussed in Section 7. Again, the emphasis has been on the assimilation of deaf people into a hearing-dominated world. Notions of normalization and assimilation are also important threads in the constructions of deafness implied by some of those who advocate integration of deaf children into mainstream schools (see the extract from Lynas and the subsequent discussion by Booth in Section 5). An alternative view of integration, underpinned by a pluralistic view of society which views Deaf people as a cultural minority group, advocates a bilingual model of integration resulting from a construction of deafness which attempts to incorporate ideas of cultural diversity.

Turning to social accounts of deafness which attempt to present the perspective of Deaf people or are written by Deaf people, it must be remembered that the perspective under discussion is not that of all deaf people. To avoid confusion and to identify the group of deaf people whose views are introduced, the terms 'Deaf' (using upper case 'D') and 'deaf' (using lower case 'd') have been used, in the articles commissioned for this book, to differentiate between those deaf people (Deaf) who belong to the Deaf community and share a common (albeit as yet not fully understood) culture, and those deaf people (deaf) who, while audiologically deaf, do not identify with Deaf culture. Previously published work included in this book does not necessarily follow this convention which really only came into common usage two or three years ago.[2]

The articulation of the Deaf construction of deafness in Britain began as recently as the 1970s. The problem of whose construction of deafness represents the Deaf perspective is addressed in Section 2. When Deaf people are viewed as a cultural minority group, the temptation arises to compare their position with that of other minority groups. It immediately becomes apparent, however, that, unlike ethnic minorities, deaf people have never shared a common specific geographical location. What they have obviously shared is a common language, and it is language which is a major focus of attention in defining Deaf community membership and culture and in attempting to establish a Deaf construction of deafness. Notions of culture which view it as a signifying system (see, for example, Geertz, 1973) reinforce the central role of language. Sign language, for so long undervalued and misunderstood (see, for example, van Uden in Section 6), has now received recognition and legitimation from academic linguists (as indicated in Section 6). By enhancing the status of the language, linguists may be seen to have enhanced the status of the native users of that language, Deaf people themselves. The linguistic perspective has encouraged a construction of deafness which values Deaf people as a cultural minority group who share a common, unique and discrete language. This cultural model of deafness can be seen to underpin bilingual approaches to deaf education and the empowerment model of social work (see Sections 5 and 7).

In attempting to characterize constructions of deafness emphasis has been placed on the importance accorded either to audiological or to social factors. An attempt has been made to indicate that it is the relative values attached to these factors and their affective evaluation which determine different ways of defining deafness. The view of Deaf people as a cultural minority does not necessarily preclude the provision and acceptance of environmental aids to facilitate access to aspects of hearing culture (see, for example, Baker in Section 4). What is important is whether deaf people are seen as a minority group within a pluralistic society, or as disabled people who, with appropriate provision, may be assimilated into a hearing world.

Notes

1 A discussion of the distinction between 'deaf' (with a lower case 'd') and 'Deaf' (with an upper case 'D') is given later in this Introduction and in Section 2.

2 This usage was proposed by James Woodward in 1982, and is discussed in Padden, C. and Humphries, T. (1988) *Deaf in America: Voices From a Culture*, Harvard University Press.

Reference

Geertz, C. (1973) *The Interpretation of Cultures*, New York, Basic Books.

Section 1
Deafness: Whose Perspective?

The papers in this section have been chosen to indicate that, in the lives and experiences of deaf people, deafness need not necessarily be a defining or salient characteristic. It is the non-deaf world which has created deafness as a subject of discourse. Both papers illustrate ways in which deafness may emerge as a topic, how a physical characteristic that is taken for granted may become a distinguishing feature. In both papers it is the views of representatives of the hearing world which create the idea of deafness as an issue. Howard, in Padden and Humphries' paper, illustrates this when he says, 'Would you believe I never knew I was deaf until I entered school?', and Groce indicates how she as a hearing author, by her methodology, created the topic:

> One of the strongest indications that the deaf were completely integrated into all aspects of society is that in all the interviews I conducted, deaf Islanders were never thought of or referred to as a group or as 'the deaf'. Every one of the deaf people who is remembered today is thought of as a unique individual. When I inquired about 'the deaf' or asked informants to list all the deaf people they had known, most could remember only one or two, although many of them had known more than that. I was able to elicit comments about specific individuals only by reading informants a list of all the deaf people known to have lived on the Island.
> (Groce, 1985, p. 4)

The deaf people living on Martha's Vineyard were not seen as a separate group by the other inhabitants. When questioned by a hearing researcher, however, lack of hearing was given as the only specific defining characteristic of the deaf people on the Vineyard. It is paradoxical that the Islanders should resort to an audiological definition since such categorizations frequently typify deficit models of deafness (see, for example, Sections 3, 4 and 5 below). Within the social context of the Vineyard, however, tl. s definition is neither stigmatizing nor does it generate attitudes incorporating notions of pathology or handicap and consequent ideas of normalization or compensation. Deafness is so integral a part of life on the Vineyard that it attracts neither attention nor moral evaluation. Despite her outmoded terminology, Groce avoids evaluating deafness as either good or bad, pathological or normal, but presents the perspective of an integrated community towards some of its members who happen to be deaf. Most people's memories of deaf people centred around events that had little or nothing to do with their inability to hear, as suggested by the following extract:

> [When we were young girls] one time we decided to walk to the general store by the road . . . And along came Mr. Jeremiah North with his horse and

wagon, and he stopped for us and we got aboard. He was a nice old man. I believe, yes, that's right, he was deaf too.
(Groce, 1985, p. 89)

Similarly, in the paper by Padden and Humphries, deaf children, while remaining within a social environment within which deafness was not perceived as different, were unaware of its presence. It is not until they came into contact with aspects of the hearing world that hearing status became a salient characteristic of identity. Padden and Humphries, writing from a deaf perspective, discuss how deaf children come to reconstruct their notions of self-identity to include deafness as a relevant feature as a result of particular encounters with hearing people.

The perspective of a researcher into deafness inevitably isolates deafness as a variable. This should not obscure the social origins of its construction as a topic.

Reference

Groce, N. (1985) *Everyone Here Spoke Sign Language: Hereditary Deafness on Martha's Vineyard,* London, Harvard University Press.

1.1 Learning to be Deaf

Carol Padden and Tom Humphries (1988)

When we began work on this book, we had collected a store of reminiscences from Deaf adults about their childhoods; many told how as young children they discovered that they could not hear sound or speech.

[. . .]

Sam Supalla once described to us his childhood friendship with a hearing girl who lived next door (this account also appears in Perlmutter, 1986). As Sam's story went, he had never lacked for playmates; he was born into a Deaf family with several Deaf older brothers. As his interests turned to the world outside his family, he noticed a girl next door who seemed to be about his age. After a few tentative encounters, they became friends. She was a satisfactory playmate, but there was the problem of her 'strangeness'. He could not talk with her as he could with his older brothers and his parents. She seemed to have extreme difficulty understanding even the simplest or crudest gestures. After a few futile attempts to converse, he gave up and instead pointed when he wanted something, or simply dragged her along with him if he wanted to go somewhere. He wondered what strange affliction his friend had, but since they had developed a way to interact with each other, he was content to accommodate to her peculiar needs.

One day, Sam remembers vividly, he finally understood that his friend was indeed odd. They were playing in her home, when suddenly her mother walked up to them and animatedly began to move her mouth. As if by magic, the girl picked up a dollhouse and moved it to another place. Sam was mystified and went home to ask his mother about exactly what kind of affliction the girl next door had. His mother explained that she was HEARING and because of this did not know how to SIGN; instead she and her mother TALK, they move their mouths to communicate with each other. Sam then asked if this girl and her family were the only ones 'like that'. His mother explained that no, in fact, nearly everyone else was like the neighbours. It was his own family that was unusual. It was a memorable moment for Sam. He remembers thinking how curious the girl next door was, and if she was HEARING, how curious HEARING people were.

When Sam discovers that the girl next door is hearing, he learns something about 'others'. Those who live around him and his family are now to be called 'hearing'. The world is larger than he previously thought, but his view of himself is intact. He has learned that there are 'others' living in his neighbourhood, but he has not yet learned that others have different ways of thinking. Perhaps others are now more prominent in his world, and his thoughts about the world now have to acknowledge that they exist in some relation to himself, but it does not occur to him that these others might define him and his family by some characteristic they lack.

In fact, in almost all the stories of childhood we have heard from Deaf children of Deaf families, hearing people were 'curious' and 'strange' but mostly were part of the background. The children's world was large enough with family and friends that the existence of 'others' was not disruptive. At the age when children begin to reflect on the world, we see an interesting positioning of the self with respect to 'others', people like Sam's playmate and her mother. Sam has not yet understood that the outside world considers him and his family to have an 'affliction'; to him, immersed in the world of his family, it is the neighbours who lack the ability to communicate.

But before long, the world of others inevitably intrudes. We can see children learning about the minds of others in stories Deaf adults tell about their childhoods. A Deaf friend of ours, Howard, a prominent member of his community, made a revealing comment to a mixed audience of hearing and Deaf people. All members of his family—his parents and brother as well as aunts and uncles—are Deaf. He told the audience that he had spent his early childhood among Deaf people but that when he was six his world changed: his parents took him to a school for Deaf children. 'Would you believe,' he said, pausing expertly for effect, 'I never knew I was deaf until I first entered school?'

Howard's comment caused the intended stir in the audience, but it was clear to us that some people thought it meant that Howard first became aware of his audiological deficiency when he was six—that he had never realized before that he could not hear sounds. But this was not his meaning at all.

Howard certainly knew what 'deaf' meant. The sign DEAF was part of his everyday vocabulary; he would refer to DEAF people whenever he needed to talk about family and friends . . . When Howard arrived at school, he found that teachers used the same sign he used for himself at home, DEAF. But it did not take him long to detect a subtle difference in the ways they used the sign.

The child uses DEAF to mean 'us', but he meets others for whom 'deaf' means 'them, not like us'. He thinks DEAF means 'friends who behave as expected', but to others it means 'a remarkable condition'. At home he has taken signing for granted as an activity hardly worth noticing, but he will learn at school that it is something to be talked about and commented on. Depending on what school a child attends, he may be forbidden to use signed language in the presence of his teachers. He will then have to learn how to carry out familiar activities within new boundaries, to learn new social contexts for his language. Skills he learned at home, such as to tell stories with detail about people and events, are not likely to be rewarded by teachers who do not know the language. His language will be subordinated to other activities considered more important, notably learning how to 'use his hearing', and to 'speak' (Erting, 1985b).

The metaphor of affliction, as it is used to describe deaf children, represents a displacement from the expected, that is, from the hearing child. Howard and Sam were used to a certain mode of exchange at home, certain ways in which Deaf friends and family acknowledge each other. But the alien organization of the school, from its hierarchical structure and its employment of hearing people to its insistence on speech, makes plain to the child that an entirely different set of assumptions is in force. Even the familiar—adults in his school whom he recognizes as DEAF—do not and cannot behave in the same ways they do in his community; their roles must change in the face of the demands of an institution that largely belongs to others (Erting, 1985a).

The child 'discovers' deafness. Now deafness becomes a prominent fact in his life, a term around which people's behaviour changes. People around him have debates about deafness, and lines are sharply drawn between people depending on what position they take on the subject. He has never thought about himself as having a certain quality, but now it becomes something to discuss. Even his language has ceased to be just a means of interacting with others and has become an object: people are either 'against' signed language or 'for' signed language. In the stories we have collected from Deaf children of Deaf parents, the same pattern emerges over and over: 'deafness' is 'discovered' late and in the context of these layers of meaning.

It is not surprising that the school is often the setting for this kind of discovery. School is not the only place where Deaf children meet others, of course, but the realization that others have different ways of thinking, and that these ways of thinking are influential in the school, is forced upon them when they arrive.

[. . .]

We have been discussing Deaf children of Deaf families, but deaf children in hearing families face an equally unusual and complementary dilemma. Compare Howard's and Sam's stories with that of Tony, a child of a hearing family who learns that, as a result of medical treatment of childhood diseases, he has become deaf at age six.

> I don't remember any one moment when I thought to myself, 'I can't hear'. Rather it was slowly assimilating a combination of different things. I had been ill for a long time. I remember the repeated visits to the doctor, until finally somehow I sensed a permanence to what had been happening to me. I remember my parents worrying about me, and at some point everyone seemed concerned about my illness. It was at that point I felt changed, and when I thought about how I was changed, my thought was: 'I'm the only one like this.'

When this child referred to himself as 'deaf', he meant an intensely individual and personal condition. The illness had affected him and no one else in his family. There were no others like himself:

I had a second cousin who was deaf but I decided I wasn't like her at all. She used her hands, she signed. I wasn't like her—I talked and I was like everyone else, except I couldn't hear. There wasn't anyone else in my hometown who was deaf, except I guess for this woman down the road we called 'mute', who lived with her sister. She didn't talk and she and her sister had this private home sign language they used with each other. I wasn't any of them.

For Tony, being deaf meant being set apart from his family and friends; he was 'deaf' and had had an 'illness'. In contrast, Sam, the Deaf child of Deaf parents, thought of being 'Deaf' not as a consequence of some event, but simply as a given. For Sam, 'Deaf' was not a term used to refer to him personally, but was just a normal way of describing himself and everyone he knew.

Another child of hearing parents, Jim, told us that his hearing loss was not diagnosed until he was almost 7 years old (his 'difficulties' were attributed to other causes). He remembered that as a child, 'I thought everyone lipread. But it always puzzled me that others seemed to lipread better than I could.' Later, when his loss was discovered, he began to wear a hearing aid, and his new teachers taught him another way of describing the difference between himself and others. He was told that the difference didn't have to do with lipreading ability; it had to do with his not being able to hear.

In contrast to Vicki and Helen [who are Deaf children of Deaf parents] who watch people's signing abilities, Jim was attentive to mouthing behaviours of the people around him, who did not sign. As a very young child he was probably not aware that he was 'lipreading', but he knew oral behaviours were important in social exchanges.

As an exercise contrasting Sam and Howard's world with that of Tony and Jim, let us imagine under what sorts of dependencies or conditions certain behaviours follow others in Deaf and hearing families. In Deaf families, people signal one another by touching or by making a movement into another's visual range. Making a small vibration on a table or the floor is also possible, and for some people in certain ranges, one can call loudly. After one person acknowledges the other, they begin to interact in other ways. They look at each other, and they use signs.

But in a hearing family, the types of behaviours used to signal one another are different. One person can move his mouth and cause another person's behaviour to change. And they do not even have to be visible to each other; someone can move his mouth and make another person come into the room. Once one person acknowledges the other, they alternate moving mouths. Sometimes they look at each other, but sometimes they do not.

We can imagine that Jim, a deaf child whose hearing family did not even realize he was deaf, must have noticed 'strange' dependencies between events and behaviours. One behaviour would suddenly be provoked, and it would not be clear to the young boy what the stimulus was. Imagine Jim sitting in a room near a door. Suddenly his mother appears, walking purposefully to the door. She opens the door, and there is a visitor waiting on the doorstep. But if the child opens the door at another time, odds are that no visitor will be there. How does the child, who does not hear the doorbell, understand what the stimulus is for the odd behaviour of opening a door and finding someone standing there? We can only guess. We know only that Jim assumed other people had powers not yet discernible to him, such as better lipreading skills.

Jim's story and the other stories we have recounted are about how children learn the significant arrangements of their worlds. Jim's theory about other people's lipreading powers is not a bad one; it is consistent with our point that his hypotheses follow from the set of assumptions held by his family about how to conduct one's life. What Jim's and the other cases have in common is that being able or unable to hear does not emerge as significant in itself; instead it takes on significance in the context of other sets of meaning to which the child has been exposed.

As a final example to drive home this point, we turn to the story of Joe, the youngest child of a Deaf family on a farm in the heart of Indiana. Joe told us, 'I never knew I was hearing until I was six. I never suspected in any way that I was different from my parents and siblings'.

It seems ludicrous to imagine a hearing child who does not know he can hear. Is a child like this unresponsive to sounds? Are we to imagine a hearing child who discovers sound at the age of six? Of course not. Joe did know about sound. He responded to sounds, and his conception of the world included sound. But in the flow of everyday life he had no cause to think about sound in anything but an incidental way. He probably thought about it as often and as consciously as children reflect on the fact that they have feet.

The key part of his comment lies in the sentence 'I never suspected I was in any way different from my parents and siblings.' This is not a case of pretended deafness; Joe did not fail to hear, but simply understood sound in a way he could reconcile with the experiences of his family. We can imagine a range of phenomena in this child's world that have double but compatible interpretations: a spoon falls and makes a sound as it hits the floor. Someone picks it up, not simply because it made a sound but because it slipped from view. The farmer goes out to milk the cows not only because they make noises, but because it is daybreak, the time set aside for milking. A door slams, air rushes into the room, and objects on the table rattle and wobble. Many sounds coincide with non-auditory events, to which Joe would have seen his parents responding. His parents' world gave him no reason to identify sound as a primary cause of events.

One might ask how a hearing child would understand a sound that had no corresponding non-auditory event. What if the door slammed in another room and his family did not respond? Would he not see this as odd, or even as a contradiction? We might imagine a moment when the child is startled by a loud noise, looks at his family, and is puzzled by their lack of response. But the child does not yet have a basis for being 'puzzled'. He does not have an alternative explanation. The most striking observation hearing children of Deaf parents make about their early years is that it never occurs to them until they are older that there is anything unusual about their abilities. For young children immersed in the world of their families, there is not yet space for contradictions.

These stories by adults about their childhood memories reveal a rare perspective on the question of how the world comes to mean what it does. The conventional belief is that there are certain immutable events, such as sound, that do not need translation and can be known directly. But Joe's story reminds us that very little is not filtered through the larger pattern of everyday life. Sound is not an entity that is free of interpretation, but something that emerges within a system of knowledge. One does not merely 'hear' thunder, but also must assimilate its place in relation to all other activity of the world, how to react to it, how to talk about it, how to know its relationship to other sounds. For both Deaf and hearing people, sound finds its place against the larger pattern of everyday life.

[. . .]

References

Erting, C. (1985a) 'Cultural Conflict in a School for Deaf Children', *Anthropology and Education Quarterly, 16,* pp. 225–43.

Erting, C. (1985b) 'Sociocultural Dimensions of Deaf Education: Belief Systems and Communicative Interaction', *Sign Language Studies, 47,* pp. 111–25.

Perlmutter, D. (1986) 'No nearer to the Soul', *Natural Language and Linguistic Theory, 4,* pp. 515–23.

1.2 Everyone Here Spoke Sign Language

Nora Groce (1985)

From the seventeenth century to the early years of the twentieth, the population of Martha's Vineyard manifested an extremely high rate of profound hereditary deafness. In stark contrast with the experience of most deaf people in our own society, the Vineyarders who were born deaf were so thoroughly integrated into the daily life of the community that they were not seen—and did not see themselves—as handicapped or as a group apart. Deaf people were included in all aspects of life, such as town politics, jobs, church affairs and social life. How was this possible? On the Vineyard, hearing and deaf Islanders alike grew up speaking sign language. This unique sociolinguistic adaptation meant that the usual barriers to communication between the hearing and the deaf, which so isolate many deaf people today, did not exist.

(From the Introduction)

[. . .]

Sign language in daily life   The community's bilingualism extended into every facet of daily life. Sign language formed an integral part of all communicative events. All informants remembered the deaf Vineyarders participating freely in discussions.

> When I used to go up to Chilmark, there were several people there who were deaf and dumb,[1] there were so many of them that nobody thought anything about it, but because I was only a boy, I was fascinated watching them and then I was wondering what they were saying. And they would have, when they had socials or anything up in Chilmark, why, everybody would go and they [the deaf] enjoyed it, just as much as anybody did. They used to have fun—we all did.

Another remembered, 'Well, wherever we met, they'd go to most everything that we'd go to around town. And in the office there in Chilmark, we went to get our mail there most days, so we'd all meet there.'

As in many small New England towns, in Chilmark the combination general store and post office was a focal point for stories, news and gossip. In the summer people gathered on the front porch, in the winter around the pot-bellied stove. Many people I talked to distinctly remembered the deaf members of the community in this situation. One man in his late eighties recalled:

We would sit around and wait for the mail to come in and just talk. And the deaf would be there, everyone would be there. And they were part of the crowd, and they were accepted. They were fishermen and farmers and everything else. And they wanted to find out the news just as much as the rest of us. And oftentimes people would tell stories and make signs at the same time so everyone could follow him together. Of course, sometimes, if there were more deaf than hearing there, everyone would speak sign language— just to be polite, you know.

Another man said, 'If there were several people present and there was a deaf man or woman in the crowd, he'd take upon himself the discussion of anything, jokes or news or anything like that. They were always part of it, they were never excluded.'

His wife remembered:

You'd go along and get your mail, or you'd buy half a pound of salt pork . . . They'd gather every night. There'd be conversations going on between these deaf people, some of them are talking, making sign language, some of them are talking to hearing people, back and forth, and it was give and take. You never thought anything about it. And even these little kids . . . knew the sign language. And these older men would stop and talk to them kids, make signs back and forth, laugh and chuckle.

Another remembered:

I learned it when I was a kid. Everybody in town knew it. Yeah, these men and women, mostly men, would be at the post office every night. There'd be six or eight of 'em, and they'd be no different than you or I. They'd mingle in with everybody—everybody knew the language. Everybody talked with 'em—just like you'd do to a person who could speak.

When they assembled right before the mail in Chilmark, for example, at night, and there would be deaf mutes there, and there would be plenty of people who could talk and hear, and they were all part of the crowd. They had no trouble, no trouble at all.

The sign language sometimes proved disconcerting to visitors who wandered into the Chilmark general store. One woman from Vineyard Haven recalled going camping up-Island as a child with her family near the turn of the century. By that time, no deaf individuals were still alive down-Island, so a young child would rarely have seen individuals speaking in signs.

That was the general store, the Chilmark general store. And we used to walk through the woods to go over there very often to telephone and get our mail, you see . . . There were all these people sitting around the store, you know, at night, the way it is with country stores. People gathered, it's a regular gathering place, social occasion. And there were several men and one young woman, there was no noise, there wasn't a sound, but they kept smiling and chuckling, so we were very much surprised and finally we realized that they were deaf and dumb. It must of been, must of been ten of them, I guess.

At least these down-Islanders were aware that deaf people lived up-Island, and they were able to piece together what was going on. But the whole town had a good laugh over the story of one summer visitor.

> Well, there was a man by the name of Joseph Walenski, who was a famous artist. I don't like his art work, but he was . . . And he came into the store one night, the post office was open as long as the store was, to buy a stamp and mail a letter. That was the meeting place for everybody in town, the deaf and dumb as well as those who weren't and, of course, everybody used the sign language, and they'd be making the signs in sign language. There would be a complete silence in there, and even those who could talk would often be silent.
> And Joseph Walenski walked in there one night, there was this assemblage of great big men, they were big, and there was complete silence, and the place was only lighted by the kerosene lamps, you know. And there were these tremendously big men—dim in the store, dim light—standing around, perfectly silent, looking at him. And he thought [they looked] aggressive. But of course they weren't, they were just, you know, making signs among themselves. He was scared to death.

I asked if all the men present that night were deaf. 'Oh no, only four of them were.'

Sign language was also used in larger groups. One man told me:

> They would come to prayer meetings; most all of them were regular church people, you know. They would come when people offered testimonials, and they would get up in front of the audience and stand there and give a whole lecture in sign. No one translated it to the audience because everyone knew what they were saying. And if there was anyone who missed something, somewhere, somebody sitting near them would be able to tell them about it.

According to a brief biography of a deaf man in the *Vineyard Gazette*'s 'Old Time Vineyarders' series, the only concession to deafness at the prayer meetings was that the deaf church members were permitted to stand at the front of the room so the audience could better see their confessions.

> An interesting demonstration of the use of sign language was formerly a common sight at village prayer meetings. Mr. Brewer, like all his family, has always been a regular attendant at religious services and on such occasions as prayer meetings, the members of his family "spoke" or offered prayers as others did. In order that the congregation might know what they "said", it was customary for them to walk to the front of the room, where they would offer their adoration in sign language.
> (*Vineyard Gazette*, 1931)

This practice seems to have occurred regularly for many years on the Island. A Vineyard clergyman called 'Reformation' John Adams mentioned a deaf man at a prayer meeting in 1821 (Adams, 1853). An account of one of the early Cottage City meetings noted: 'Most soul-stirring of all is to see a deaf and dumb sister speak in signs of the goodness and wonderful works of God' (Hough, 1936, p. 40).

Several informants recalled that at town meeting a hearing person would stand at the side of the room and translate the often lengthy and frequently heated discussions into sign language so that all the deaf people could follow it. Because sign language was known so widely, no one individual was singled out as translator, although those with deaf family members probably filled this role more often.

In fact, there was little need for translators on a day-to-day basis. Almost everyone who had even occasional contact with people from West Tisbury and Chilmark could speak 'well enough to get by', including the postmaster, delivery clerks from down-Island stores, and the doctor from Vineyard Haven (a nephew of two deaf men and a grandson of two others). If someone who could not speak the language came up-Island, any nearby hearing person was pressed into service. Presumably, this was also true down-Island as well until the middle of the nineteenth century.

The only regular event for which deaf Vineyarders needed some assistance seems to have been the Sunday church sermon. Most of them attended church regularly, and a spouse or other relative usually translated. One informant remembered that the hearing wife of a deaf man 'used to sit side of him in church and give him the sermon. She'd sit there and her hands were flying all the time, and he was getting every word of the sermon . . . She moved her hands just about the same as a person would if they were knitting a sock, just down in her lap.' Another couple would 'sit way up in front and he'd sit partly around in the pew and she'd interpret every word about the sermon. And he'd shake his head sometimes, and he'd shake his head "no", he didn't agree. She never missed a thing. She gave him the whole thing.' An elderly woman reported:

> My son came home with a friend . . . from off-Island, who was studying for the ministry. The news got around that my son had brought home a minister, so he was . . . invited to speak in church that Sunday. And he said he would. Well, Mr B. was deaf and dumb and he and his family always sat in one of the front pews. She'd always preach the whole sermon to him in deaf and dumb sign. So this ministry student, he preached and when we come back home, I asked him how he thought it went. 'All right' he said, 'except there was one lady in the front pew who was awfully nervous, couldn't keep her hands still.' I explained and he thought that was wonderful, he was very flattered.

Signing by hearing Islanders Hearing members of the community were so accustomed to using signs that the language found its way into discussions even when no deaf people were present. Where speaking was out of place, as in church or at school, hearing people often communicated in sign. Such stories as the following were common:

> Fred and I sat across the aisle from each other in school. His grandfather was deaf, so he could talk real good, and the teacher, she was from off-Island, she'd always yell 'Stop talking.' If she'd of said 'Stop communicating,' she'd of had us there, but as it was, we'd just say, 'We're not talking' and go on doing it.

Ben and his brother could both talk and hear, but I've seen them sitting across from each other in town meetings or in church [when they were both old men], and telling each other funny stories in sign language . . . I remember the last time I ever saw Ben in one such assembly, and he was not feeling good . . . And he was telling Ernest that he wasn't feeling well, and telling how he didn't feel well, in sign language.

One woman remembered her in-laws from up-Island, who were hearing and who had no close relatives who were deaf. 'They'd make the signs, or very often, they'd use a sign to say something—well, it was just kind of reflex, like scratch your head, you know. They were so in the habit of doing it. They'd transfer back and forth between speaking and sign language.' Another man recalled seeing signs used 'all the time, at the post office, or around the beach. I spent all my time then, as I do now, around the beach, and particularly if there was a group of men there and they were about to discuss something that was either your family affair or they didn't want to get too involved in, they'd stop talking with tongues, turn around, and make signs.'

Signs were also used when distance made it impossible to be heard. One man remembered, 'Jim had a shop down on the shore of Tisbury Pond, and his house was a ways away, up on the high land. When Prudy, his wife, wanted to tell Jim something, she'd come to the door, blow a fish horn, and Jim would step outside. He'd say, "Excuse me, Prudy wants me for something," then she'd make signs to tell him what she needed done.'

Another recounted, 'I have seen Jonathan and Sally, I have actually seen them on a windy day talking to each other in deaf and dumb language when they could just as well have spoken. Sally was on our side of the fence—come to see me about something—and they could of perfectly well talked, but they would of had to raise their voices.' One lady recalled often seeing her hearing father standing on a windy cliff and signing his intentions to fellow fishermen on the shore below.

These practices were noted in newspapers. In the *Vineyard Gazette* (1933), a reporter who had grown up in Chilmark referred to this practice, then still current. 'This sign language is often used in conversing at long distances, both by deaf-mutes and others who find it a convenience. Raising the arms until they stand out from the body or above the head, Mr North [a deaf man], and his wife, for instance, can carry on conversations at a distance far beyond the range of the human voice.'

The *Boston Sunday Herald* (1895) reported:

Nowhere else in the world could you see such singular pantomimes as are carried on daily from Chilmark back doors. Suppose you live in a lonely farm house and your nearest neighbor is an eighth of a mile away. Your men folk in both houses are fisherfolk, and so you have spyglasses. You go to your door at eleven, say, in the morning. Your neighbor is at hers. You signal to her in the sign language with your glass some question about the catch or the take from the lobster pots or a bit of womanly gossip and then you put your glass to your eye and she waves to you with her glass her reply.

Sign language was also used by fishermen in boats on the open water. One man recalled, 'Fishermen hauling pots outside in the Sound or off Gay Head, when they would be heaven knows how far apart, would discuss how the luck was running—all that sort of thing. These men could talk and hear all right, but it'd be too far to yell.' Another man, originally from off-Island, remembered his first exposure to the use of sign language:

> I do know that my father-in-law and his brother [both hearing] used to converse when they'd pass in boats [in sign language]. I remember one time we were out there in the Bight, and this is when I had first started coming to Martha's Vineyard, the first or second trip. He said, 'There's Zeno,' and he went on to tell how many lobsters he had in the hold, which string was doing well, what wasn't, so forth and all this stuff. We were probably a hundred, a hundred fifty yards apart. They'd hold their hands up here [above their heads], where they'd be clearly seen.

One off-Island woman recalled, 'One time, my husband was out on a fishing boat, a pleasure boat with one of the regular fishermen, and when he came in, when this fisherman came in, he made deaf and dumb language signs to the people on the shore, to a certain man on the shore, because he wanted him to understand how many fish he had.'

Since the Islanders turned to fishing long after sign language seems to have come into regular use on the Vineyard, it is unlikely that the language was developed for maritime use. Signs for boats, fishing equipment, marine life, and so forth must have been added to the original language. However, it seems to have been a particularly effective means of communication on the water and was regularly used there, as well as on land.

As in other bilingual communities, use of the language was a way to delineate who was and who was not a member of the community. Island people frequently maintained social distance from off-Islanders by exchanging comments about them in sign language:

> My husband had a friend, and when they were grown men, they were in New Bedford, getting their boats repaired—and they were always full of mischief. So they would get on the electrics [electric trolley cars] and go uptown. And just to cause trouble, one would sit on one end of the car and one would sit down at the other, and they'd make funny remarks about fellow passengers and discuss plans. And my husband said people would look at them. I believe they thought they were crazy! They used to think it was very funny.

Two young hearing up-Island men went to visit the daughters of a family who had come to the Vineyard for the summer.

> I believe I told you about Jonathan, going off with somebody there to a house over near the brick yard when they were young men, before they were married. The man with him made some sort of a sign to him in the sign language, and he made a sign back and these girls immediately assumed that Jonathan was deaf and dumb. Since they'd heard that there were people down there like that, they simply assumed that he was.

Jonathan was a great character, so he and this friend carried on throughout the evening, and in the process of the evening, the girls told the friend how sorry they were for Jonathan and how handsome he was. Things like that. And they finally were ready to leave. Of course, his friend was doing all the translating by hand. When they were ready to leave, why Jonathan got his hat and coat on, and then he says: 'Jeese, it was a lovely evening.' He would tell that story and laugh.

Jonathan's father and grandfather were deaf. Although the girls were mistaken in assuming he was deaf, it was his initial communication in sign language that caused them to make that mistake.

What linguists call code-switching from speech to sign also seems to have occurred. I was told:

People would start off a sentence in speaking and then finish it off in sign language, especially if they were saying something dirty. The punch line would often be in sign language. If there was a bunch of guys standing around the general store telling a [dirty] story and a woman walked in, they'd turn away from her and finish the story in sign language.

Perhaps the following anecdote best illustrates how integral sign language was to all aspects of life:

My mother was in the New Bedford hospital—had a very serious operation. And my father went over in his boat and lived aboard his boat and went to the hospital to see her every single night. The surgeon, when he left him in her room, said they mustn't speak, father couldn't say a word to her. So he didn't. But they made signs for about half an hour, and mother got so worked up, they had to send father out, wouldn't let him stay any longer.

[. . .]

As with all other aspects of Island life, in socializing no one made any distinctions between deaf people and hearing people. No one was able to give me an example of social activities in which only the deaf participated. Unlike the mainland, where various deaf clubs and activities are the centre of social interaction for many deaf people, the Vineyard activities were attended by both the deaf and the hearing. It was not simply that the hearing Islanders welcomed the deaf into their midst; the deaf Islanders apparently made no attempt to set up activities independent of their hearing family, friends and neighbours. If a deaf Islander wanted to entertain only other deaf individuals, he or she probably would have had to exclude spouse, siblings, children, best friends, or immediate neighbours, all of whom would have been hurt.

There were some close personal friendships between deaf Islanders, but none of them were friends exclusively or primarily with other deaf persons. Close friendships were based on whom one grew up with or who lived nearby. Nor does it seem that deaf Islanders maintained ties with deaf individuals living off-Island whom they knew from Hartford. And they did not participate in state or national deaf organizations, which are important social links for many deaf men and women on the mainland. As far as can be ascertained, deaf Islanders did not perceive themselves as a distinct social group.

[. . .]

[Note

1   It should be noted that in using the outdated terms, 'deaf and dumb' and 'deaf mute', the people of Martha's Vineyard did not intend to imply the negative connotations that we now associate with such terminology.]

References

Adams, J. (1853) *The Life of 'Reformation' John Adams, an elder of the Methodist Episcopal Church*, (written by himself, 2 vols.) Boston, MA, George C. Rand.

Boston Sunday Herald (1895) *Mark of Chilmark, Deaf and Dumb in the Village of Squibnocket*, 20 January.

Hough, H. B. (1936) *Martha's Vineyard, Summer Report, 1835–1935*, Rutland, V. T. Tuttle.

Section 2
Defining the Deaf Community

The papers in this section are concerned not only with ideas of deafness but also with the problem of what constitutes a community. What factors, for example, allow us to ascribe the social cohesion of a community to a group of people? How important are geographical location and face-to-face interaction? What factors should be used in differentiating between those deaf people (Deaf) who are members of a deaf community and those deaf people (deaf) who are audiologically deaf but who may choose to work and socialize with hearing people? Is competence in sign language a *sine qua non* for membership of the deaf community?

In addressing these issues, the papers in this section present a range of responses. Although all the authors agree that not all deaf people belong to the Deaf community, their answers to the question of whether all members of the Deaf community are deaf vary according to the criteria they adopt for defining 'community'. Padden's emphasis on geographical location permits the inclusion of non-deaf people as members of a deaf community. Higgins and Lawson, on the other hand, seem to suggest that although degree of deafness may be irrelevant, a person must have at least some hearing loss, however minimal, to be eligible for membership.

The concept of Deaf community is intimately related to that of Deaf culture. Padden distinguishes between a deaf community which can have hearing members and a Deaf cultural group whose members are Deaf but, much more importantly, share cultural values and a specific language. For Padden, not all members of deaf communities subscribe to Deaf culture. Higgins, Lawson and Ladd, however, view the sharing of Deaf cultural values as an integral part of Deaf community membership. This is reflected in the importance they attach to sign language competence and use in defining who belongs to a Deaf community.

In popular use, the term 'culture' is often used for what might perhaps be termed cultural productions. These include literature, drama and the visual arts. It is perhaps interesting that very little is written about Deaf cultural production, though Ladd addresses this issue briefly.

Many current definitions of culture emphasize symbols. Geertz, for example, says of culture:

> . . . it denotes an historically transmitted pattern of meanings embodied in symbols, a system of inherited conceptions expressed in symbolic forms by means of which men *(sic)* communicate, perpetuate, and develop their knowledge about and attitudes toward life.
> (Geertz, 1973, p. 89)

Such an approach often leads to a stress on the importance of language in constituting culture. Hermeneutical approaches to culture also place language in a paramount position. An emphasis on language pervades current discussion of Deaf culture which often seems to be more concerned with the medium of communication rather than with its products.

The term 'culture' in sociological discourse encompasses not only the symbols but also the beliefs and values of a particular group of people. Whether Deaf people share common beliefs and values, and what these might be, has not as yet been fully explored, although insights may be gained through an examination of the changes which have taken place in the language of deafness as Deaf people themselves have become active in defining their own situation. For example, the sign for DEAF which previously indicated 'deaf-and-dumb' now indicates only deafness; and the use of the thumb extended hand-shape, with its connotations of good or correct, as part of the sign for HEARING, has now been changed to a more neutral hand-shape using an extended index finger. Related to this is a rejection by the Deaf community of the spoken language term 'hearing-impaired' to refer to Deaf people.

The cultural model of deafness, which underpins the early papers in this section, may be contrasted with the pathological/deficit models discussed in subsequent sections of this book, which stress the importance of hearing loss. (This distinction is discussed further in Brien's paper.) Thus, the papers in this section emphasize social rather than audiological construc-tions of deafness, and characterize Deaf people as a minority group who share a common language and cultural values. This section presents early attempts to define deafness from within a Deaf perspective, and perhaps indicates the beginning of a Deaf construction of deafness.

Reference

Geertz, C. (1973) *The Interpretation of Cultures*, New York, Basic Books.

2.1 Outsiders in a Hearing World

Paul Higgins (1980)

[. . .]

Membership

Deafness is not a sufficient condition for membership in deaf communities, though some degree of hearing impairment is a necessary condition, which I examine later. Deafness does not make 'its members part of a natural community' (Furth, 1973, p. 2). Membership in a deaf community must be *achieved*; it is not an ascribed status (Markowicz and Woodward, 1978). Membership in a deaf community is achieved through (1) *identification* with the deaf world, (2) *shared experiences* that come of being hearing impaired, and (3) *participation* in the community's activities.[1] Without all three characteristics, one cannot be nor would one choose to be a member of a deaf community.

Identification

A deaf community is in part a 'moral' phenomenon. It involves a 'sense of identity and unity with one's group and a feeling of involvement and wholeness on the part of the individual' (Poplin, 1972, p. 7).

A deaf woman, hearing-impaired since childhood, dramatically described her realization in her late teens and early twenties that she was part of the deaf world:

> I didn't think I was very deaf myself. But when I saw these people (at a deaf organization) I knew I belonged to their world. I didn't belong to the hearing world. Once you are deaf, you are deaf, period. If you put something black in white paint, you can't get the black out. Same with the deaf. Once you are deaf, you're always deaf.

While it is problematic both physiologically and in terms of identification that 'once you are deaf, you are always deaf', the woman's remarks express her commitment to the deaf world.[2] Whether members dramatically realize it or not, what is important is their commitment to and identification with the deaf. Other members, who attended schools and classes for the deaf since childhood and continued their interaction in the deaf world as adults, may, upon looking back, find no dramatic moment when they realized that they had become part of a deaf community.

Members of the deaf community feel more comfortable with deaf people than they do with the hearing. They feel a sense of belonging. A young deaf woman explained:

> At a club for the deaf, if I see a deaf person whom I don't know, I will go up to that person and say, 'Hi! What's your name?' I would never do that to a hearing person.

Again, when I asked a deaf couple how they felt about hearing people,

> . . . the wife answered that she likes to be with her *own* people. According to her husband, though, she can get along well with the hearing. Her speech is understandable, and her husband feels that she is a good lipreader. He recalled that one day he was across the street conversing with a neighbor, but could not understand him. His wife, looking through the window, did.

Most deaf individuals cannot lipread that well—nor, probably, can this wife on most occasions. As she said herself, the neighbour's speech seemed so clear that time. What is important, though, is her desire to be with her *own* people. This identification with other deaf people is the foundation for membership in the deaf community. Based on this identification, members of a Jewish synagogue for the deaf donated items to a bazaar run by a Lutheran church for the deaf, rather than to a synagogue for hearing Jews.

Identification with the deaf world can momentarily unite people who are otherwise complete strangers. Deaf Americans who travel abroad are often cordially received by members of deaf clubs in foreign countries. While my hearing companions and I were travelling on the subway in Paris, a group of deaf Japanese tourists noticed that we were signing to one another. When it is noisy, signing often comes in handy. While we had difficulty communicating with one another due to the (sign) language barrier, the deaf Japanese tourists were quite obviously pleased to meet some American people who they thought were deaf. (They never did realize that we were able to hear.)

Not all deaf or hearing-impaired people, though, identify with the deaf world. Those who lost their hearing later in life through an accident, occupational hazard, or presbycusis (i.e. the ageing process) do not seek to become members of deaf communities.[3] Rather, as Goffman (1963) notes, they are likely to stigmatize members of deaf communities in the same way that those with normal hearing stigmatize them. Others, impaired from birth or from an early age, may never have developed such an identification. They are likely to have had hearing parents and were educated in schools for the hearing or in oral schools for the deaf (which I will discuss later). Some may participate in activities of deaf communities, but are not members. They are tolerated, though they are not accepted, by the members. While audiologically they are deaf, socially they are not.

A hearing-impaired man, who participates in a religious organization for the deaf but is not part of the deaf community, explained his self-identity in the following way:

> In everyday life I consider myself a hearing person. [His hearing-impaired wife interjected that she did too.] I usually forget it that I have a hearing problem. Sometimes I'm so lost [absorbed] in the hearing world, I mean I don't even realize I have a hearing problem. It seems automatic. I don't know

what it is. I feel I'm hearing people to the deaf and hearing. I don't feel hearing-impaired not even if I have a hard time to understand somebody. Still I don't feel I'm deaf because I couldn't hear you or understand you.

The same man remarked:

> I was deaf for a few days. My ears blocked up. That was [a] scary moment for me. I was completely deaf. I was walking and it was completely quiet. I tried talking on the phone. I used my amplifier all the way up. It didn't work too much. And I was deaf. My wife used to call me and I didn't hear her call me. Nothing! I could talk and that's why I was still hearing. I could talk even if I couldn't hear a thing.

Hearing-impaired people like this man and his wife are often a source of both ill feelings and amusement for members of deaf communities. They are a source of ill feelings because their behaviour does not respect the identity of the deaf community. Thus, this same hearing-impaired man was severely criticized for having someone at a board meeting of a religious group interpret his spoken remarks into sign language, rather than signing himself. His failure to sign was interpreted as an insult to the members of the deaf community who served on the board. As I explain later, signing skill and communication preference are indications of one's commitment to the deaf community. Those who are opposed to signing or who do not sign are not members of the community.

They are a source of amusement for trying to be what members of deaf communities feel they are not, hearing. A deaf couple were both critical and amused at the attempt of the same hearing-impaired man's wife to hide her deafness. As they explained:

> A hearing woman who signs well came up to her [the wife] at a religious gathering, and assuming that she was deaf, which she is, began to sign to her. The wife became flustered, put her own hands down and started talking.

Such hearing-impaired people serve as examples that members of deaf communities use in explaining to others what their community is like and in reaffirming to themselves who they are. These hearing-impaired people help to define for the members the boundary of their community and their identity as deaf people. The members reject the feelings of these 'misguided' hearing-impaired people—feelings which deny their deafness. And in rejection, the members affirm who they are and what their community is.

Shared experiences
In developing an identification with the deaf world, members of deaf communities share many similar experiences. These experiences relate particularly to the everyday problems of navigating in a hearing world and to being educated in special programmes for the deaf.

[. . .]

Since childhood, members of deaf communities have experienced repeated frustration in making themselves understood, embarrassing misunderstandings, and the loneliness of being left out by family, neighbourhood acquaintances, and others. Such past and present experiences help to strengthen a deaf person's identification with the deaf world. A *typical* instance of these experiences, remarkable only because it is so routine, was described by a deaf man who speaks well:

> Most of my friends are deaf. I feel more comfortable with them. Well, we have the same feelings. We are more comfortable with each other. I can communicate good with hearing people, but in a group, no. For example, I go bowling. Have a league of hearing bowlers. Four of them will be talking, talking, talking and I will be left out. Maybe if there was one person I would catch some by lipreading, but the conversation passes back and forth so quickly. I can't keep up. I just let it go; pay attention to my bowling. Many things like that.

Or as the same deaf man explained when I asked him during an interview, two months later, 'What are your feelings about hearing people?':

> Well, funny. With my good speech and lipreading ability I don't care to mix with hearing people. I've been deaf all my life. But I never feel comfortable with hearing people. I could if it's a one-to-one basis, but in a group I'm out. And I don't want to be put in a situation, an embarrassing situation [where] I don't feel comfortable. That's why I don't do it.

I went on, 'You told me once you went bowling with hearing people. How was it? Did you feel included?' His response was:

> No. No. I enjoy bowling with the deaf more, even though most of them are [pause] not on my level, my intellectual level, I mean. They have ability, but were never given a chance to learn. So I never give them any feeling that I am superior to them.

What comes through so clearly in this man's remarks is a mixture of his feelings of belonging with fellow members of the deaf community and the uneasiness of interacting with the hearing. That uneasiness, which is part of the shared experiences of being deaf, is a basis for identification with the deaf world as well as a factor which further strengthens identification with the deaf world.

However, to be a member of a deaf community one need not actually be deaf. Some members have lesser degrees of hearing impairment. As children, though, they were processed through educational programmes for the deaf. These children were not necessarily mislabelled, though certainly some were. Rather, many times no local programmes for 'hard of hearing' children or children with less severe impairments were available. Children with various degrees of impairment, ranging from mild to profound, were educated together. Nowadays more specialized educational programmes exist, but, still, children with widely varying hearing losses are educated (often properly so) in the same programme. Through such processing, these children developed friendships with deaf children and an identification with the deaf. As adults, they moved comfortably into deaf communities. With amplification, these members of deaf communities are often able to use the telephone successfully, if somewhat haltingly. Some converse with hearing people reasonably well. Yet, due to that childhood processing in programmes for the deaf, these hearing-impaired people choose to live their lives within deaf communities. Audiologically they are not deaf; socially they are (Furfey and Harte, 1964, 1968; Schein, 1968).

Other members of a deaf community may have once been deaf, but through surgery or fortuitous circumstances they have regained some hearing. Though no longer severely hearing-impaired, they remain active in the deaf community where their identity as a person developed. A dramatic case is that of a now slightly hearing-impaired man. He went to the state school for the deaf in Illinois. His childhood friends were deaf. During World War II, though, he regained much of his hearing from working in a munitions plant. The loud blasts from testing the bombs apparently improved his hearing. Consequently, his speech also improved. Only his modest hearing aid indicates that he has a slight impairment. However, his wife is deaf, most of their friends are deaf, and he is active in a state organization for the deaf. When I asked, 'As your speech got better, did you continue to associate with your deaf friends in . . . [town]?' he explained:

> Oh, yeh, I'm more involved with the deaf community now than I was back then [during World War II]. To me they are still my family. I feel more at home when I walk into a room with 1,000 deaf people more so than walking into a room with 1,000 hearing people, non-deaf. I feel at home. I can relate to them. We had something in common—our childhood, our education, our problems, and all that.

That communality of experience and identity is the basis for belonging to the deaf community. Some who are audiologically deaf lack it. Others who are no longer deaf or never were profoundly hearing-impaired possess it. Without it, one cannot be nor would one choose to be a member of the deaf community.[4]

Since membership in deaf communities is based on shared experiences of being deaf and identification with the deaf world, it is difficult for hearing individuals to be members of such communities. In general, those who are not outsiders are unlikely to be members of communities of outsiders. Though it is not impossible, heterosexuals are unlikely to be members of the gay community and whites are unlikely to be members of the black community (Warren, 1974, pp. 150–1). A deaf woman put it simply: 'Hearing people are lost in the deaf world, just as deaf people are lost in the hearing world.' Another deaf woman, married to a hearing man whom I have met and who signs quite well, explained:

> Even though my husband signs well enough to communicate with the deaf, he

isn't really comfortable among them. Some of my friends accept him. Others, who don't know him as well, don't. At a club he might be signing, and some deaf don't know that he is hearing. When they learn that he is hearing and that he is my husband, they say, 'Good! You sign well.' But he doesn't really feel comfortable with the deaf. I wonder how a hearing person could feel comfortable.

Hearing people, as indicated by these two deaf women and by other members of the community, are not part of the deaf community. Marrying a deaf individual is not sufficient for obtaining membership in the community. Again and again I was told by deaf respondents that they knew of no hearing people who were members of the community, though specific hearing people that they knew from work or childhood might be their friends.

Two hearing women, one with a deaf daughter and the other with a deaf sister, were pointed out to me by some deaf Jews as active participants in religious and social functions of deaf Jews. They seemed to be accepted within this more limited group of deaf people. Yet neither one claimed to be members of the community. They were friends, particularly of some deaf Jews, but they were not members. One of the women noted that when deaf people who do not know her learn that she is hearing, they immediately slow their signing to her. Some deaf, when signing to hearing people, switch to signed English rather than use American Sign Language (Markowicz and Woodward, 1978). . . . signed English is used in formal occasions, whereas American Sign Language is used among fellow members of the deaf community. Manoeuvres like these by the deaf are an indication that the hearing person is not fully one of them.

Outsiders are often wary and resentful of those from the dominant world—blacks of whites, gays of straights, and so on. Likewise, deaf people are sceptical of hearing people's motives and intentions. A deaf man remarked: 'When a hearing person starts to associate with the deaf, the deaf begin to wonder why that hearing person is here. What does that hearing person want?' When a 'hard of hearing' woman, who for years had associated exclusively with the hearing, started a North Shore club for the deaf, her motives and behaviour were questioned by some of the deaf members. I was warned myself by two deaf leaders to expect such scepticism and resistance by members of the deaf community. I encountered little in my research, but having deaf parents and clearly establishing my intentions probably allayed members' suspicions.

Outsider communities, though, may grant courtesy membership to 'wise' people who are not similarly stigmatized (Goffman, 1963). These individuals are 'normal', yet they are familiar with and sympathetic to the conditions of outsiders. For example, gay communities grant courtesy membership to 'wise' heterosexuals: heterosexual couples or single females known as 'fag hags' (Warren, 1974, p. 113). Researchers are often granted that status. Yet that courtesy membership represents only a partial acceptance by the outsiders of the 'normals'.

Some hearing individuals are courtesy members of deaf communities.

They may be educators, counsellors, interpreters, or friends of the deaf. Often they have deafness in their families: deaf parents, siblings, children, or even spouses. Yet their membership is just that, a courtesy, which recognizes the fundamental fact that no matter how empathic they are, no matter that there is deafness in their families, they are not deaf and can never 'really' know what it means to be deaf.

Participation

Active participation in the deaf community is the final criteria for being a member. Participation, though, is an outgrowth of identification with the deaf world and of sharing similar experiences of being hearing-impaired. In that respect, then, it is the least important characteristic for being a member of the deaf community. Yet the deaf community is not merely a symbolic community of hearing-impaired people who share similar experiences. It is also created through marriages, friendships, acquaintances, parties, clubs, religious organizations, and published materials. The activities provide the body of the community, whereas the identification and shared experiences provide the soul.

[. . .]

Notes

1 See Padden and Markowicz (1975) for a similar conception of the Deaf community.

2 Most 'coming out' among homosexuals, a process of defining oneself as gay, seems to occur in interaction with other homosexuals. Gays too seem to feel that being gay is a permanent condition (Dank, 1971; Warren, 1974).

3 I met no one nor heard of any member of the Community who lost their hearing after the age of twenty. Though such members surely exist, they are few. The identity of those who lose their hearing after adolescence is already fully established as a hearing person. Entrance into the deaf world is usually not sought, even when a successful adjustment to one's impairment is made.

4 Warren (1974, pp. 154, 161) argues that while secrecy and stigmatization lead many homosexuals to the gay community, identity as a gay person and membership in the gay community is fundamentally an existential choice.

References

Dank, B. M. (1971) 'Coming out in the Gay World', *Psychiatry, 34*, pp. 180–197.

Furfey, P. H. and Harte, T. J. (1964) *Interaction of Deaf and Hearing in*

Frederick County, Maryland, Washington, DC, Catholic University of America Press.

Furfey, P. H. and Harte, T. J. (1968) *Interaction of Deaf and Hearing in Baltimore City, Maryland,* Washington, DC, Catholic University of America Press.

Furth, H. G. (1973) *Deafness and Learning: A Psychosocial Approach,* Belmont, CA, Wadsworth.

Goffman, E. (1963) *Stigma: Notes on the Management of Spoiled Identity,* Englewood Cliffs, NJ, Prentice Hall.

Markowicz H. and Woodward, J. (1978) 'Language and the Maintenance of Ethnic Boundaries in the Deaf Community, *Communication and Cognition, 11,* pp. 29–38.

Padden, C. and Markowicz, H. (1975) 'Crossing Cultural Group Boundaries into the Deaf Community', presented at the *Conference on Culture and Communication,* Temple University, Philadelphia.

Poplin, D. E. (1972) *Communities: A Survey of Theories and Methods of Research,* New York, MacMillan.

Schein, J. D. (1968) *The Deaf Community: Studies in the Social Psychology of Deafness,* Washington, DC, Gallaudet College Press.

Warren, C. A. B. (1974) *Identity and Community in the Gay World,* New York, John Wiley.

2.2 The Role of Sign in the Structure of the Deaf Community

Lilian Lawson (1981)

[. . .]

Deaf people are separated from the hearing society around them, and from the culture that belongs to that society, because of a physical feature: lack of hearing. They therefore belong to a minority group. Deafness means that speech and hearing cannot be the primary means of group social interaction. However, the desire to belong to a group, the desire for social contact, is no less strong in deaf people than it is in normal hearing people. Deafness isolates deaf people from the social group of which they would otherwise be members because of their residence and work, and is also the main cause of the formation of special social groupings of deaf people. Such groups have existed from at least the introduction of special education in Britain in the last century. At that time the medium of instruction was sign language, or at least a manual communication method.

The sign language of schools for the deaf has the flexibility and expressiveness typical of any language used for the natural communication of daily thoughts, feelings and needs of a close-knit group of people. Pupils leaving a school for the deaf continue their association with each other and with pupils from other deaf schools in different parts of Britain. The means by which they carry on that interchange of thought, so necessary for full social interaction, has always been the language of signs. Thus, sign language, namely British Sign Language (BSL), while undergoing growth and evolution, has become a vital part of the culture of the British deaf.

It is the pleasure gained from mixing with other deaf people that makes one remain a member of the deaf 'in-group'—the British deaf community. So powerful is the attraction of social interaction with deaf people that others, on making contact with the deaf but who have no skill in BSL, learn to sign and become members of the community. These latecomers are the post-lingually deaf, orally educated deaf and deaf people who are educated in schools for the hearing.

The British deaf community is held together by such factors as self-identification as a deaf community member, language, endogamous marital patterns, and numerous national, regional and local organizations and social structures . . . These factors have been defined as responsible for the formation of the American deaf community (Croneberg, 1976; Markowicz, 1979; Woodward, 1975, 1978). Not all hearing-impaired and deaf individuals belong to the deaf community; some prefer to identify themselves with the larger 'hearing world' and try to belong to that group. The deaf community comprises those deaf and hard-of-hearing individuals who have a common language, common experiences and values, and a common way of communicating with each other and with hearing people. A person's actual degree of hearing loss (audiometric deafness) is not important in determining that individual's identification with and acceptance by the deaf community, though some loss of hearing must have occurred at a fairly early stage. The principal identifying characteristic appears to be a native knowledge of sign language. For the deaf in Britain it is BSL, just as it is American Sign Language (ASL) for the deaf in America and so on.

Members of the deaf community usually attend special schools for the deaf. A large number of these schools are residential institutions where deaf pupils eat, sleep, study and play together—isolated from their hearing counterparts. After leaving school, deaf people tend to work together at those limited places which employ deaf adults. Most of the adult deaf marry within the deaf community. Throughout their school and adult years the deaf are also drawn together by numerous sporting opportunities (e.g. sports meetings of the SDASA and the BDASA),[1] regional meetings (e.g. BDA[1] council meetings), school reunions, social activities such as those arranged by the local deaf clubs, etc. The result is that the deaf have formed a cohesive and mutually supportive community.

The majority of deaf people have two hearing parents. As these parents use a language (spoken English) that the deaf child can neither hear nor consequently use with much fluency, communication with family members is limited. It is at school among peers that most personal and social information develops (sharing occurs and close relationships are established), all through a language specially shaped for the eyes rather than the ears (visual/manual channel), and a language passed on by deaf parents whose deaf children then teach other deaf children how to use the language.

At the heart of every community is its language. This language embodies the thoughts and experiences of its users and they, in turn, learn about their culture or heritage and share in it together through their language. Thus deaf people achieve this through British Sign Language.

From the above it may be inferred that attitudinal deafness (self-identification as a member of the deaf community and identification by other members as a member) appears to be the most basic factor in determining membership of the deaf community. Attitudinal deafness is associated with appropriate language use. The language situation in the British deaf community can best be described as a diglossic[2] continuum between BSL and English.

[. . .]

The attitudes of native signers towards the use of BSL or the status of BSL in the deaf community tend to be more positive than those of non-native signers. Among native signers, the deaf children of deaf parents and deaf children who learned to sign when very young at deaf schools, there is a more favourable feeling towards the use of 'pure' BSL in schools for the deaf. However, the attitude of some deaf signers who have excellent competence in English and who became deaf at the age of about 6 years or upwards, tends to be one of repugnance towards the use of BSL in schools and they have referred to it as a 'dumb language' or a 'stupid non-language'. Disapproval is also shown by some deaf signers who learned to sign upon entering a deaf club and these deaf people usually cannot use the 'pure' BSL variety because they did not acquire BSL when they were very young. They may nevertheless admit that BSL is the native language of the deaf community in Britain and also that its usage is a powerful cohesive bond resulting in unrestricted and relaxed exchanges of thoughts, ideas and feelings between members of the deaf community.

Generally all deaf signers assume that BSL is used only at home or in deaf clubs while a formal variety of BSL, such as Signed English, is preferable to BSL as the medium for formal conversation with hearing people and for platform interpreting at conferences, meetings, churches and lectures. This is because they have been told, for too long, by teachers and others in authority that signing is disgraceful and must not be used in public. It is naturally bewildering for many deaf signers to be informed now that BSL is a real language consisting of proper signs, previously thought improper, in contrast to the kind of signs (including borrowed English and initialized signs) which were considered superior by the hearing social workers and missioners of the deaf and some teachers for the deaf. However, most native signers are opposed to the notion of hearing educationalists inventing or creating signs specifically for classroom teaching or borrowing words from English which are supposed to have no equivalent in the BSL vocabulary. Such invented signs are 'for', 'the', 'a', 'of', the 'to be' verbs, and the 'to do' verbs. These signs are regarded by the native signers as odd or even ridiculous.

[. . .]

Diglossia serves important functions in the deaf community by maintaining social identity and group solidarity. No overt attempts by hearing people should be made to change the social situation of the deaf community as they, being outside this community, do not share the values and experiences common to the members of the deaf community. Plans that hearing people evolve for deaf people are often totally inappropriate as a result of cultural differences and, therefore, if bilingual education is promoted solely by hearing people, it will probably fail. No social changes (and bilingual education is a social change), should be attempted without adequate knowledge of all the possible social ramifications involved. Sociolinguistic studies of the local deaf communities are absolutely necessary, and these studies must include the consideration of the attitudes of deaf people, deaf parents and deaf schoolchildren towards the local and/or standard language varieties used; towards diglossia; and identification of the local sign varieties in use.

Since research into BSL has begun so recently, we can look forward to exciting developments. It is to be hoped that these developments will promote the full and active participation of all deaf people in both the British deaf community and in British society as a whole.

[Notes

1   SDASA: Scottish Deaf Amateur Sports Association.
   BDASA: British Deaf Amateur Sports Association.
            (These are now both incorporated into the BDSC
            British Deaf Sports Council.)
   BDA: British Deaf Association.
   NUD: National Union of the Deaf.

2   Diglossia: two different varieties of a language used in different situations. It is argued that, in British Sign Language, there is a form more closely related to English and used in formal situations, and a form which exploits the visual medium which is used in more informal situations (Deuchar, 1977).]

References

Croneberg, C. (1976) 'The Linguistic Community', in Stokoe, Casterline and Croneberg, (eds.) *A Dictionary of American Sign Language,* Silver Spring, MD, Linstok Press.

Deuchar, M. (1977) *British Sign Language,* London, Routledge, Kegan Paul.

Markowicz, H. (1979) 'Sign Languages and the Maintenance of the Deaf Community' paper presented at the *NATO Symposium on Sign Language Research,* Copenhagen.

Woodward, J. C. (1975) 'How you Gonna get to Heaven if You Can't Talk with Jesus: The Educational Establishment versus the Deaf Community', paper presented at the annual meeting of the *Society for Applied Anthropology,* Amsterdam.

Woodward, J. C. (1978) 'Some Sociolinguistic Problems in the Implementation of Bi-lingual Education for Deaf Students', paper presented at the *Second National Symposium on Sign Language Research and Teaching,* San Diego.

2.3 The Modern Deaf Community

Paddy Ladd (1988)

[. . .]

The British Sign Language community today

. . . How can one describe the community's life in dry statistics and data? But, come to that, how can one describe it in words? Perhaps the life, bustle and laughter when deaf people get together and have the chance to use their language in full flow is best left to the imagination. Notable scenes in deaf culture include the standing joke of the club committee trying to push people out at closing time, and crowds standing around in the street signing for a good hour afterwards. Or of people of all ages staying up half the night together, telling jokes and stories (a major part of deaf culture), signing songs or poems or playing sign language-based games. Or of a regional rally, where a town centre is taken over by sign language for a weekend, and people from all over the country greet old schoolfriends across the street on their morning promenade.

At present there are over 200 clubs throughout the United Kingdom, and a survey of one such club revealed that 58 per cent of the members attended at least weekly (70 per cent of the men and 48 per cent of women). The rest of the time, unless one has a deaf spouse, is spent effectively in the hearing, English-speaking world which builds up a steady pressure that simply has to find release in being with other British Sign Language users. In addition, there is a strong national identity, as many people keep up old school contacts and, in so doing, make many others, which in turn are maintained. One classic example is the way news travels around the community. Information can go from one end of the country to the other and back again in a matter of days, despite the lack of access to the telephone.

In many cases there is an international consciousness too. It is much easier for signers from different countries to grasp and adapt to each others' visual messages, than for two speakers to create a common tongue. There is considerable international traffic between the different deaf communities, with individuals launching themselves into foreign lands and banking on making deaf contacts to make the trips successful.

Hearing members of the deaf community

Many people are surprised to learn that hearing people can be part of the British Sign Language community. But if one realizes that hearing children of deaf parents will often have BSL as their first language and English as their second, it begins to make sense. For many, deaf-club life is part of their Saturday night childhood, whether or not they stay members and work in deaf-related occupations as adults. In addition, deaf people have hearing brothers and sisters and, as the teaching of British Sign Language spreads, one can anticipate an increase in the number of siblings, as well as parents and workmates, who will learn the language enough to take part in the community.

[. . .]

Deaf culture, art and history

All languages develop creative forms, using metaphors, puns, symbols and so on, both to express new ideas, which in turn get built on and developed further, and also through simply playing with the language. If a language is severely oppressed, however, these creative forms can be lost, and it can contract down to a very functional level, simply serving everyday needs.

Something similar has happened to British Sign Language during this century. New signs are still developed, but it is only recently that the upturn in pride in the language has started to produce signs which express new ideas as a result of playing with old ones.

There are a number of ways in which the community currently expresses itself artistically. The one most taken for granted, storytelling, is in fact the one which has survived best. Drama is popular, but as yet has little to do with reflecting deaf people's language and culture. The other three, signed poetry, signed songs and cabaret, have only just started to develop again, but if recent American experience is anything to go by, they could become crucial not only in restoring deaf pride, but in capturing the attention of the hearing public.

[. . .]

The Deaf revival

In the past 10 years, there has been a revival in the strength of the British Sign Language community, which has taken several forms. In 1976, a number of deaf people, impatient with the lack of self-advocacy, formed the National Union of the Deaf (NUD). Although this organization has remained small, it has provided the impetus for deaf people once again to take charge of their own affairs, and has significantly influenced a number of important trends.

In 1974, the British Deaf Association started to speak out more vociferously for sign language, and in 1981 became more of an active campaigning body than before. In 1982 they produced a manifesto asking for official recognition of British Sign Language as a native British language, and made clear to the hearing world deaf people's aspirations to greater equality. In 1983, the first ever major lobby of the House of Commons took place, and in 1985, in conjunction with the National Union of the Deaf, a series of campaigns took place at the International Conference of Education of the Deaf in Manchester which formed the most successful fightback seen this century.

Inspired by developments in America, and encouraged by the advocacy of the organizations above, several schools have reverted back to using sign language in the classroom. These changes started with Signed English, but British Sign Language itself is beginning to find acceptance once more. The previous climate of fear is beginning to be replaced by one of happy cooperation between parents, teachers and the deaf community. However, there are few indications that deaf people are being encouraged to train as teachers, although more are now being accepted as classroom assistants in schools.

Sign language research

Few things changed people's thinking on this issue so radically and so fast as sign language research. Inspired by William Stokoe's work on American Sign Language, teams in Edinburgh and Bristol examined British Sign Language and found it was indeed a language, and one of greater complexity than had ever been suspected. By simply declaring that British Sign Language *was* a language, people's conceptions changed. Deaf people officially had something positive and attractive which made them equal to hearing people; deafness was not just viewed as being about the *loss* of something. And the difference in the way hearing people perceived deaf people's intelligence and ability can be measured by considering what must have been the previous image held—that signs were just monkey gestures used by a group of sub-humans who did not even have a language. Indeed the change has immense potential, for now the deaf community has a way of measuring the degree of respect they are or are not getting from society, by the degree to which it accepts their means of communication. Now the developing philosophy is 'Accept me—accept my language'.

In 1983, the Swedish government officially recognized Swedish Sign Language as a native language of Sweden. This has set a crucial world precedent, a goal for other deaf communities to strive for in order to achieve political recognition as a distinct sociocultural group rather than as a scattering of disabled individuals requiring state charity.

Other changes that have resulted from the linguistic recognition of BSL include:

(i) The deaf community can now be identified as a linguistic minority, rather than as individual handicapped people whose problem is the inability to hear sounds, and who are themselves a problem. This has made the issue a question of discrimination against a language-using group, and society's attitude has become the problem. Indeed, there is ongoing pressure from the National Union of the Deaf to get the United Nations to place sign languages under the protection of rulings on linguistic minorities (and thus prevent the abuses of oralism from re-occuring).

(ii) Inadequacies of teaching and interpreting methods have become much easier to identify now that British Sign Language is seen as a bona fide language, and we can look forward to an era of improved professional standards.

(iii) Greater prominence has been given to grass-roots British Sign

Language users, especially the deaf of deaf parents, rather than the previous models, who were people with good oral or English skills, and who were usually deafened people whose commitment to the deaf world was often equivocal.

(iv) Although welfare work had always included interpreting, little attention had previously been given to the subject. Once British Sign Language was formally acknowledged, and deaf people began to take more of an active role in their own and society's affairs, the demand for interpreters mushroomed, and whole areas of previous neglect came to light. These included the absence of interpreters in higher education, in the workplace, at social functions and so on. Although there are still far too few interpreters, and most of the work is still done almost on an *ad hoc* basis, we seem to be entering an age where this will become a major profession. It has been interesting to note that once an interpreter is present at a meeting of hearing people, interest in the deaf suddenly shoots up, and a host of issues emerge. It is interesting also to speculate how much more prominent in the public eye deaf people would have become, but for oralist policies driving British Sign Language underground. More sobering is the realization that the developments described above have come just in time, for in recent years there have been further changes in educational policy that, if unopposed, could bring the deaf community close to extinction.

The oralist responses

Oralist policies continue to place deaf children into hearing schools, either in groups in Partially Hearing Units, or alone in 'individualized integration'. These moves, backed by the Warnock Report[2] and the 1981 Education Act, have resulted in deaf schools all over the country being closed, including some which had started to use sign language. So far has this gone that the Department of Education and Science no longer even recognizes that there is such a thing as a category of 'deaf children' placing them instead into the category 'Children with special needs'. Encouraged by this, local authorities have started to cut expenditure on deaf education, the irony being that if *proper* integration programmes with interpreters, etc. were set up, it would actually be *more* expensive than deaf school education.

In the early 1980s, medical people started to devise cochlear implant surgery, which, although highly experimental in nature, has been performed on many deaf children in America and Europe. The media, ready as ever to treat deafness in science-fiction terms, gave these operations massive publicity, creating false hopes in parents and deaf teenagers alike. Once again, the oralist idea of 'getting rid of deafness' has been put back on the agenda, and the recent improvements of deaf life are once again facing severe threats.

The media and the BSL community

Once the deaf community had been driven underground, hearing people's images of deafness had to be obtained from the media. The latter insist upon seeing deafness in terms of something that can be 'overcome', and give prominence to a select few oral deaf people who succeed in behaving like hearing people by, for example, playing musical instruments, ballet dancing, having cochlear implants, and so on. Interestingly, this was the case right back at the beginning of oralism, when even *The Times* had declared that 'Deafness is abolished'.

In 1976, however, the National Union of the Deaf, recognizing that the key to the community's survival was in being seen on television, began to campaign for regular programmes in BSL. A pilot programme was made in 1979 for BBC Television's *Open Door*, aptly named *Signs of Life*, and a joint campaign thereafter with the British Deaf Association, called the Deaf Broadcasting Campaign, resulted in the establishment of the magazine programme *See Hear* in 1981. This has been followed by programmes on ITV and Channel 4, through which the image and status of British Sign Language users and their community has grown apace.

Despite the media influence of oral deaf models, there has nevertheless remained in the general public a fascination for sign language, one that we can trace right back in history . . . . This came together with the spread of BSL in the media in the 1980s, to produce a new peak, a televised teaching series *British Sign Language*.

In the final analysis then, in a future where the struggle for survival of the British Sign Language community has intensified on both sides, the readers of this book, with their committed interest in the language and its people are in an interesting position. For the first time, the hearing public on a wide scale are active participants in the struggle for final recognition or obliteration of the deaf community and British Sign Language.

[Notes

1   This paper was published originally in Miles, D. (1988) *British Sign Language: A Beginner's Guide,* which accompanied the BBC Television series *British Sign Language*, first Broadcast on BBC 1 in Spring 1988.

2   The Warnock Report: Special Educational Needs, Report of the Committee of Enquiry into the Education of Handicapped Children and Young People. HMSO, May 1978.]

2.4 The Deaf Community and the Culture of Deaf People

Carol Padden (1980)[1, 2]

[. . .]

The *Dictionary of American Sign Language*, published in 1965 by Bill Stokoe, Carl Croneberg and Dorothy Casterline, was unique for at least two reasons. First, it offered a new description of sign language based on linguistic principles. Second, it devoted a section to the description of the 'social' and 'cultural' characteristics of Deaf[3] people who use American Sign Language.

It was indeed unique to describe Deaf people as constituting a 'cultural group'. Professionals in the physical sciences and education of deaf people typically describe deaf people in terms of their pathological condition: hearing loss. There are numerous studies which list statistics about the types, ranges and aetiologies of hearing loss and how these physical deficiencies may subsequently affect the behaviour of deaf people. But rarely had these professionals seriously attended to other equally important aspects of Deaf people: the fact that Deaf people form groups in which the members do not experience 'deficiencies' and in which the basic needs of the individual members are met, as in any other culture of human beings.

Deaf people have long recognized that their groups are different from those of hearing people; in the 'Deaf world', certain behaviours are accepted while others are discouraged. The discussion of the 'linguistic community' of Deaf people in the *Dictionary of ASL* represented a break from a long tradition of 'pathologizing' Deaf people. In a sense, the book brought official and public recognition of a deeper aspect of Deaf people's lives: their culture.

When I re-read the book, as I do from time to time, I am always appreciative of the many insights that I find about the structure of American Sign Language and the culture of Deaf people.

The Deaf community

We commonly hear references to the 'deaf community'.[4] The term has demographic, linguistic, political and social implications. There is a national 'community' of deaf people who share certain characteristics and react to events around them as a group.

[. . .]

The term has been used in two restricted ways—either meaning only those persons who are audiologically deaf, or those persons who are a part of the culture of Deaf people. But it is clear that Deaf people work with and interact with other people who are not Deaf, and who share the goals of Deaf people and work with them in various social and political activities. Earlier definitions of 'deaf community', such as Schein's study of the Washington, DC deaf community in 1968, included only those persons who are audiologically hearing impaired. I propose a definition which differs from earlier ones:

> A deaf community is a group of people who live in a particular location, share the common goals of its members, and in various ways, work toward achieving these goals. A deaf community may include persons who are not themselves Deaf, but who actively support the goals of the community and work with Deaf people to achieve them.

. . . a deaf community has not only Deaf members, but also hearing and deaf people who are not culturally Deaf, and who interact on a daily basis with Deaf people and see themselves as working with Deaf people in various common concerns.

The culture of Deaf people, however, is more closed than the deaf community. Members of the Deaf culture behave as Deaf people do, use the language of Deaf people, and share the beliefs of Deaf people toward themselves and other people who are not Deaf.

[. . .]

The culture of American Deaf people
I will turn now to a discussion of some identifying characteristics of the American Deaf culture. My descriptions here are based first on intuition—my own understanding of how I grew up as a child of Deaf parents and how I interact with other Deaf people. I also consulted a number of books and articles written by Deaf people and have found several ideas and concerns repeated throughout these writings. I have picked out some of the more frequently occurring comments Deaf people make about themselves or their lives and have placed them in a framework of culture and cultural values. Some of the books I found helpful in explaining concerns of Deaf people are: Leo Jacobs' *A Deaf Adult Speaks Out* and W.H. Woods' *The Forgotten People*. The *Deaf American* magazine is another good source of information about issues that concern Deaf people.

Deaf people
What does it mean to be Deaf? Who are Deaf people?
Deaf people can be born into the culture, as in the case of children of Deaf parents. They begin learning the language of their parents from birth and thus acquire *native competence* in that language. They also learn the beliefs and behaviours of their parents' cultural group. When they enter schools, they serve as cultural and linguistic models for the larger number

of deaf children who do not have Deaf parents and who become a part of the culture later in life.

Being Deaf usually means the person has some degree of hearing loss. However, the type of degree of hearing loss is not a criterion for being Deaf. Rather, the criterion is whether a person identifies with other Deaf people, and behaves as a Deaf person. Deaf people are often unaware of the details of their Deaf friends' hearing loss, and, for example, may be surprised to learn that some of their friends can hear well enough to use the telephone.

But the most striking characteristic of the culture of Deaf people is their cultural values—these values shape how Deaf people behave and what they believe in.

Cultural values
What are some examples of values held by Deaf people?

Language Certainly an all-important value of the culture is respect for one of its major identifying features: American Sign Language. Not all Deaf individuals have native competence in ASL, that is, not all Deaf individuals have learned ASL from their parents as a first language. There are many individuals who become enculturated as Deaf persons and who bring with them a knowledge of some other language, usually English. While not all Deaf people are equally competent in ASL, many of them respect and accept ASL, and more now than before, Deaf people are beginning to promote its use. For Deaf people who prefer to use ASL, the language serves as a visible means of displaying one of their unique characteristics. While use of ASL sets the Deaf person apart from the majority English-speaking culture, it also belongs to Deaf people and allows them to take advantage of their capabilities as normal language-using human beings.

[. . .]

Speaking There is a general disassociation from speech in the Deaf culture. Some Deaf people may choose to use speech in community activities that involve non-Deaf people, such as mixed parties, parent education programmes, or while representing the community in some larger public function. But on the cultural level, speaking is not considered appropriate behaviour. Children who are brought up in Deaf culture are often trained to limit their mouth movement to only those movements that are a part of their language. Exaggerated speaking behaviour is thought of as 'undignified' and sometimes can be interpreted as making fun of other Deaf people.

[. . .]

Social relations As with any minority group, there is strong emphasis on social and family ties when family members are of the same culture or community. Carl Croneberg commented on this fact in the *Dictionary of ASL*. Deaf people consider social activities an important way of maintaining contact with other Deaf people. It has frequently been observed that Deaf people often remain in groups talking late, long after the party has ended, or after the restaurant has emptied of people. One reason is certainly that Deaf people enjoy the company of other like-minded Deaf people. They feel they gain support and trusting companionship from other Deaf people who share the same cultural beliefs and attitudes.

[. . .]

Stories and literature of the culture   The cultural values described in this paper are never explicitly stated; there are no books that Deaf children read to learn these values. Deaf children learn them through the process of training in which other Deaf people either reinforce or discourage their comments and actions. And these values are found among the symbols used in the literature of the culture. The play, *Sign me Alice* by Gil Eastman is a good example, or the poetry of Dot Miles in *Gestures: Poetry in Sign Language*, and many other unrecorded stories or games.

[. . .]

Entering into the culture of Deaf people
An interesting perspective on being Deaf comes from deaf people who are going through a process of becoming Deaf and are beginning to assimilate the values of Deaf people. In a study that Harry Markowicz and I did several years ago, we described the conflicts that these people experience. For many people who grow up as part of the culture of Hearing people, they think of themselves as hearing people with a hearing loss. But when they encounter the new and different culture of Deaf people, they find that not all of their beliefs and values will be accepted. They experience a conflict between what they have always believed and what they must accept when they are with other Deaf people. Their success in becoming full members of the culture of Deaf people depends on how they are able to resolve the conflicts they experience.

As an example of a conflict, a deaf person may value her speaking ability and may have always spoken when communicating with other people. But now she learns that speaking does not have the same positive value with Deaf people that it has with hearing people. Even though some Deaf people can hear some speech, and some speak well themselves, speaking is not considered usual or acceptable behaviour within the cultural group. The deaf person finds that she must change the behaviour that she has always considered normal, acceptable and positive.

[. . .]

Finally, an important behaviour to learn is what to call yourself. In hearing culture, it is desirable to distinguish between degrees of hearing loss. 'Hard-of-hearing' is more valued and indicates that the person is closer to being hearing and is more capable of interacting on an equal basis with other hearing people. However, 'deaf' is viewed more negatively and usually carries the implication that the person is difficult to communicate with, or may not speak at all.

Thus, a deaf person is more likely to be avoided if he calls himself 'deaf'. But, among Deaf people, the distinctions between hearing loss are not considered important for group relations. 'Deaf' is not a label of deafness as much as a label of identity with other Deaf people. A person learning to interact with other Deaf people will quickly learn that there is one name for all members of the cultural group, regardless of the degree of hearing loss: Deaf. In fact, the sign DEAF can be used in an ASL sentence to mean 'my friends', which conveys the cultural meaning of 'Deaf'. Although Deaf people recognize and accept members that are audiologically hard-of-hearing, calling oneself 'hard-of-hearing' rather than by the group name is interpreted by some Deaf people as 'putting on airs', because it appears to draw undue attention to hearing loss.

The existence of conflict brings out those aspects of the culture of Deaf people that are unique and separate from other cultural groups. It also shows that the group of Deaf people is not merely a group of like-minded people, as with a bridge club, but a group of people who share a code of behaviours and values that are learned and passed on from one generation of Deaf people to the next. Entering into Deaf culture and becoming Deaf means learning all the appropriate ways to behave like a Deaf person.

[. . .]

[Notes

1   We felt it important to include this paper because of its significance and relevance to the situation in the UK. However, because of our constraints on word length we have had to make drastic cuts to it. Most of the cuts are of material more specifically relevant to the situation in the USA.

2   *The Deaf Community and the Culture of Deaf People* draws from Carol Padden's earlier work with Harry Markowicz on the cultural boundaries within the Deaf community, as well as from her own experiences as a Deaf child of Deaf parents.]

3   I will use here a convention adopted by a number of researchers where the capitalized 'Deaf' is used when referring to cultural aspects, as in the culture of Deaf people. The lower case 'deaf', on the other hand, refers to non-cultural aspects such as the audiological condition of deafness.

4   As will be explained in a later section, the 'deaf community' as described here is not a cultural entity; thus the capitalized Deaf adjective will not be used to describe it. This differs from earlier treatments of the deaf community such as those found in Markowicz and Woodward (1975), Padden and Markowicz (1976), and Baker and Padden (1978).

References

Baker, C. and Padden, C. (1978) *ASL: A Look at its History, Structure, and Community,* Silver Spring, MD, TJ Publishers, Inc.

Deaf American, Silver Spring, MD, National Association of the Deaf.

Eastman, G. (1974) *Sign Me Alice: A Play in Sign Language,* Washington, DC, Gallaudet College.

Jacobs, L. (1969) *A Deaf Adult Speaks Out,* Washington, DC, Gallaudet College Press.

Markowicz, H. and Woodward, J. (1975) Language and the maintenance of ethnic boundaries in the Deaf Community. Paper presented at the *Conference on Culture and Communication,* held at Temple University, 13–15 March 1975.

Miles, D. (1976) *Gestures: Poetry in Sign Language,* Northridge, CA, Joyce Publishers, Inc.

Padden, C. and Markowicz, H. (1976) 'Cultural conflicts between hearing and Deaf communities', in *Proceedings of the Seventh World Congress of the World Federation of the Deaf,* Silver Spring, MD, National Association of the Deaf.

Schein, J. (1968) *The Deaf Community,* Washington, DC, Gallaudet College Press.

Stokoe, W. C., Croneberg, C. and Casterline. D. (1965) *Dictionary of American Sign Language,* Washington, DC, Gallaudet College Press. Second publication, 1976, Silver Spring, MD, Linstok Press.

Woods, W. H. (1973) *The Forgotten People,* St. Petersburg, FL., Dixie Press.

2.5 Is There a Deaf Culture?

David Brien (1981)

[. . .]

Is there a deaf culture? By culture I mean a distinctive way of life—the customs, habits, ideas, beliefs, institutions, etc. which a particular group, through a shared language, hold in common. The existence of a deaf culture presupposes the existence of a deaf community. It would seem that one must first define that community (its membership, boundaries, etc.) before one can be in a position to describe the actual shared assumptions, practices, beliefs, etc., which comprise the culture. However, the relationship between the two may not be so easily disentangled. In what follows I argue that the two are experienced as inseparable: facets of a single entity.

It is an approach which is most concisely presented by Baker and Cokely (1980) (to whom I am indebted in that I have drawn in particular from their work in defining the deaf community). They observe that although many different definitions of the deaf community have been suggested in recent years these may be reduced to two types:

1 *Clinical – Pathological:* definitions of the deaf community which accept as given that the 'behaviour and values of the hearing majority (be taken) as the "norm", and then focus(es) on how deaf people deviate from this norm'. It is an approach which may be characterized as seeking to 'repair' deaf people so that they might become as 'normal' as possible. Baker and Cokely conclude that it is the approach traditionally associated with the 'majority of hearing people who interact on a professional basis with deaf people'.

2 *Cultural:* definitions which focus on the common language, shared experiences etc. which characterize a particular group of people, who in addition, in this case, 'happen to be deaf'. It is a view which conceives of the deaf community as a separate cultural group with 'its own values and language' which should be accepted as such. If such definitions are accepted, the appropriateness of redefining the deaf as a 'minority' group, rather than a 'handicapped' group, becomes apparent.

The distinction that Baker and Cokely are making between the two categories (clinical – pathological and cultural) may be clarified if we examine the individual definitions which they allocated to each category. Under the clinical – pathological there are a number of definitions from studies which are probably familiar to you. Jerome Schein in *The Deaf*

Community (1968) defines the deaf community as 'an audiologically definable group of persons whose hearing loss is sufficient to interfere with, but does not preclude the normal reception of speech'. Myklebust *The Psychology of Deafness* (1960) and Davis and Silverman *Hearing and Deafness* (1960) are two amongst a number of publications which define the deaf community as 'a group of hearing-impaired persons who have learning and psychological problems due to their hearing loss and communication difficulties'. In an article in the *Deaf American* entitled 'Deafness and Minority Group Dynamics', Vernon and Makowsky (1969) provided the following definition: 'a minority group composed of hearing-impaired persons who are treated in certain ways by the hearing majority'. The use of the term 'minority group' (despite its negative orientation) suggests that this definition might more appropriately be seen as straddling the divide between the two categories being distinguished (clinical – pathological and cultural), than listed under the clinical – pathological. However, as with each of the others, it grants to the single characteristic 'hearing loss' a master status, one which precludes the inclusion of any positive conception of deaf people within the definition. It may be summarized as the 'deaf as deficient' approach. In contrast, Baker and Cokely list the following definitions of the deaf community under cultural: the first, taken from *Sound and Sign* by Schlesinger and Meadow (1972), describes the deaf community as 'a group of persons who share a common means of communication (American Sign language) which provides the basis for group cohesion and identity'. In a paper presented at the Seventh World Congress of the World Federation of the Deaf, Padden and Markowicz (1976) used the following: '[a] group of persons who share a common language and a common culture'.

The contrast in orientation (between the cultural and the clinical – pathological) is obvious. The cultural provides a way to call into question the deeply entrenched view that profound deafness is to be associated automatically with disability, and thereby, inability. In a society which sought to accommodate rather than assimilate difference, to maximize potential rather than reify differences as unacceptable, the position of deaf people would indeed be different.

[. . .]

The work of William Stokoe (1960, 1972) and other linguists (see for example, Klima and Bellugi, 1979; Brennan, Colville and Lawson, 1980; and Woll, Kyle and Deuchar, 1981) has demonstrated that the individual sign languages of the deaf are indeed proper languages (and not constructions based on an inadequate grasp of oral languages, as was once suspected). It is this which has provided the catalyst for the change in focus implicit in the cultural definition of the deaf community. In summary, it seeks to draw attention to what deaf people actually do instead of what they do not; in particular, it focuses on how deaf people communicate rather than how they do not. It enables deaf people to be seen as other than 'handicapped', and therefore other than 'deficient'—at present the prevailing view in society. To continue to accept the clinical – pathological based definitions as the most appropriate descriptions of the deaf community available, is to limit the lives of deaf people through an ignorance that is no longer excusable.

In my introduction, I suggested that culture and community may be understood as facets of a single entity. This is illustrated in various studies which seek to define the boundaries of the community, and in so doing, the membership of the community. The differences which appear in the literature revolve around two types of definition. The definition given above is contrasted with a looser, more elastic use of the term 'community', and the view that the low incidence of deafness does not permit selectivity (in any vigorous sense) of membership. The two approaches are not, however, necessarily contradictory, as will be seen.

In that not all deaf people seek membership, or have it bestowed upon them, it is an achieved status. Minimally, three basic requirements have to be met (or 'achieved'). Higgins (1980) identifies these as:

1   An identification with the deaf world.

2   Shared experience of being deaf (e.g. attendance at a residential school).

3   Involvement with other members of the community.

Carol Padden (1980) incorporates these factors into a definition which distinguishes between members of the deaf community and those (a restricted group) she describes as 'culturally' deaf (for whom culture and community are a single entity). . . Padden defines the local community as 'a group of people who live in a particular location, share the common goals of its members, and in various ways work towards achieving these goals. A deaf community may include people who are not themselves deaf but actively support the goals of the community, and work with deaf people to achieve them'. The culturally deaf she identifies as those who 'behave as deaf people do, use the language of deaf people and share the beliefs that deaf people have about themselves and about those who are not deaf'. In distinguishing between the deaf community and the culturally deaf, Padden draws attention to the different variants of sign language in use within the community. These are illustrated in Figure 1: a continuum, with at either end a 'Sign Language' whose grammatical structure is totally different from the other. The language of the culture is British Sign Language, and its use acts as an effective cultural boundary; that is, access is only available through British Sign Language. When in communication with those who, in Padden's terms, are part of the outer community (e.g. hearing people who work with the deaf), deaf people usually use some form of Pidgin Sign English reflecting their acquaintance (if any) with English.

Figure 2 is taken from Baker and Cokely (1980) and provides a more detailed consideration of what it is that defines membership. They identify four 'avenues' by which membership may be achieved, and define them as follows:

1   Audiological: refers to hearing loss, and is therefore, by definition, an avenue of entry unavailable to hearing people.

2   Political: the ability to exert influence on matters which directly affect the deaf community.

3   Linguistic: the ability to use and understand British Sign Language. Fluency does appear to be related to the level of acceptance one may hope to achieve. In that the values of the community are transmitted by its language, the need for fluency is self evident.

4   Social: the ability to participate satisfactorily in the social functions of

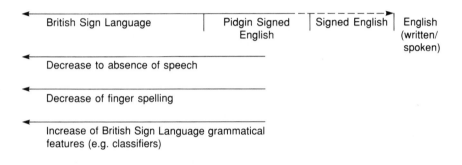

Figure 1   Sign language continuum[1] (after Lawson, 1980)

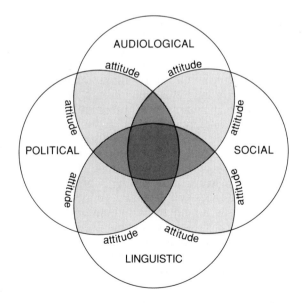

Figure 2   Avenues to membership in the deaf communities (after Baker and Cokely, 1980)

the community. It means being invited to such functions, feeling at ease whilst present, and having friends who are themselves members. This ability may presuppose other factors, such as competence in sign language.

It is apparent from such an analysis that being a member of the community is not granted as a consequence of any single factor but rather, in Baker and Cokely's words, 'a complex process in which certain skills (linguistic), activities (social and political), and realities (hearing loss) are weighed' in relation to the individual's basic identification with the community. By having access through at least two of the avenues you may be said to be a member of the community according to this definition.

[. . .]

I wish to turn next (briefly) to what it is deaf people themselves obtain from the community. The short answer is normality. The reality which has the greatest influence on the lives of deaf people has so far escaped attention—that deaf people pass most of their existence in a hearing world.

As Higgins (1980) explains, the existence of the deaf community, and the identity of deaf people, is a consequence of deaf people's experience in that hearing world. The promise of oral education, that the born profoundly deaf person would be able to pass, at best, as a slightly deficient example of a hearing person, has not come to pass. It is this failure, and the unwillingness, so far, of the majority in society to learn to sign, that necessitates the existence of the deaf community.[2] Its existence, in the form of its institutions, etc., is not the consequence of exclusion from hearing society alone, but arises in equal part from a desire to have its own alternative structures to those of hearing society. In that they mirror those of hearing society it may be argued that this conceals a desire for integration which goes unstated. However, as Higgins stresses, it (the deaf community) is a consciously developed alternative from which the problems of communication and interaction with non-signing hearing people are excluded. Through interaction with others, the individual is able to develop an awareness and acceptance of self. Through participation in the various organizations that make up the community, (the British Deaf Association, deaf club, sports club, etc.), individuals are able to acquire a sense of self-esteem which may be impossible to develop within the hearing world. Each may draw on the experiences of others to compensate for any lack of general information. In a community in which so many experiences and expectations are shared, the fact that 85–90% of deaf people take a deaf spouse is unsurprising. In summary, as Higgins (1980) has noted, the deaf community represents a most complex response to the threat of social isolation and the difficulties of communication, which the deaf person experiences in the wider community. Its culture comprises 'a range of activities which are sufficiently powerful to nullify, for the majority of deaf people, the negative experiences of daily life'. By 'sealing off' those aspects of their lives that really matter, deaf people have made the existence of a positive deaf identity possible.

[. . .]

Notes

1 Based on Lawson, L. (1980) 'Is British Sign Language the Language of the Deaf?', Paper presented at the *British Deaf Association Triennial Congress,* Scarborough, June. 1980.

[2 Kannapell, B. (1977) in a section of Brien's paper not included here is quoted as saying:

> It is important to understand that American Sign Language is the only thing that we have that belongs to Deaf people completely. It is the only thing that has grown out of the Deaf group. Maybe we are afraid to share our language with hearing people. Maybe our group identity will disappear once hearing people know American Sign Language. Also, will hearing people dominate Deaf people more than before if they learn American Sign Language?]

References

Baker, C. and Cokely, D. (1980) *American Sign Language: A Teacher's Resource Text on Grammar and Culture,* Vol. 1, Maryland, T. J. Publishers Inc.

Brennan, M. Colville, M. and Lawson, L. (1980) *Words in Hand: A Structural Analysis of the Signs of British Sign Language,* Moray House College, Edinburgh, BSL Project.

Davis, H. A. and Silverman, S. (1960) *Hearing and Deafness,* New York, Holt, Rinehart and Winston.

Higgins, P. (1980) *Outsiders in a Hearing World: A Sociology of Deafness,* London, Sage Publications.

Kannapell, B. (1977) 'The Deaf Person as a Teacher of American Sign Language', in *National Symposium on Sign Language Research and Teaching,* 1977, Washington, DC, National Association of the Deaf, and quoted in Baker and Cokely (1980).

Klima, E. and Bellugi, U. (1979) *The Signs of Language,* London, Harvard University Press.

Myklebust, H. (1960) *The Psychology of Deafness,* New York, Grune and Stratton.

Padden, C. (1980) 'The Deaf Community and the Culture of Deaf People', in Baker, S. and Battison, R. (eds.) *Sign Language and the Deaf Community: Essays in Honour of William Stokoe,* Washington DC, National Association of the Deaf.

Padden, C. and Markowicz, H. (1976) 'Cultural Conflicts between Hearing and Deaf Communities', in *Proceedings of the Seventh World Congress of the World Federation of the Deaf,* Washington, DC, National Association of the Deaf.

Schein, J. (1968) *The Deaf Community: Studies in the Social Psychology of Deafness,* Washington, DC, Gallaudet College Press.

Schlesinger, H. and Meadow, K. (1972) *Sound and Sign,* Berkeley, CA, University of California Press.

Stokoe, W. (1960) 'Sign Language Structure', in *Studies in Linguistics Occasional Papers 8,* Buffalo, University of Buffalo Press.

Stokoe, W. (1972) *Semiotics and Human Sign Language,* New York, Humanities.

Vernon, M. and Makowsky, B. (1969) 'Deafness and Minority Group Dynamics', *The Deaf American 21, 11,* pp. 3–6.

Woll, B., Kyle, J. and Deuchar, M. (1981) *Perspectives on British Sign Language and Deafness,* London, Croom Helm.

Section 3
Psychological Perspectives: Understanding Difference or Different Understandings?

In contrast to previous papers which have attempted to understand aspects of deafness by taking Deaf people's own perspectives seriously, and which have tried to understand deafness from 'within', the present section introduces studies of deaf people from 'outside', from the perspective of a well established, powerful, non-deaf, professional discourse. In cognitive psychology, the impetus for the study of deaf people came from attempts to understand the cognitive functioning of hearing people. Hearing people provided the standard or norm against which the (almost invariably negative) effects of a sensory impairment or deficit could be measured. Until recently psychological perspectives of deafness have been dominated by a deficit model underpinned by audiological definitions of hearing loss. Within cognitive psychology deaf people have provided a natural experimental group; by using a sensory impairment, deafness, as the independent variable, psychologists have attempted to measure dependent variables. Deafness has been viewed as the absence of hearing and deaf people as linguistically deficient:

> . . . a number of new studies with deaf subjects have been reported. It seems that psychologists are beginning to realise the opportunity offered by the presence of linguistically deficient persons to test theories about the influence of language on various cognitive activities which are here subsumed under the word 'thinking'.
> (Furth, 1971, p. 58)

Quigley and Paul summarize this approach but indicate that it need not inevitably carry a negative evaluation of deafness, albeit implicit. Kyle's paper, in emphasizing the importance of process rather than result in cognitive studies, moves away from a deficit model of deafness towards a non-evaluative model of difference, towards a pluralist psychology.

The deficit model, with its negative connotations, has been pervasive in the area of clinical psychology. Descriptive studies of the personality characteristics of deaf people in the 1960s and 1970s suggested that deafness had a negative influence on personality development. Rainer and Altshuler (1967) described deaf people as egocentric, rigid, impulsive and lacking in insight. Myklebust (1960) suggested that they were aloof, disengaged and isolated from other people. The paper by Lane in this volume provides a detailed and systematic critique of such studies. However, the influence of this work so pervaded the mental health field that a specific mental health problem became attributed to deaf people and was labelled 'surdophrenia'. Although this notion has now been largely discredited, partly because it locates the problem within the individual rather than within social interaction, it nevertheless persists in the psychiatric literature about deaf people (cf. Denmark and Adams, 1988).

As deaf people become more actively involved in the construction of a psychology of deafness the sensory deficit model with its negative connotations is being replaced by a more complex pluralistic model.

References

Denmark, J. and Adams, J. (1988) 'Surdophrenia', in Taylor, I. (ed.) *The Education of the Deaf—Current Perspectives,* London, Croom Helm.

Furth, H. (1971) 'Linguistic Deficiency and Thinking: Research with Deaf Subjects 1964–69', *Psychological Bulletin, 76, 1,* pp. 58–77.

Myklebust, H. R. (1960) *The Psychology of Deafness*, New York, Grune and Stratton.

Rainer, J. D. and Altshuler, K. Z. (1967) *Psychiatry and the Deaf,* Washington, DC, US Department of Health, Educational Welfare.

3.1 Cognition and Language

Stephen Quigley and Peter Paul (1984)

[. . .]

Two questions have engaged the interest of researchers in the areas of cognition (thinking) and language, and resolution of these questions has practical significance for teachers, clinicians and other practitioners with deaf children and adults. First, there is theoretical and practical significance to knowing whether quantitative or qualitative differences exist between deaf and hearing people on various aspects of cognitive functioning such as memory, perception, creativity and so forth. If certain differences do exist, they might indicate limitations on deaf persons' abilities to acquire particular cognitively based skills that are acquired readily by hearing people (such as reading), or they might dictate that in order to acquire those skills different developmental and teaching approaches need to be used with deaf children than are used with hearing children. Second, study of the cognitive and language functioning of deaf individuals might shed light on the persistent philosophic and scientific question of whether there is a relation between language and thought and if there is, what is the nature of it. Is language dependent on thought; is thought dependent on language; are the two mutually dependent; or are they mutually independent? This question, too, has practical significance. For example, if language is dependent on thought (cognition), then any differences or deficits in cognitive development will likely affect language acquisition.

Pintner and a group of colleagues, starting in the 1910s, were among the first to study these questions (and the psychology of deafness) in a systematic way with deaf people, and their resulting research conclusions led to the first of three positions that have been taken on the first question. This was that deaf people were intellectually inferior to hearing people and showed definite deficits in various aspects of cognitive functioning (Pintner and Reamer, 1920; Pintner, Eisenson and Stanton, 1941). It is important to note that most of the tests used by these investigators were paper-and-pencil tests which often required verbal manipulation and verbal responses in the English language. Much of the historical development in the study of cognitive functioning of deaf people is a history of increasingly successful attempts by investigators to devise truly non-verbal tests of cognition. The goal is to assess the deaf person's performance on cognitive tasks, such as sequential memory, without the involvement of language. This is extremely difficult because of the pervasive influence of language in most of human behaviour, but as attempts to accomplish it have been increasingly successful, differences between deaf and hearing persons in various cognitive abilities have tended to decrease and often to disappear.

The theoretical position of Pintner and his colleagues was dominant until the 1940s when it was challenged by the formulations proposed by Mykelbust (1960). Myklebust interpreted a series of studies by him and a number of his students as showing that there are quantitative similarities but qualitative differences between deaf and hearing individuals when verbal factors in cognitive and intellectual tasks are controlled. The types of differences found by Myklebust and his students led him to conclude that on global measures (e.g. total score on IQ tests such as the [Wechsler Intelligence Scale for Children] WISC) deaf individuals equalled hearing individuals, but that the profiles of deaf and hearing individuals on specific abilities differed. That is, deaf and hearing persons performed differently on the various subtests of such tests as the WISC. Similar findings were revealed on tests of a variety of cognitive functions such as memory and creativity. The findings led Myklebust to conclude that deaf individuals were more concrete and less abstract cognitively than hearing individuals. He further concluded that the basic experiences of deaf people are altered as a direct consequence of hearing impairment and that all subsequently developed behaviours are also altered, thus making the deaf person inherently different from the hearing person in many ways. Myklebust proposed the 'organismic shift hypothesis' to explain these alleged inherent differences of deaf people.

The third stage of this historical perspective is the one that seems to prevail today—that deaf people are intellectually and cognitively similar to hearing people in all important abilities. Rosenstein (1961), Furth (1966) and Vernon (1967) have taken the position that few if any differences exist between deaf and hearing individuals in cognitive functioning. This position is based on a substantial body of research conducted by numerous individuals (mostly in the 1960s and 1970s), some of which is discussed in this chapter. It is now generally accepted by researchers that any differences that do exist between deaf and hearing individuals on cognitive abilities are the result of environmental or task influences rather than being inherent in deafness. Quigley and Kretschmer (1982, p. 51) categorized these task influences as: '1) the inability of the researcher to properly convey the task demands because of language differences or deficits on the part of the subject, 2) implicit bias within the solution of the task, or 3) general experiential deficits (including verbal language and communication in general) on the part of the subjects'.

The second question posed, concerning the relationship between cognition and language, has also had various answers at different historical stages. The early position (known as the language dominant position) was that language was primary and that thinking (beyond early and primitive stages) took place in language. This position is exemplified by the linguist Sapir (1958) who states that:

> It is quite an illusion to imagine that one adjusts to reality without the use of language and that language is merely an incidental means of solving specific problems of communication or reflection . . . we see and hear and otherwise

experience as we do because the language habits of our community predispose certain choices of interpretation.
(Sapir, 1958, p. 162)

In this view, the child's linguistic development is determined largely by experience with language, and language accounts for the acquisition of concepts that are expressed within it (Quigley and Kretschmer, 1982). The opposing (and the presently prevailing) view is the cognitive dominant hypothesis which proposes that basic perceptual and cognitive development precedes language and provides the basis or underpinning for linguistic development. Language, in this view, is a natural extension or subset of the previously developed cognitive process.

The present evidence does not appear to support the language dominant hypothesis (also known as the Whorfian hypothesis). Studies of hearing children by numerous investigators (notably Piaget and his followers) and of deaf children (notably Furth and his colleagues) have shown that much perceptual and cognitive development takes place prior to language development and also concurrently but independently of early language development. In Piaget's view,

A symbolic function exists which is broader than language and encompasses both the system of verbal signs and that of symbols in the strict sense . . . it is permissable to conclude that thought precedes language . . . language is not enough to explain thought, because the structures that characterize thought have their roots in action and in sensorimotor mechanisms that are deeper than linguistics.
(Piaget, 1967, pp. 91–2)

Although the present weight of empirical evidence does not seem to support the language dominant (Whorfian) hypothesis, a number of recent investigators have presented a weaker version of this hypothesis (Cromer, 1976; Schlesinger, 1977; McNeill, 1978). This weak form of the Whorfian hypothesis suggests that although language does not dictate thought, it can and does influence thought. The evidence for this position comes primarily from linguistic intuitions rather than from direct studies of cognitive and linguistic development. It has been pointed out, for example, that there are certain distinctions made in languages, such as gender and verb transitivity, that are language specific, and do not have real world correlates or referents.

It is not the purpose of this chapter to analyse in depth the enduring question of the relationship between thought (cognition) and language. The present weight of evidence in favour of the cognitive dominant hypothesis is accepted. Interest in the issue and in the comparative cognitive functioning of deaf and of hearing individuals is concerned with how it, and more importantly the data collected in pursuing it, can illuminate the problem of language development in deaf individuals. This interest is centred in two questions. First, how does the cognitive development of deaf individuals compare with the cognitive development of hearing individuals? Second, what are the internal symbolic mediators of thought in deaf people?

[. . .]

Present resolution of the enduring question of the relationship between language and cognition (thought) seems to favour the primacy of basic cognitive processes with language being dependent on them. Perception, attention, memory and other abilities need to develop appropriately to ensure the adequate development of the abstract thinking processes and language on which educational development is largely based. Deficits or problems in the development of basic cognitive processes will be reflected in problems of language development and ultimately in most academic educational areas. This is why the work of psychologists such as Piaget and others with hearing children, and Furth and others with deaf children, have major implications for teachers and clinicians.

While the language/cognition question seems at this stage to have been resolved in favour of the primacy of cognition, the question of how deaf individuals compare with hearing individuals on cognitive tasks seems to have been resolved in favour of equality of performance; however, this should be treated with caution. It has long been obvious from the successful social and occupational functioning of deaf individuals that the Pintner position of deficits in the general cognitive and intellectual functioning of deaf people is untenable. As greater control has been exerted over the variables that influence studies of cognitive abilities, especially verbal language, differences between deaf and hearing individuals have decreased, and in some cases disappeared. They have not disappeared in all areas, however. Some differences continue to be found on various Piagetian tasks and in areas such as sequential memory which are important to language and educational development. There is a tendency to assume that even greater experimental control will eventually eliminate those differences also. But the possibility that they are true differences should also be entertained. This is particularly true of linguistically codable materials where studies have consistently shown deaf people to have shorter memory spans than hearing people (Lichtenstein, 1983).

It does not follow from the acceptance of true differences between deaf and hearing individuals in some cognitive areas, that *inferiority* in cognitive, linguistic and educational development will inevitably follow. Knowing the nature and effects of any true differences allows developmental and educational programmes to be shaped to capitalize on the differences. For example, if deaf people do perform as well as, or better than, hearing people on tests of spatial memory, but less well on tests of sequential memory, and if these are true differences, there are several implications for educational practice. First, since hearing is an efficient processor of temporal–sequential input (such as auditory language), while vision is more efficient at processing spatial information, ASL might have some advantages over spoken language as the initial linguistic input for at least some deaf children. ASL makes use of motion and position in space to convey some concepts that depend on temporal–sequential transmission in spoken language. This might be particularly true in connected discourse where certain syntactic constructions might be heavily dependent on temporal–sequential storage in short-term memory. According to the work of Lichtenstein, this type of processing of information is important in comprehending embedded or interrupted syntactic constituents such as sentences with medial relative clauses (e.g. The boy who kissed the girl ran away) which require integration of information from the beginning and end of a sentence for proper understanding. Deaf persons have great difficulty in understanding the spoken and written forms of such syntactic constructions (Quigley, Smith and Wilbur, 1974), yet it is possible that the constructions can be readily understood through ASL where they are conveyed in terms of space, movement and facial expressions. ASL might be uniquely adapted to capitalize on the cognitive differences between deaf and hearing individuals by using space and motion where spoken language uses time for the same purpose.

A second implication in the same area is that manually coded English systems might have some advantage over spoken language in that, like ASL, they make the individual units of language (words) more visible than does speech, but they might have the same disadvantage as speech in connected discourse in that they rely on time rather than space as an important element in syntactic transmission. A third in this chain of implications derived from possible differences between deaf and hearing individuals in spatial and temporal–sequential memory is that teachers and clinicians, in order to teach deaf children the language of the core society, need to know some of the basic ideas of cognition and the comparative performances of deaf and hearing children in various cognitive abilities.

References

Cromer, R. (1976) 'The Cognitive Hypothesis of Language Acquisition and its Implications for Child Language Deficiency', in Morehead, D. and Morehead, A. (eds) *Normal and Deficient Child Language,* Baltimore, University Park Press.

Furth, H. (1966) *Thinking Without Language: Psychological Implications of Deafness,* New York, Free Press.

Lichtenstein, E. (1983) *The Relationship Between Reading Process and English Skills of Deaf Students,* Rochester, NY, National Technical Institute for the Deaf.

McNeill, D. (1978) 'Speech and Thought', in Markova, I. (ed.) *The Social Context of Language*, New York, Wiley.

Myklebust, M. (1960) *The Psychology of Deafness,* New York, Grune and Stratton.

Piaget, J. (1967) 'Language and Thought from the Genetic Point of View', in Elkind, D. (ed.) *Six Psychological Studies*, New York, Random House.

Pintner, R., Eisenson, J. and Stanton, M. (1941) *The Psychology of the Physically Handicapped*, New York, Crofts.

Pintner, R. and Reamer, J. (1920) 'A Mental and Educational Survey of Schools for the Deaf', *American Annals of the Deaf, 65*, pp. 451–72.

Quigley, S. and Kretschmer, R.E. (1982) *The Education of Deaf Children*, Baltimore, University Park Press.

Quigley, S., Smith, N. and Wilbur, W. (1974) 'Comprehension of Relativized Sentences by Deaf Students', *Journal of Speech and Hearing Research, 17*, pp. 325–41.

Rosenstein, J. (1961) 'Perception, Cognition and Language in Deaf Children', *Exceptional Children, 27*, pp. 176–284.

Sapir, E. (1958) 'Language and Environment', in Mandelbaum, D. (ed.) *Selected Writings of Edward Sapir in Language, Culture and Personality*, Berkeley, University of California.

Schlesinger, I. (1977) 'The Role of Cognitive Development and Linguistic Input in Language Acquisition', *Journal of Child Language, 4*, 153–69.

Vernon, M. (1967) 'Relationship of Language to the Thinking Process', *Archives of General Psychiatry, 16*, pp. 325–33.

3.2 Looking for Meaning in Sign Language Sentences

Jim Kyle (1983)

[. . .]

I want to describe an experiment whose outcomes I can only partly explain, but which throws some light on the question of what sort of language Sign is, and how we might describe the sentences it produces. The need for such a study arises because when deaf people retell an event from their experience, it seems incredibly rich in imagery, and leads me to the prediction that a deaf viewer of a signed story is generally better able to replicate the story than a hearing person who has heard the same story retold in speech. There is a complex qualitative difference in language used. Deaf people appear to be very accurate in their story, while hearing people tend to infer the outcomes of the story.

The study

The study of recall in speech and in sign is an attempt to examine the complexity of sign grammar when viewed from above, that is from the meaning of the story. The stimulus used was a 1920s' silent movie. The film lasts three minutes and consists of three main episodes.

Episode 1

Husband, wife and mother-in-law at home, when the doorbell rings. A postman brings an 'Invitation for One' to a notorious dance-hall. The wife is shocked and returns the ticket to the postman. But, the husband secretly obtains the ticket and pays the postman for his trouble.

Episode 2

Husband leaves the house supposedly to go to the boxing, but goes to the dance hall where he enjoys himself with another woman. Unfortunately they win a Charleston contest which is being broadcast live to his wife and mother-in-law at home. His name is announced over the air.

Episode 3

He returns home and tries to creep into the house, sporting an unexplained black eye. He is accepted back into the family.

The story is inconsequential in a way which allows modification of its meaning and makes it necessary for organizational processes to work on the retelling of it.

The story was shown individually to deaf and hearing people, and they were asked to retell the story immediately, and again after one hour. The deaf people signed to a deaf researcher and the hearing people spoke to a hearing researcher.

Rumelhart (1975) suggests some simple principles for writing down the schema of a story which allow it to be divided into *episodes* and *events*. Using an approach derived from Kintsch (1977) these events may then contain a number of propositions each of which contribute a unit of meaning which can stand alone—they consist of a relational term and one or more arguments. In this interpretation, for English they consist of units with at least a verb and implied subject—'the bell rang' or 'he gave her a ticket'; while for sign they consist of units containing an action or attribution which constitutes an identifiable advancement of meaning (from a deaf transcriber's point of view) and would tend to be translated as a proposition in English—'MAN-GO' (the man is going) and 'MAN-GONE' (the man has gone) (Figures 1 and 2.)

The comparisons are therefore of spoken and signed versions of the same silent film, considered as the communication of a story from one language user to another.

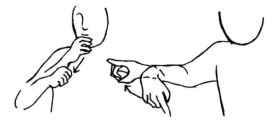

Figure 1   MAN-GO

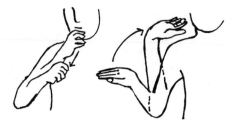

Figure 2   MAN-GONE

Participants

There were six hearing and six deaf people in this initial examination of recall. The hearing people were secretarial staff in the University aged 30–58. The deaf people were filmed in different locations around the UK. Their ages ranged from 31–63. They all had been deaf from an early age and had hearing parents. All had severe to profound hearing losses. A seventh deaf and seventh hearing person provided a commentary of the film.

Procedure

For the deaf people the task was introduced at the beginning of a session involving a series of sign language tasks. Each person was shown the silent film, and then introduced to a deaf researcher (the same one each time) who supposedly had not seen this film. They were asked to describe what they had seen in as much detail as they could. Their narrative was video-recorded. Approximately one hour later, they were asked to retell the story (without warning), and again this was video-recorded.

In exactly the same way, the hearing people were individually shown the film then asked for an immediate recall and a recall approximately one hour later. The stories were told to a hearing researcher. Audio recording was made.

Recordings of commentaries of the film, that is, simultaneous descriptions of the film's content, were made one in Sign by a deaf viewer, and one in speech by a hearing viewer. These, when transcribed, were used to estimate the propositional content of the story, in speech and Sign. It is possible to divide these commentaries into eighty-five propositions for speech, and 111 propositions in Sign. The reason for the larger amount of grammatical construction in Sign I think relates to the main issue of how information is structured in the language. There is no doubt that the level of accuracy of these accounts and the propositional content is determined by the individuals involved. Qualitatively, there appears to be a difference in the type of propositions used, and it is this which is most interesting. However, it is accepted that there are serious problems in analysis of this data which make the determination of propositions in the surface structure of speech as well as of Sign, extremely difficult. The study claims only to be an initial examination of what is a highly complex, but possibly extremely rich area.

Examination of the data

Inevitably, the data is very complex and we are only in the initial stages of finding a description for it. The purpose is to examine to what extent the schema or the overall plan used for description differs between deaf and hearing people, and whether this affects or explains the difference in language structure.

There are three major divisions in the story descriptions: episodes, events and propositions. Our examination of deaf and hearing recall therefore revolves around these divisions. By taking a number of hypotheses for analysis we can begin to attempt some answers.

Hypothesis 1

Deaf people and hearing people differ in their descriptions of the story because of different perceptions of the world.

There is no support for this hypothesis. All deaf and hearing people reported the main episodes in the story accurately, also the eighteen main events in both recalls to the same extent. Comparing hearing people's propositional recall to that of the hearing commentary, we find an average of 28 per cent propositions recalled accurately after one hour, for deaf people's signed recall the figure is 29 per cent in comparison to a deaf commentary. These findings reflect a similarity in the process of recall at least at the schema level, and a similarity in the capacity for recall.

Hypothesis 2

Deaf and hearing people differ markedly in the structure of the language production, due to the capacities of the language itself.

Certainly, there are differences between the two commentaries: 111 propositions in sign compared to eighty-five in speech. These indicate individual differences to some extent, and I do not wish to belabour these actual figures; nevertheless, they provide a yardstick for estimation. However, it is the content of the commentaries which is more interesting. There were twenty-five one-sign sentences as Stokoe (1980) has defined them (23% of the total). These include examples such as:

MAN SAY NO–*RIVALRY*–WOMAN SAY STAY
Where 'rivalry' consists of alternative upward and downward movement of [both] hands, meaning they disputed who was to go to the door (Figure 3).
and
MAN PANIC–*HOLD* – NO SEND US
Where 'hold' consists of [both] hands held in neutral space, meaning 'he held the ticket' (Figure 4).

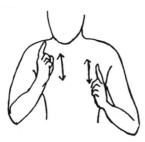 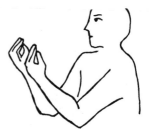

Figure 3   RIVALRY   **Figure 4**   HOLD

There were four propositions (5%) in the spoken version which were incompletely specified in a way similar to the one-sign sentences. These examples include:

Who is it? – *Ah, the postman* – So now he . . .
and
. . . sending the postman away – *pretending* – that he is as. . .
So there are features in each of these commentaries where there are these different mechanisms at work.

Ten per cent of the propositions in sign contained reduplication, while there were no such instances in speech. In addition, there were instances of non-grammatical listings which should not occur in a language such as BSL (Bellugi, 1980).
e.g. WALK – CREEP – APPROACH (Figure 5).

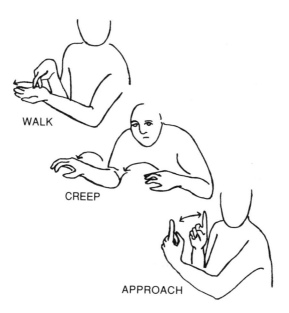

Figure 5 WALK–CREEP–APPROACH

However, it might be expected that these features are highlighted in a commentary where there is little time to organize the meaning and the temporal element has to be specified by reduplication. If these differences between speech and sign exist in recall after an hour, then perhaps we have to consider the existence of a different structure. Tables 1 and 2 contain transcripts and glosses of a short extract of the participants' recall after one hour.

Table 1   Transcripts of spoken recall of one event after one hour

1   So you next see him on a dance floor and he is dancing a Charleston with some much larger woman than he is.

2   Then the scene switches to the very glamorous Cafe Royale where all the ladies in their beautiful flapper dresses and the men are having a wonderful time and in fact our friend Walter McNab is engaged in a Charleston contest with a young lady of perhaps dubious repute.

3   And actually he goes to this night club that he's got tickets for: there he does the Charleston with some young lady.

4   . . . because he has been at the Cafe Royale all this time—dancing and having a good time.

5   He goes to the Cafe Royale and involves himself in a dance competition, the object of which is to dance the best Charleston. His partner, one Tessa McNab, and he have a high old time.

6   . . . and off he goes—but he goes to the Cafe Royale. He gets there and is dancing on the floor with the large tall woman doing the Charleston and everyone around at the sides clapping their hands and cheering them on . . .

Clearly the spoken versions represent a re-organized view of the event with only Transcript 6 capturing the actual occurrences in the event.

Table 2   Sign glosses of recall of one event after one hour

1   WENT TO DANCE ENJOYED HIMSELF WITH WOMAN ENJOYED.

2   HUSBAND DANCE OTHER WOMAN DANCE MUSIC . . . CLAPPED GOOD.

3   REALLY HE WENT TO c.a.fe. r.o.y.a.l.e. ENJOYED HIMSELF DANC-ING WITH GIRL DANCE c.h.a.r.l.e.s.t.o.n. *MIME.*

4   NEXT in c.a.f.e. r.o.y.a.l.e. (STANDING) PEOPLE PEOPLE CLAPPED (STANDING) PEOPLE WEARS SAME BOW (ties) DRESS DRESS UP COUPLE MAN WITH ANOTHER WOMAN DANCE *MIME* DANCE c.h.a.r-.l.e.s.t.o.n. d.a.n.c.e. *MIME* DANCE *MIME* GOOD CLAPPED GOOD.

5   NO – DANCE MAN DANCED MAN DANCED WITH c.h.a.r.l.e.s.t.o.n. DANCE WITH WOMAN.

6   i.t. i.s. DANCE h.a.l.l. DANCE HUSBAND ENJOYED HIMSELF WITH OTHER WOMAN ENJOYED.

Even without transcription of body movement, I think it is easy to see the differences in the signed version which support the points in the commentary. These deaf versions capture the richness of the event in a way which is not presented in English.

The question is how this qualitative difference in production can be used to give any insight into sentence construction in Sign. One might describe the signed versions as the reporting of events rather than a rephrasing of the story, and the signers appear to use an event structure rather than a 'reorganization', which normally occurs in spoken English versions.

If sign language tends to report events rather than inferences, we should find an event structure within the recall which most closely reflects the event structure of the original story.

Hypothesis 3
Deaf people in Sign reflect the original events more closely than do hearing people in English.

Examining the actual order of retelling of the story events, we find that in the spoken version, 17 per cent of all propositions recalled were in a different position from the chronological order as reflected in the commentary; only 5 per cent of sign propositions were in different chronological position.

This supports the idea of the re-ordering apparent in the spoken version which is an outcome of the process fitting the recall to an overall predetermined schema. The signed version seems more related to the actual events themselves.

Table 3   Simultaneous commentaries on one event from the story

---

Speech
> Oh, now he's on the dance floor with a rather tall dolly bird
> very busy doing the Charleston
> There were a lot of people
> watching them
> just the two of them on the floor
> doing the Charleston
> really quite agile

Sign
> MAN AND WOMAN DANCE IN h.a.l.l.
> ALL PEOPLE WATCH THEM
> CHARLESTON DANCE
> DANCE
> ALL CLAP CLAP CLAP
> DANCE DISCO-DANCE
> SHOW DANCE DANCE DANCE

Table 3 has the commentary transcripts for both deaf and hearing, and one can see the obvious similarities in the two. If we then compare the transcripts from Tables 1 and 2 with these, we see that speech produces different recall after one hour, while Sign retains much of the original event structure as described in the commentaries.

We expect this to occur in English, as it is a medium which allows subjects to interpret the task so as to produce inference as an outcome of remembering. There is considerable evidence on this: for example, Bransford and McCarrell, 1975. However, we can now make a weak claim at least that Sign is more likely to be event-structured in representation, and that production is likely to reflect the original events. This does not mean it is iconic or purely visual imagery, since the signs are arbitrary and not transparent. However, there is obviously a large *imaginal* element which is particularly apparent in Sign.

Discussion

At least in this pilot study, sign language when used in narrative differs from speech, not in context or meaning, nor capacity for recall, but in the way the events are reported. It tends to be *more literal* of the original happenings, *more imaginal* in presentation and *deviates much less* from the original sequence of events. This leads to an event-based description where there is less need of explicit referents (as subjects and objects of sentences). As a result, there are increased uses of what deaf transcribers call 'mime' and there is a considerable occurrence of one-sign sentences and propositions. At its simplest, one might say *the Sign task is imaginal*, while *the Speech task is referential; Sign uses an event structure*, while *English creates a different propositional network*.

[. . .]

It is true that when deaf people tell a story they do something very different from hearing people. We are only beginning to be aware of the methods available to describe such complex issues among languages. I think, however, that some understanding of these processes is essential to our knowledge and use of sign language.

Acknowledgements

I would particularly like to thank Gloria Pullen and Jennifer Ackerman for their considerable work and advice on this study.

This research was supported by the DHSS grant JR/212/8 for the project 'Sign Language Learning and Use'.

References

Bellugi, U. (1980) 'Clues from the Similarities between Signed and Spoken Language', in Bellugi, U. and Studdert-Kennedy, M. (eds) *Signed and Spoken Language: Biological Constraints on Linguistic Form*, Berlin, Verlag Chemie.

Bransford, J.D. and McCarrell, N.S. (1975) 'A Sketch of a Cognitive Approach to Comprehension', in Weimer, W.M. and Palmero, D.S. (eds) *Cognition and the Symbolic Processes*, Hillsdale, NJ, Lawrence Erlbaum Associates.

Kintsch, W. (1977) 'On Comprehending Stories', in Just, M.A. and

Carpenter, P.A. (eds) *Cognitive Processes in Comprehension*, Hillsdale, NJ, Lawrence Erlbaum Associates.

Rumelhart, D.A. (1975) 'Notes on a Scheme for Stories', in Bobrow, D.G. and Collins, A. (eds) *Representation and Understanding*, New York, Academic Press.

Stokoe, W.C. (1980) 'The Study and Use of Sign Language', in Schiefelbusch (ed.) *Non-speech Language and Communication*, Baltimore, University Park Press.

3.3 Surdophrenia

The psychic consequences of congenital or early acquired deafness

Some theoretical and clinical considerations

Terje Basilier (1964)

Our standardized textbooks on psychiatry contain little or nothing about the psychic consequences of congenital or early acquired deafness. The reason might be that the number of genuinely deaf persons is so small that psychiatrists very seldom receive deaf persons with psychiatric syndromes for therapy.

[. . .]

Numerically the deafened and hard of hearing exceed the genuinely deaf, and it is on the basis of this larger patient group Kraepelin has formed the classical syndrome: 'Der Verfolgungswahn der Schwerhörigen'. With this conception in mind, psychiatrists have a tendency to think that there is a direct proportionality between the degree of hearing loss and the degree of persecution ideas. This proves not to be true. The fact that deaf persons often seem to carry aggressive tendencies towards the hearing society around them has another and more easily understandable reason: we who hear represent a challenge to the deaf, and because of our failing capacity in helping the deaf, we represent their handicap. If everybody was deaf, there would be no such problem of mutual communication.

Which consequences for the mental development of a child may it have never to have experienced the oral contact of spoken language with his fellow-beings—a contact that we who hear take as granted—never to have heard the consoling voice of his mother, or never to have had chance to play with his own voice, and thus never been able to gain verbal identification with his parents? The problem is even more serious because so many deaf people have visual defects,—even deafblindness. The most renowned of them, Helen Keller, has expressed that deafness—not blindness—was her gravest handicap.

[. . .]

The American psychiatrist David Farber has the opinion that, while the hearing child takes his parents' language as a part of the identification process, the non-verbal proceedings play an essential role in the corresponding process in the deaf child. By imitating the movements of his parents the deaf child may be able to identify with his parents. Farber says that the difficulties in teaching language to a deaf child is not so much a question of the child's lack of hearing, as of the failing capacity of the pedagogues in utilizing the deaf child's particular qualities and needs. He describes how deaf patients have a tendency to repeat themselves in signs during the conversations, and he interprets this so: the movements of the signs give the deaf person a sort of pleasure (an experience of identity?). Bodenheimer (1963) thinks that 'Der Mensch muss sich selbst hören, muss sich aber nicht sehen, um sich zu bestätigen' (i.e. the man must hear himself, not see himself, to confirm himself). While we confirm ourselves by hearing our own voices during the conversation, the deaf persons may experience something of the same sort by the view and proprioceptive sensations of their own signs. When deaf children do their homework or read letters from home, they very often go through the topic with the corresponding manual signs. All children express things to each other with their whole bodies, (body language)—and even hearing children make use of natural signs until they have learned oral language in their homes or surroundings. The deaf child, however, goes through a verbal vacuum period from age 3–8, and in these years they will carry on with pantomime and natural signs in communication. If these deaf children go to a kindergarten for deaf and hard of hearing where the old motto: 'Sit on your hands' prevails, the word-needy deaf child may be thrown into a serious crisis. Many pedagogues have the opinion that the use of natural signs restrains the acquiring of oral language. According to their theory, the child should be stimulated to read from the lips and not to make use of the non-verbal communication methods. The deaf child has not yet learned lipreading, and, at the same time, he is not allowed to employ his spontaneous and most adequate way of expression. Their parents are also told that all gesturing must cease. Sharoff (1959) has clearly pointed out how great a rejection it must be for the child who suddenly finds all his attempts to communicate with his parents denied him. Sharoff tells about a father who went into the bedroom where he thought the child was already asleep and found the boy lying in bed practising signs and the alphabet. As soon as the child saw the father, he stopped. Feelings of guilt had perhaps already been attached to the only communication method mastered by the child, and thus the child came into conflict with his interpersonal relationship—with its need of sufficient emotional contact. From these reflections it should be legitimate to ask whether it is the hearing loss *per se* or the multidimensional influences that follow with deafness which give the deaf person special characteristics. The hearing society and several of its pedagogical systems have tried to foster the young deaf into our oral world without any ideas of the violence used against the nature of deafness by the enforced restriction of communication.

The American investigators Mendelson, Siger and Solomon (1960) have tried to explore the perceptual and symbolic processes occurring in the dreams of students with congenital or acquired deafness. Twenty-six deaf college students were interviewed, and it was found out that the dreams of the deaf students were distinctly different from the dreams of the hearing. The differences resided in greater vividness, depth of spatial dimension, brilliant colours and greater frequency of recall. The character-

istic differences were most marked in the congenitally deaf, and least
marked in those with deafness acquired after age 5. Objections to the
results may be urged out from the theories of personality structure and
reaction types to colour, form and movement, as, for instance, shown in
Ratleff's (1958) Rorschach investigations regarding the selection of the
deaf college students. Anyhow, the results appear to be in correspondence
with the clinical experience: that many deaf persons seem to have a rather
weak superego structure. The vividness and frequency of dreams in the
deaf are, for one thing, explained by the investigators as a possible weak
dream censor and impaired superego structure. Many experts think that
the development of the superego is intimately associated with auditory
experiences in the first five so-called magic years of a child's life.
Mendelson *et al.* set off abundant evidence of superego structuring in the
deaf population, as, for example, 'the appearance of primitive signs in
affectively-toned dreams of the congenitally deaf indicates introjection and
subsequent displacement of very early non-verbal superego material'.

Myklebust (1960) has found that a sensory deprivation, such as early
deafness, may bring about organismic effects and that there might emerge
a characteristic profile of personality. The pattern is described as 'one of
lack of apprehension, worry and concern with onself, and the manifestation of obliviousness in regard to the true circumstances'. They have a
feeling of 'severe isolation and detachment with aggressive, almost
desperate attempts to compensate and thereby maintain interpersonal
contact'! This attitude is the diametrically opposite to that of the hard of
hearing and deafened in higher year groups, where the occurrence of
'Verfolgungswahn' is more frequent and intelligible because of their
increasing loss of contact with the environment of sound. The deaf,
however, is steadily improving contact in every particular.

In the discussion of his Rorschach observations, Sharoff points out how
'it is important to avoid misinterpretation with respect to some signs of
thought disorder usually considered indicative of schizophrenia. Deaf
persons in general "by the nature of their defect" tend to think in vaguely
wholistic and concrete terms. Hence, a thought disorder may be strikingly
simulated in their written communications, which often show a fragmented, confused and primitive quality. Without knowledge of the specific
language handicap of the deaf, these written communications might
suggest the kind of thought pathology seen in chronic schizophrenia'.

Something that may have a scaring effect regarding deaf persons is that
when they are under severe psychic stress and are not able to express
adequately what they think and feel, they may react in excitement
explosions or abnormal single reactions.

[. . .]

It is important to stress that the normal deaf citizens seem to be
ordinarily happy family members who are stable in their work and who
have a tendency to take the days as they come. Some deaf who have had
special training from early childhood on have reached far and even

received academic degrees. Our experiences are that congenital or early acquired deafness may give a certain personality structure—a surdophrenia—and that deaf persons with nervous reactions are in need of specialized psychiatric service.

References

Bodenheimer, A.R. (1963) 'Was lehrt uns der Verfolgungswahn der Schwerhörigen als Paradigma der Psychosen?', Schweiz, *Archiv Neurol., Neurochir, Psychiat, 91*, p. 129.

Farber, D. *Language Attainment in the Pre-school Deaf Child*, Article for the Pedagogical Staff at Galluadet College, Washington, DC.

Mendelson, J.H., Siger, L. and Solomon, P. (1960) 'Psychiatric Observations on Congenital and Acquired Deafness: Symbolic and Perceptual Processes in Dreams', *American Journal of Psychiatry 116*, p. 883.

Myklebust, H.R. (1960) *The Psychology of Deafness*, New York and London, Grune and Stratton.

Ratleff, A. (1958) *Form, farve og Emotioner* (Form, Colour and Emotions), Copenhagen, Nyt Nordisk Forlag Arnold Busk.

Sharoff, R. (1959) 'Enforced Restriction of Communication, its Implications for the Emotional and Intellectual Development of the Deaf Child', *American Journal of Psychiatry, 116*, p. 443.

3.4 Is There a 'Psychology of the Deaf'?

Harlan Lane (1988)

[. . .]

I have reviewed journal articles and books on the 'psychology of the deaf' from the last 20 years, and I have assembled a list of the good and bad characteristics of deaf people according to the authorities. It, too, is a dismaying list—all the more so as it is presented as the outcome of extensive and impartial scientific testing with well-known instruments such as the Scholastic Aptitude Test, the Minnesota Multiphasic Personality Inventory (MMPI), the Rorschach test, and others. This is how the experts portray deaf children and adults to the young men and women who are in training to become their teachers, counsellors, doctors, and so on. The list describes the deaf client that the experienced practitioner imagines is seated across the table: socially isolated, intellectually weak, behaviourally impulsive, emotionally immature.

The list of traits attributed to deaf people is inconsistent: they are both 'aggressive' and 'submissive'; they are 'naive/shrewd, detached/passionate, explosive/shy, stubborn/submissive, and suspicious/trusting'. The list is, however, consistently negative: nearly all the traits ascribed, even many in pairs of opposites, are unfavourable.

[. . .]

I propose to examine the hypothesis that the trait attributions [see Table 1] made by the 'psychology of the deaf' reflect not the characteristics of deaf people but the paternalistic posture of the hearing experts making these attributions. Thus, the education and counselling of deaf children and adults may rest on no more sound foundation than a set of paternalistic stereotypes. The alternate hypothesis is that these attributions are by and large true of deaf people; they are the reliable and valid results of test administrations; they capture ways in which deaf people as a group differ from hearing people more than the individuals in either group differ among themselves. Only in this case may a valid claim be made that there is indeed a 'psychology of the deaf'.

[. . .]

Table 1 Some traits attributed to deaf people in the professional
literature

Social	Cognitive	Behavioural	Emotional
Admiration	Conceptual	Aggressive	Anxiety (lack of)
(depends on)	thinking poor	Androgynous	Depressive
Asocial	Concrete	Conscientious	Emotionally
Clannish	Doubting	Hedonistic	disturbed
Competitive	Egocentric	Immature	Emotionally
Credulous	Failure externalized	Impulsive	immature
Disobedient	Failure internalized	Initiative lacking	Empathy (lack of)
Conscience weak	Insight poor	Interests few	Explosive
Dependent	No introspection	Motor development	Frustrated easily
Immature	No language	slow	Irritable
Irresponsible	Language poor	Personality	Moody
Isolated	Mechanically inept	undeveloped	Neurotic
Morally	Naive	Possessive	Paranoid
undeveloped	Reasoning restricted	Rigid	Passionate
Role-rigid	Self-awareness poor	Shuffling gait	Psychotic
Shy	Shrewd	Stubborn	reactions
Submissive	Thinking unclear	Suspicious	Serious
Suggestible	Unaware	Unconfident	Temperamental
Unsocialized	Unintelligent		Unfeeling

The psychology of the deaf

. . . Is there, as the hearing establishment maintains, a body of scientific knowledge concerning the psychology of deaf children and adults? Are the trait attributions trustworthy? Can this information be used to screen students, develop curricula, prepare teaching materials, train teachers and design environments?

An examination of the studies that gave rise to the trait attributions in Table 1 reveals grave recurrent flaws: test administration is unclear and unreliable; test language is incomprehensible to the testee; test scoring is undependable and radically open to examiner bias, undermining test reliability and validity; test content is unrelated to deaf experience and schooling, and test norms are absent or inappropriate; finally, subject populations are inadequately characterized and controlled.

Test administration

The first problem of test administration, according to some investigators, is set: The deaf schoolchild or adult may be unfamiliar with the procedures and format of standardized testing such as reading items on the test form, encoding them as letters or numbers, marking responses on a separate answer sheet, self-pacing and following printed directions. However sophisticated deaf clients may be in test taking generally, they cannot know what is required by the particular test confronting them; they are commonly baffled and the examiner is forced somehow to convey what needs to be done without dropping any hints on how to do it (Levine, 1971; Trybus, 1973; Vernon and Ottinger, 1981; Watson, 1979).

Some specialists believe that group testing of deaf clients is ruled out by the dual problems of set and communication (Heller and Harris, 1987; Vernon, 1968, 1976). The examiner commonly resorts to ad hoc pantomime which is undependable, often unclear and incomplete. A hearing group and a deaf group taking the Wechsler Intelligence scale (WISC) following pantomime instructions both scored five points less than a hearing control with English administration, so the investigators suggest that five points be added to all deaf WISC scores (Graham and Shapiro, 1953; Goetzinger and Proud, 1975; support this conclusion). The manner of administering intelligence tests to deaf children can account for a change in score of two standard deviations (Dillon, 1980).

Consistent and clear administration of personality tests is even more problematic. For example, when the Sixteen Personality Factor test (16PF) was administered with written English designed for low-literate adults and again with a manual-language videotape, the results were so poorly correlated that the investigators concluded the two forms were not equivalent (Dwyer and Wincenciak, 1977). When using clinical instruments such as the Rorschach and the Thematic Apperception Test (TAT) with deaf subjects, it is difficult to know whether they understand the instructions or not. Many of those tested simply describe what is in the TAT picture. Others give rather little verbal output to either test (Rainer and Altshuler, 1967). Clearly, there is a dilemma in administering to deaf people tests standardized on hearing people: If the procedures are changed, the norms are invalidated; if they are not, the results are even more invalid (Heller and Harris, 1987).

Test language

Since deaf test-takers in America frequently are not fluent in English, they not only fail to understand test instructions thoroughly, invalidating the results, but they also fail to understand the test content itself, as most tests are presented in written English, and in rather high-level English at that. Nevertheless, psychologists continue to administer such tests to deaf subjects, to report the inevitably anomalous results in the scientific literature, and to misclassify deaf children as, for example, learning disabled (Levine, 1981; Orr, De Matteo, Heller, Lee and Nguyen, 1987). When Rudner (1978) performed an item analysis of deaf and hearing responses on the Stanford Achievement Test, he found twenty-six items markedly biased against deaf students and these all fell into six categories—not of knowledge but of language use: conditionals (if, when); comparatives; negatives (not, without); inferentials (should, could, because, since); pronouns (it, something); and long passages. Quigley and Kretschmer (1982) conclude that reading level is the primary determinant of achievement in all the academic areas of the test; Moores (1982) finds its validity highly questionable.

[. . .]

The outcomes of many personality tests are even more dependent on the English-language skills of the deaf subject. One authority estimates that the testee must have a 10th-grade knowledge of English to take most personality tests meaningfully (Montgomery, 1978; Smith, 1986, estimates 8th grade conservatively for the MMPI). Yet the average deaf school leaver has only a 4th-grade command of English, and only one deaf student in ten reads at 8th-grade level or better (Quigley and Kretschmer, 1982; Wolk and Allen, 1984). Even if merely a 4th grade reading level is necessary, half of the test respondents must frequently be answering on whim. Thus, professionals should reject the results of most personality testing done with deaf people, and with it many of the unfavourable attributions I reported earlier.

[. . .]

Test scoring

Examiner bias, the belief that the deaf person cannot be normal in cognition and behaviour, that 'common sense considerations would suggest that the deaf would have an increased risk of developing schizophrenia' (Lebuffe and Lebuffe, 1979, p. 299), has also operated to invalidate the psychological literature on deafness. To aggravate the problem of bias, a child or adult who is acting up and who also does not respond to English commands represents a double threat to the examiner, parent, or teacher (Hoyt, Siegelman and Schlesinger, 1981; Meadow, 1981). When the assessment of the deaf person is subjective, as it is with rating scales, checklists and interviews, a biased examiner can unwittingly influence the scores and therefore invalidate the results. Nevertheless, just such subjective scoring methods are used by the TAT, the Rorschach, the Vineland Social Maturity Scale, the Bender-Gestalt, and many more tests whose findings make up the literature on the 'psychology of the deaf'.

[. . .]

Test content and norms

Scores are assigned to deaf children by teachers, examiners, or parents using a rating scale: or the children themselves, unclear as to the procedures and the meanings of the questions, docilely answer test items as best they can. Now their answers must be referred to a normative set of answers to obtain a raw score, and the raw score must be referred to a normative distribution for interpretation; however, such data are generally unavailable or inappropriate (Holm, 1987). Personality tests, for example, are weighted with items selected to detect evidence of personality deviance among the hearing. When the scoring system designed for hearing people is applied to deaf people, the results often have little validity. A host of items on the MMPI patently presuppose hearing ('I would like to be a singer'; 'At times I hear so well it bothers me') while others are more subtly biased ('I enjoy reading love stories'; 'In a group of people I would not be embarrassed to be called upon to start a discussion or give an opinion about something I know well'). Perhaps a fourth of the items are inappropriate. Should it count as paranoid if a deaf person confirms that

'People often stare at me in restaurants' when indeed they do generally eye his signing?

Although it is a major source of the literature on the 'psychology of the deaf', the MMPI suffers from all the invalidating weaknesses cited—difficult to administer, to read and to interpret, with content and norms inappropriate to deaf people, it should never have been used with this population, and certainly the reuslts should not have been published (Smith, 1986; Zieziula, 1982). Nearly all of the other tests whose results constitute the literature of the 'psychology of the deaf' have likewise not been revised for and standardized on deaf populations.

Subject populations

Finally, I will note that the research on the 'psychology of the deaf' commonly fails to characterize and distinguish its subject populations, reporting average performances of extremely heterogeneous groups and obscuring important differences in performance. This, too, is a paternalistic error, regarding all members of a minority as fundamentally alike. Commonly obliterated in the research are the following population variables for which there is evidence of substantial effects (Schildroth and Karchmer, 1986): sex, age, race, and social class; cause, extent, and nature of hearing loss: age at onset of hearing loss; hearing status of the parents: mode of communication used at school, at home and with peers; type of schooling received; command of oral and written English; minority group membership; presence of physical or mental handicaps prior to and following deafness; and familial mental health.

The common failure to screen subjects on these characteristics, often because treatment assignments are made by the schools or parents and not by the researchers, has two nefarious consequences for research. First, the heterogeneity of an amorphous deaf population on the one hand and of a hearing population on the other makes it particularly unlikely that differences between deaf and hearing subjects can be discovered that are large compared to the average differences among individuals within the two groups; thus, there can be no confidence in the apparent trend if one is uncovered. Second, unless the make up of the samples is known and controlled by the experimenter, it is unclear to which populations, if any, the results may be generalized. When Schlesinger (1985) concluded from the Berkeley school ratings that 'deaf school-age children' are five times more emotionally disturbed than their hearing peers, she was assuming that a residential school sample was representative of the national population, which is decidedly not the case (Ries, 1986). Research that fails to determine, not to say control, the characteristics of its test samples is uninterpretable and without value for educational policy, whatever the validity of the test instruments.

Conclusions

Because the literature on the 'psychology of the deaf' is so gravely flawed by weaknesses in test administration, language, scoring, content, norms and subject groups, many in the professions serving deaf people have sounded the alarm that the field is improperly lending the weight of science to common stereotypes. More than a decade ago, Bolton (1976) wrote: 'Valid procedures for personality assessment of deaf children and adults are lacking . . . All research studies are suspect' (p. 8). Shortly thereafter. Chess and Fernandez (1980) concurred: 'The judgment as to whether the deaf child has specific deviant personality characteristics is still inconclusive' (p. 656). Moores (1982) dismissed the literature of the 'psychology of the deaf' in his textbook: 'For the most part, inappropriate tests have been administered under unsatisfactory conditions and results have been compared with unrealistic norms' (p. 146). And, most recently, this indictment appeared in the *Journal of Rehabilitation of the Deaf*: 'Professionals who work closely with deaf people have responded to the inconsistencies between these biases and their own experience with deaf people by writing off the whole field of testing' (Holm, 1987, p. 15).

Deaf people have their apologists who remind us that the typical deaf child grows up with severely impoverished communication at home and at school. They argue that the maladaptive responses of parents and teachers are the cause of deaf children's deviant cognition and behaviour (cf. Moores, 1982; Schlesinger, 1987). Some investigators suspect the cause may be undetectable lesions of the central nervous system that accompanied the child's loss of hearing (Vernon, 1969). Before these explanations are debated, however, researchers must be sure there is something to explain and must know some of its reliable characteristics to constrain their explanations. If there are characteristic psychological consequences of deafness, however, they have yet to be established.

There is no psychology of the deaf. It is, in fact, not clear that there *can* be one. The term may inevitably represent the pathologizing of cultural differences, the interpretation of difference as deviance. There is no 'psychology of Blacks', or 'psychology of Mexican-Americans', although there are Black studies programmes that treat Black history, culture, dialect, literature and so on, as there are courses in deaf history, culture, language and literature.

Attempts to articulate the psychology of a minority group play into the hands of oppressors who manipulate them for their own ends. Neither the blatant shortcomings of the research on the 'psychology of the deaf', nor the incongruity of its findings with the achievements of countless deaf people, nor the cries of alarm have inhibited the proliferation of hasty studies purporting to show the character flaws of deaf children and adults. Perhaps the perceived incompetence of deaf people is not the result of research on the 'psychology of the deaf' but its cause. This interpretation has a disturbing parallel with the stages of colonial racism set out by Memmi (1966): (a) discover differences; (b) valorize them to the advantage of the colonizer and the disadvantage of the colonized; and (c) absolutize them, affirming that they are definitive, and act to make them so.

How did such a tragedy occur in the professions serving deaf people, at great cost in human suffering, scholarly effort and federal funds? Why does much of the research in this field not meet elementary standards of scientific rigour? I believe it is because social science research is a social institution itself. As a hearing activity devoted to characterizing the deaf minority, it came under the sway of the basic tenet of hearing–deaf relations in our society, paternalism. Hearing experts, commonly ignorant of the language, institutions, culture, history, mores and experiences of deaf people, could only be guided in the first instance by the stereotypes to which we have all been acculturated.

I submit that when their investigations tended to confirm these seemingly logical a priori beliefs, they pursued them and published them without niggling, as it seemed, about procedural details. To show that the relations institutionalized between two groups are paternalistic is to reveal ways in which social structures operate to the detriment of both parties. There are, of course, individuals who try by their actions and statements not to behave paternalistically, but it is in the nature of things that they can be only partially successful. Probably a distinction should be made between voluntary and involuntary paternalism. And not all individuals and groups are voluntarily paternalistic, nor paternalists to the same degree.

How can research on deaf children and adults be protected from the structural paternalism that dictates the training of professional people, the funding of their research, their access to subjects, publication, and so on? The single most effective remedy, it seems to me, would be to involve deaf people themselves at all levels of the undertaking. A strategy is needed to recruit and train many more deaf principal investigators. Researchers must turn preferentially to the deaf community for advisors and collaborators in research design and implementation, for assistance in data collection and analysis, and for guidance in interpretation of results. Africans contribute to social science research on Africa with cogency, originality and insight, and they hold their non-African colleagues to account. The old paternalism of the European Africanists is no longer tenable. Should it not be the same with studies of deafness?

References

Bolton, B. (ed.) (1976) *Psychology of the Deaf for Rehabilitation Counsellors,* Baltimore, MD, University Park Press.

Chess, S. and Fernandez, P. (1980) 'Do Deaf Children Have a Typical Personality?', *Journal of the American Academy of Child Psychiatry, 19,* pp. 654–64.

Dillon, R.F. (1980) 'Cognitive Style and Elaboration of Logical Abilities in Hearing-Impaired Children', *Journal of Experimental Child Psychology, 30,* pp. 389–400.

Dwyer, C. and Wincenciak, S. (1977) 'A Pilot Investigation of Three Factors of the 16PF Form E, Comparing the Standard Written Form with an Ameslan Videotape Revision', *Journal of Rehabilitation of the Deaf, 10,* 17–23.

Goetzinger, C.P. and Proud, G.O. (1975) 'The Impact of Hearing

Impairment Upon the Psychological Development of Children', *Journal of Auditory Research, 15,* 1–60.

Graham, E. and Shapiro, E. (1953) 'Use of the Performance Scale of the WISC with the Deaf Child', *Journal of Consulting Psychology, 17,* pp. 396–8.

Heller, B.W. and Harris, R.I. (1987) 'Special Considerations in the Psychological Assessment of Hearing Impaired Persons', in Heller, B.W., Flohr, L.M. and Zegans, L.S. (eds) *Psychosocial Interventions with Sensorially Disabled Persons,* pp. 53–7, Orlando, FL, Grune and Stratton.

Holm, C.S. (1987) 'Testing for Values with the Deaf: The Language/ Cultural Effect', *Journal of Rehabilitation of the Deaf, 20,* 7–19.

Hoyt, M.F., Siegelman, E.Y. and Schlesinger, H.S. (1981) 'Special Issues Regarding Psychotherapy with the Deaf', *American Journal of Psychiatry, 138,* pp. 807–11.

Lebuffe, F.P. and Lebuffe, L.A. (1979) 'Psychiatric Aspects of Deafness', *Primary Care, 6,* pp. 295–310.

Levine, E.S. (1971) 'Mental Assessment of the Deaf Child', *Volta Review, 73,* pp. 80–105.

Levine, E. (1981) *Ecology of Early Deafness,* New York, Columbia University Press.

Meadow, K.P. (1981) 'Studies of Behaviour Problems of Deaf Children', in Stein, L.K., Mindel, E.D. and Jabeley, T. (eds) *Deafness and Mental Health,* (pp. 3–22), New York, Grune and Stratton.

Memmi, A. (1966) *Portrait du Colonisé,* Paris, Pauvert.

Montgomery, G. (1978) 'Towards a Viable Surdotherapy: Mental Hygiene in Schools', in Montgomery, G. (ed.) *Of Sound and Mind,* Edinburgh, Scottish Workshop, pp. 75–8.

Moores, D. (1982) *Educating the Deaf* (2nd edn), New York, Houghton Mifflin.

Moores, D.F. (1986) 'Public Education: Implications for the Deaf Community', in Rosen, R. (ed.) *Life and Work in the 21st Century: The Deaf Person of Tomorrow, Proceedings of the 1986 NAD Forum,* Silver Spring, MD, National Association of the Deaf, pp. 33–42.

Orr, F.C., De Matteo, A., Heller, B., Lee, M. and Nguyen, M. (1987) 'Psychological Assessment', In Elliott, H., Glass, L. and Evans, J.W. (eds) *Mental Health Assessment of Deaf Clients: A Practical Manual,* San Diego, CA, College Hill, pp. 93–106.

Quigley, S. and Kretschmer, R. (1982) *The Education of Deaf Children,* Baltimore, MD, University Park Press.

Rainer, J.D. and Altshuler, K.Z. (1967) *Psychiatry and The Deaf,* US

Department of Health, Education and Welfare, Social and Rehabilitation Service, Washington, DC, US Government Printing Office.

Ries, P. (1986) 'Characteristics of Hearing-Impaired Youth in the General Population and of Students in Special Education Programs for the Hearing-Impaired', in Schildroth, A.N. and Karchmer, M.A. (eds) *Deaf Children in America,* San Diego, CA, College Hill, pp. 1–32.

Rudner, I. (1978) 'Using Standard Tests with the Hearing-Impaired', *Volta Review, 80,* 31–40.

Schildroth, A.N. and Karchmer, M.A. (eds) (1986) *Deaf Children in America,* San Diego, CA, College Hill.

Schlesinger, H. (1985) 'Deafness, Mental Health, and Language', in Powell, F., Finitzo-Hieber, T., Friel-Patti, S. and Henderson, D. (eds) *Education of the Hearing-Impaired Child,* San Diego, CA, College Hill, pp. 103–19.

Schlesinger, H. (1987) 'Effects of Parentlessness on Dialogue and Development. Disability, Poverty and the Human Condition', in Heller, B.W., Flohr, L.M. and Zegans, L.S. (eds) *Psychosocial Interventions with Sensorially Disabled Persons,* Orlando, FL, Grune and Stratton.

Smith, D. (1986) 'Mental Health Research Enters Realm of Linguistics,' *Research at Gallaudet,* Fall, pp. 3–5.

Trybus, R. (1973) 'Personality Assessment of Entering Hearing-Impaired College Students Using the 16PF Form E', *Journal of Rehabilitation of the Deaf, 6,* pp. 34–40.

Vernon, M. (1968) 'Fifty Years of Research on the Intelligence of the Deaf and Hard of Hearing', *Journal of Rehabilitation of the Deaf, 1,* pp. 1–11.

Vernon, M. (1969) *Multiply-handicapped Deaf Children: Medical Educational and Psychological Considerations,* CEC Research Monographs, Washington, DC, The Council for Exceptional Children.

Vernon, M. (1976) 'Psychological Evaluation of Hearing-Impaired Children,' in Lloyd, L. (ed.) *Communication Assessment and Intervention Strategies,* Baltimore, MD, University Park Press, pp. 195–223.

Vernon, M. and Ottinger, P. (1981) 'Psychological Evaluation of the Deaf and Hard of Hearing', in Stein, L.K., Mindel, E.D. and Jabaley, T. (eds) *Deafness and Mental Health,* New York, Grune and Stratton, pp. 49–64.

Watson, D. (1979) 'Guidelines for the Psychological and Vocational Assessment of Deaf Rehabilitation Clients', *Journal of Rehabilitation of the Deaf, 13,* pp. 25–57.

Wolk, S. and Allen, T.E. (1984) 'A Five-Year Follow-up of Reading Comprehension Achievement of Hearing-Impaired Students in Special Education Programs', *Journal of Special Education, 18,* 161–76.

Zieziula, F.R. (1982) *Assessment of Hearing-Impaired People,* Washington, DC, Gallaudet College Press.

Audiology and Technology: From Description to Prescription

In this section we have not attempted to do justice to the range of audiological knowledge and techniques. Our aim has been not to provide an overview of current audiological theory or practice but to indicate an important aspect of the audiological construction of deafness which has pervaded professional and lay perceptions. This is essentially a scientific view of deafness within which measurement has a paramount role. It is this 'objective' approach to deafness which we wish to characterize: the idea that hearing loss can be measured objectively and degree of deafness inferred.

The view of deafness as the absence of hearing, which dominated the early psychological perspective discussed in the previous section, also characterized medical and audiological perspectives which viewed deafness as pathology. These may be contrasted with the social definitions of deafness discussed in Sections 1 and 2. Deafness is viewed as impaired hearing and the audiologist is concerned to identify and measure the extent and nature of what a client/patient can hear, with a view to compensating for hearing loss through amplification. It would be unusual for a hearing loss to be diagnosed and no hearing aids provided.

The first paper in this section provides a brief introduction to pure tone audiology. The paper by Noble indicates that the basis of audiological measurement, audiological zero, is itself a social construction. Noble maintains that audiologists have regarded as normal a level of hearing which commonsense notions would regard as highly acute.

We have provided examples of two contrasting applications of technology which reflect differing approaches to deafness. Tucker and Nolan's article on hearing aids reflects a view of deafness as impaired hearing and the use of technology to facilitate normalization. Baker's paper, on the other hand, views Deaf people as a cultural minority group and provides an example of technology used to facilitate access to aspects of the dominant culture. He also advocates a role for deaf people in the development of appropriate technology.

4.1 Basic Acoustics

Barry McCormick (1988)

Sound is defined as any pressure variation (in air, water or some other medium) that the human ear can detect. The human hearing system has evolved to respond to a wide range of sounds in the environment but it functions at its peak of sensitivity to those sounds in the human speech range.

Sound can be characterized by three main features, namely, intensity, frequency and duration. Intensity is perceived as loudness and frequency as pitch and these, together with the ability to comprehend speech, are the main characteristic features which we attempt to check in simple forms of hearing tests. There are other complex interactions which can be measured in more sophisticated diagnostic hearing tests, for example temporal processing (time relationships) and frequency resolution (or separation). Consideration of these is, however, beyond the scope of this [article] because simple 'screening' methods have not yet been devised for measuring these characteristics in a form suitable for routine application with babies and children.

Returning to basics, sound is produced by vibrations and these vibrations may be characterized by their rapidity and force (or pressure) which, in turn, will determine the pitch and loudness of the sensation produced in the hearing system. The picture can begin to unfold by taking each of these in turn.

Pitch

The young healthy normal ear can perceive as pitch a wide range of frequencies from approximately 20 pressure variations per second (20 Hertz or Hz) at the lower end up to 20,000 pressure variations per second (20 kHz) at the upper limit (Table 1). Pressure variations outside these ranges do exist, of course, but they do not stimulate the hearing pathway of man. Viewed in physical terms they have a frequency but are not perceived as having a pitch for man. Bats, for example, can perceive vibrations up to 120 kHz and dolphins extend the range even further up to 150 kHz. A relatively limited range of frequencies available to man is actually used in speech and most of the sounds in speech occur in the frequency range from 250 Hz up to 8 kHz. This range can be reduced even to 500 Hz–4 kHz without producing any serious deterioration in the clarity of speech. The piano offers a useful reference for the frequency scale with the lowest note having a frequency of 27.5 Hz and the highest note having a frequency of 4,186 Hz. Middle C has a frequency of 256 Hz.

Table 1   Frequency spectra (approximate)

Man	20 Hz– 20 kHz
Dog	15 Hz– 50 kHz
Cat	60 Hz– 65 kHz
Dolphin	150 Hz–150 kHz
Bat	1 kHz–120 kHz
Piano	30 Hz– 4 kHz

For convenience, only certain frequencies are used for hearing measurement purposes and these are chosen such that each is taken as either double or half the adjacent value. The lowest frequency of interest for speech and hearing purposes is usually 125 Hz and subsequent ones are taken at octave intervals above this, the octave being a doubling of frequency. The frequency scale appears as follows:

125 Hz, 250 Hz, 500 Hz, 1 kHz, 2 kHz, 4 kHz, 8 kHz

Higher frequencies above 8 kHz may occasionally be considered and also mid-octave intervals such as 750 Hz, 1.5 kHz, 3 kHz and 6 kHz may sometimes be of interest.

Loudness

The human ear is responsive to a wide range of sound pressures and the difference between the pressure of the quietest sound which can be heard and the loudest sound which can be tolerated is several million-fold. To accommodate this vast range of values on a convenient scale with simple notation a logarithmic scale is used with a basic unit known as the decibel (dB).

[. . .]

For convenience (although adding to confusion) different decibel scales are used according to the area of interest. Such scales include the dB(A), dB(B), dB(C), dB(D), dB(Hearing Level or HL) and dB(Sound Pressure Level or SPL) scales. The reason why such a range of scales exists is that the human ear is not equally sensitive to all frequencies and this sensitivity changes as the sound pressure increases. For quiet sound the human ear is most sensitive in the frequency range between 2 kHz and 5 kHz and is least sensitive at extremely high and low frequencies. For louder sounds the differences in sensitivity are not so great. The different decibel scales attempt to characterize the way this sensitivity changes. The scales used almost exclusively for hearing screening purposes are the dB(A) and dB(HL). dB(A) is used when a sound level is being measured in a room setting and dB(HL) is used when sounds are presented through earphones. The two scales differ by 4dB or so depending upon the frequency of the sound in question with the dB(A) values being higher numerically. The reference value of 0dB ISO (International Organization for Standardization) corresponds to the quietest level at which young healthy normally hearing subjects can just hear a sound on two out of three of the occasions when it is presented. This is an average value and it is possible for some individuals to hear at even quieter levels of − 10 dB or even − 20 dB.

An introduction to the pure tone audiogram

The pure tone audiogram is a convenient chart for recording the threshold levels at which an individual listening through standard earphones can hear different frequencies known as pure tones (because they contain a single or pure frequency of pressure variation). The basic audiogram scale configuration is shown in Figure 1. The frequency scale covers the range from 125 Hz up to 8 kHz along the horizontal (abscissa) axis and the vertical (ordinate) hearing-level scale covers the range from − 20 dB(HL) (ISO) up to 120 dB(HL) (ISO). To establish the audiometric threshold at each frequency it is necessary to follow a standard procedure and it is not appropriate to discuss this fully in the context of an introduction to a screening system. [In the original McCormick goes on to provide examples of audiometric configurations which characterize a range of hearing losses. Unfortunately, limitations on space prevent them being reproduced here.]

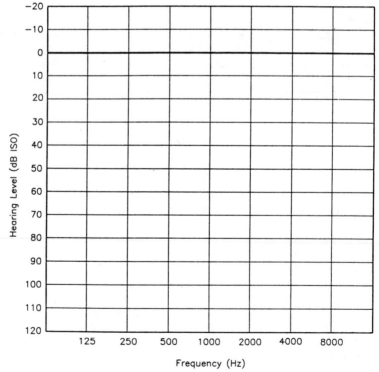

Figure 1   The audiogram

4.2 Assessment of Impaired Hearing

William Noble (1978)

[. . .]

The meaning of 'normal'
In this text the term *normal* has been used as a shorthand way of describing levels at threshold for tones or speech that are not elevated beyond certain recognized limits. Where possible I have avoided use of the term altogether for two major reasons. First, the term has connotations of 'proper', 'correct', etc., and its use in place of *hearing* (as opposed to *deaf* or *partially deaf*) perpetuates the evaluative labelling that adheres to the latter states. It is only hearing people who are 'normal'; deaf people are thus 'abnormal'. It is time such evaluative descriptions were done away with, so that 'hearing' can be recognized as having a different but no lesser or greater status than 'deaf'.

The other reason for trying to avoid the use of *normal* is because the term refers to a person's response on tests. One's hearing is 'normal' if the level at threshold is at or around 0 dB on an audiogram. The bulk of this [article] is taken up with a rather convoluted exploration of this state of affairs. Let me point out from the start that application of the term *normal* to the audiogram trace begs the question about that trace's validity in differentiating hearing from partially hearing listeners . . . Traditionally, *normal* refers to zero level at tonal threshold, hence it applies as a label not broadly to people who hear but quite narrowly to people who hear tones at very low output levels. If we bracket, for the moment, the issue of validity and take it that this capability (hearing acuteness) is a sufficient measure of hearing capacity in general, then it follows that *normal* applies only to people with highly acute hearing. This application of the term is fitting, in that *normal* means *not deviating from a standard*. But the term *normal* also means *ordinary* or *as a rule*. The question then is, can audiometric zero function as a 'normal standard'? Does it represent *ordinary* hearing? I will show, after a necessarily circuitous critique, that a certain zero level no longer in use can be taken to represent an 'ordinary standard' for hearing, but that the currently used zero represents highly acute and hence non-normal hearing.

[. . .]

In the next section, there is a review of work that has been carried out to establish the so-called 'normal threshold of hearing' and a discussion of why there is a difference in average normal thresholds, despite the tight constraints on the investigations, between the old United States standard and virtually all other normal standards.

[. . .]

Audiometric zero

Origin of the 'normal' zero

According to Davis (1970), when the first commercially produced audiometer was designed in the 1920s, the standardization of output was to have been based on acoustic zero (0 dB = 20 μP). But E.P. Fowler, the otological consultant involved, was adamant that the instrument should fulfil a diagnostic-assessment function and that zero output should represent 'normal' hearing. Fowler figured quite prominently in the early days of audiology, and this surely must be the worst conceptual legacy he has bequeathed to the field. The zero level on the early audiometer was accordingly fixed at the average threshold level of listeners at the Bell Telephone Laboratory. Other manufacturers may or may not have used this reference in constructing audiometers over the next 15 years or so, but they all fixed the zero output along the same conceptual lines. It then required the results of a vast survey of the population to provide a standard to which all manufacturers could reliably adhere.

The former United States 'normal' zero (ASA, 1951)

In 1938, results were reported which had been obtained as part of the monolithic 1935–1936 National Health Survey organized by the United States Public Health Service (USPHS). The Hearing Study Series was directed by W.C. Beasley. A representative sample of about 9,000 people from the United States populace had their levels at various tonal thresholds determined. The threshold levels of those who reported 'no noticeable difficulty with hearing' (N = 4662) were taken as the data pool for 'normal' threshold of hearing in that country. Actually, according to Beasley (1957), the distributions of the 'normal' threshold results were controlled for skewness by use of model values after the results had been trimmed so as to exclude audiograms 'exceeding a 20 dB variation for all frequencies, with reference to the average characteristic of the distributions with skewness eliminated from the distributions for high frequency tones (Beasley, 1957, p. 669)'. Quite what this means is unclear. In the same paper (p. 665), it is taken by Davis and Usher (1957) to mean results from people in whom threshold level at any frequency was more than 20 dB above the mean. Harris (1954), however, states that data were from people 'whose air conduction audiograms for both ears did not exceed a variation of 20 dB (p. 930)'.

Whatever was done, the effect was to eliminate extreme values from the data pool. By this procedure, the original 'normal' sample of 4662 people was reduced to 1,242. A further constraint was placed on data from this smaller group, namely use of threshold values only from the 'better' (lower threshold level) ear, or from both ears if they showed the same values. The surprisingly high attrition rate (from 4,662 to 1,242) is perhaps explicable by the fact that the values under consideration were drawn from people of all ages (8 to 76 years), hence in the older groups levels at threshold at higher frequencies varying by more than 20 dB from threshold level at other frequencies (or from the group mean) would be fairly common. The feature of age structure is one we will return to presently. Its being left uncontrolled in the 'screened' sample of 1,242 people has created no small confusion regarding the final composition of the USPHS survey 'normal' sample. An age-stratified analysis was reported, but using the data from the original 4,662 listeners. These data, as Harris (1954) points out, do not coincide with the data base of the later standard adopted in the United States. That standard is based on the data from the 1,242 persons remaining after the screen. Nonetheless, the age-stratified data from the 4,662 listeners have been taken by other authors as 'normal' values (Spoor, 1967; Sunderman and Boerner, 1950).

In 1939, according to Watson and Tolan (1949), Beasley's screened 'normal' values were adopted by the National Bureau of Standards. But while subsequent investigations produce results in confirmation of that standard (Watson and Tolan's own data, for example), according to these same authors, data from the New York World's Fair of 1939 (Steinberg, Montgomery and Gardner, 1940) and from Bunch (1943) seemed to provide average values up to 10 dB lower than the USPHS survey 'normal' values. Despite these apparent discrepancies, the American Standards Association (1951) adopted the USPHS survey data as the specification for audiometers.

It is at this point that the water becomes a little murky. ASA (1951) clearly states (p. 7, paragraph 1.2) that 'normal threshold' is defined as the modal value of the level at threshold in normal ears of people *aged 18–30 years,* to be taken for these purposes as the level observed in the USPHS survey of 1935–1936. The appearance of an age range of 18–30 years in ASA (1951) is a puzzle. It is beyond dispute that ASA (1951) is based on the screened sample of 1242 listeners in the USPHS survey and that their ages ranged from 8 to 76 years. However, as I stated earlier, the older contingent in that sample would doubtless have formed the bulk of the people screened out of the original group of 4,662, but no clues as to the age structure of the screened sample are publicly available. What remains is a strange discrepancy in age range between ASA (1951) and USPHS survey (1938).

In spite of this curious puzzle, it seems clear that the USPHS survey was carefully conducted and results (giving rise to an ASA specification) were painstakingly treated. As from 1939, with the adoption of the survey standard by the United States National Bureau of Standards (Watson and Tolan, 1949), and certainly from 1951, American audiometers conformed with the 'USPHS zero'. These instruments were both exported and used in the United States, and it was supposedly the dissatisfaction voiced by otologists in the United Kingdon and Europe, to the effect that the 'normal zero' was too high, which led to the search for a new standard.

The former British 'normal' zero (BSI, 1954)

Two independent but co-operating research teams in the United Kingdom set about determining threshold values in highly selected young people. Their reports (Dadson and King, 1952; Wheeler and Dickson, 1952) showed results that agreed almost perfectly with each other and disagreed quite markedly with the American standard. It was undoubtedly the similarity of two independent data sets that silenced any argument against setting up a new British standard. The data of the two teams confirmed the Anglo-European complaint that ASA (1951) 'zero' was at too high a level. The mean difference across the usual audiometric frequencies between ASA (1951) and the British data was about 10 dB.

Naturally, as soon as the British standard was established (British Standards Institution, 1954), British audiometer manufacturers had to conform to it. In Germany, a separate standard midway between British and American was established, and indeed in many countries different zero levels have been used, apparently covering a considerable acoustic range. The International Organization for Standardization has finally produced a document (1964) which supposedly provides a single international zero (R 389) . . . The point in [the] present context is that ISO 'zero' conforms more to British than to American zero. Furthermore, independent investigation by many subsequent authors has tended to confirm the British standard rather than the American, ASA (1951) is now defunct, and the new American National Standards Institute (1969) specification is ISO R 389 (1964).

Following publication of the British Standard (1954), a considerable amount of agonizing took place to try to account for the discrepancy between American and British results. This culminated in a meeting held under the auspices of the Armed Forces–National Research Council Committee on Hearing and Bioacoustics (CHABA). Davis and Usher (1957) edited synopses of the papers delivered by various authoritative persons at this meeting, as well as providing their own observations. One of the contributors to the symposium was none other than Dr W.C. Beasley, the man whose data formed the ASA (1951) zero. While it would perhaps put the wrong light on proceedings to say that Beasley was 'grilled' at the meeting, it would be fair to say he was called upon to try to account for the discrepancy between American and British results. Despite all this effort, no satisfactory explanation for the difference was forthcoming.

The controversy about the former Anglo-American mismatch

Readers may ask why the whole business should not be let subside into history while attention is turned to the problem of establishing a reliable international audiometric zero that will do away with all discrepancies.

To such readers I can only bow and seek indulgence to unfold what to me has been an illuminating inquiry into the Anglo-American controversy. In addition, the reason I propose later in this section for the difference between the USPHS and other data bears critically upon the central theme of this book [in which this article originally appeared]; namely the valid assessment of hearing ability. I think it is irrelevant what value zero takes on the audiometer; but it is not irrelevant to inquire why one value is thrown over in preference for another.

Finally, had there been no follow-up scrutiny of the Anglo-American difference, and of the USPHS survey in particular, I would have more contentedly dismissed the difference with a shrug of 'who knows why?' But the fact is, after fairly intensive limelighting of survey and data—of a kind that would probably embarrass a great deal of audiological survey-type research—no fault could be found, no convincing explanation made for the difference.

The 'survey–laboratory' myth   To be sure, Davis (in Davis and Usher, 1957), when summing up, produced an explanation for the difference as lying within a difference in the attitudes of both audiologist and listener to the measurement task. Supposedly this attitude is more serious-minded in 'laboratory–research' studies (the British approach to normal hearing determination) than in 'survey–clinical' studies (the American approach). This 'explanation' is simply drawn out of the air, no evidence for it having been adduced anywhere in the body of the report. A highly illuminating comment on it comes from Harris (1954). He reports that Davis *et al.* (1947) had produced the 'laboratory–survey' distinction upon reporting seemingly higher levels at threshold in listeners tested by the 'survey–clinical' approach than in those tested by the 'laboratory–research' approach. But Harris notes that the reference zero for data by the two procedures was different and that there was in fact a negligible difference between the two sets of results produced by Davis *et al.* Harris states (1954) that data of his own show no difference between 'survey' and 'laboratory' contexts. It is instructive that Davis (in Davis and Usher, 1957 and Davis,1970) goes on relying on this non-existent distinction.

A final and very important point needs to be emphasized. The ASA (1951) standard is apparently isolated from other survey results. But according to Harris (1954) once again, when earphone calibration differences are correctly accounted for, data from the New York World's Fair, for example, are in quite close agreement with the USPHS survey results. The ASA (1951) standard is not necessarily out on its own.

The only reasonable conclusion to be drawn at this stage, in light of the quite intense inquiry into the conduct and conditions of the USPHS survey, is that the Anglo-American difference is a real one, not explicable by some flaw in one programme or another.

This conclusion stands despite the remarks of Glorig, Quiggle, Wheeler and Grings (1956) and Glorig (1958). These authors showed that the USPHS survey results are in close agreement with results from the 1954 Wisconsin State Fair (Glorig, 1958) whereas results from the 1955 Wisconsin State Fair (Glorig, 1958) are more in accord with the British standard data. Glorig *et al.* (1956) and Glorig (1958) point out that the 1954 Wisconsin procedure was less strict, more hurried, etc. than the 1955 procedure. Without claiming anything one way or the other, the authors allow the implication that the USPHS survey procedure is somehow akin to that of the 1954 Wisconsin State Fair, whereas the British study has more in common procedurally with the 1955 fair. No evidence backs up the former claim, and the conclusion that the USPHS survey result is attributable to the same sloppy procedure as occurred in the 1954 Wisconsin State Fair cannot be made. Apart from the fact that this method of argument, relying on implication without proof, is quite inadmissable, Beasley (1940) provides the following refutation:

> Careful attention was given to securing reliable measurements on each subject. For over one-half of the 9324 subjects studied. . . . two complete sets of audiograms were obtained for both ears by air conduction and by bone conduction for both the ascending and descending approach to threshold. For the remainder of the subjects, one complete set of audiograms was obtained for the ascending and descending approach to threshold. Although more time than was really necessary was devoted to the audiometric tests, it is considered that the higher degree of reliability resulting from this procedure fully compensated for the additional time spent in testing (Beasley, 1940, p. 117).

The final point to be made is that ASA (1951) and BSI (1954) zeros do not reflect an actual difference in hearing threshold acuity between the two national groups. Subsequent American study has confirmed the British data. There must be some other explanation.

The politics of 'normal' hearing   I prefer to take a circuitous route to an alternative explanation because it is important to include in this discussion a consideration of the consequences of using a 'louder' or 'softer' audiometric zero. It was stated by Davis and Usher (1957) that growing dissatisfaction in Europe with American audiometric zero led to new investigations of normal hearing. Why should it trouble otologists in Europe to have a 'loud' zero? Because, it would be argued, the audiometer is relied upon as an instrument to allow discrimination of normally hearing from hearing-impaired persons. If zero is taken to represent the normal standard, then the higher its acoustical level the greater the chances of non-normally hearing listeners slipping through the screen.

[. . .]

If the aim of audiometry is to try to detect people with impairments of hearing, a strict standard of normal will facilitate the task, a liberal standard will not. It makes otological sense, then, to push for a strict standard. But does it? The only place a strict standard actually makes sense is in the armed forces and certain other occupations that demand good hearing. Only in these will there be concern to separate those with good hearing from those with possible impairments. In all other circumstances, there is no need for such vigilance. Clients in a clinical setting seek the services of otologists presumably because they recognize that something is wrong with their hearing, and diagnosis of the complaint is then the prime issue, the location of audiometric threshold is of secondary concern. It is only conceivably in situations where good hearing is an occupational requirement that precautions are needed to reduce the likelihood of the inclusion of partially deaf persons. And of course a strict standard cuts two ways: while it may block more of those with partial deafness, it also blocks more with good hearing. Many more people than need be will be excluded from occupations if a strict standard operates. Although it could be argued that this is unfortunate but necessary if one wants to exclude people who cannot hear well, of course this is true only if reliance is placed on audiometric measurement in the first place.

The whole problem emerges because, despite the USPHS data, the otological and audiological world has taken it that a given audiometric level actually corresponds to a given experienced hearing level when . . . no such state of affairs can be said to exist.

Nonetheless, given this presumption, however dubious, the argument presumably runs that 'normal' hearing is audiometrically defined as X dB. Observations of $X + n$ dB presumably are derived from those with non-normal hearing. More than occasionally, X dB will also be observed in those with non-normal hearing, but rarely will $X - n$ dB occur in such folk. A standard of 'normal' at $X - n$ dB is desirable, then, to ensure reliable exclusion. The question then becomes how to gain such a standard.

There are ways of ensuring that only persons with low acoustic levels at threshold are included in a standardization sample, hence providing legitimately strict normalizing levels. The basis of selection would be such as to exclude persons of certain socioeconomic background, age, occupation, and clinical otological state. The effects of noise exposure, childhood middle-ear infection, ageing, and minor 'attenuative' states of the outer ear (wax, scarring, etc.) all contribute to a raising of sound level at threshold. Standardization samples, with one exception, have always been carefully stripped of such cases. That exception, of course, is the USPHS survey. A *report* of normal was sufficient for inclusion in that group.

[. . .]

If one subscribes to the view that 'normal' hearing is merely related to but not identical with 'good' hearing, then it comes as no surprise that ASA (1951) zero is higher than any other. The assumption that elevation of threshold is a sign of reduction of hearing ability necessarily leads to the conclusion that elevation of threshold must imply a departure from *normality* when of course all that it may mean is a departure from *good*. One might still *report* normality of hearing because, of course, normality of hearing can mean anything from good hearing to adequacy of hearing for one's general life purposes.

We can see an immediate general implication of this argument, namely that what I assert about my hearing is ignored in favour of what I do in response to the tests of an audiologist. In the determination of normal hearing, we witness the conflict between functional tests and self-report. We see too, in the 'good-to-adequate' concept, one reason why there is lack of correspondence between self-report and functional test.

Let me make it clear once again that I care little which acoustic level is used as audiometric zero. What I am concerned to show is the interest being served by determination of a strict standard and the means adopted to legitimate such a standard. I wish to show further that, although strict standards may fulfil a discriminative function, they should not be taken to represent the universe of 'normal hearing'. Wheeler and Dickson (1952) recognized this in presenting the data which largely dictated the British standard. Their description of the thresholds as representing 'normal *good hearing*' (my italic) is an acknowledgment that the standard typifies not the norm of hearing but an extreme aspect of that norm.

Why has this seemingly simple explanation of the Anglo-American difference not been recognized before? For the reason, I think, that the concept of 'self-reportedly normal' has not been realized as different from the concept of 'otologically normal'. Researchers have so closely identified the audiogram trace with the state of a person's hearing that a self-report of 'normal' has come automatically to mean 'audiometrically in and around 0 dB'.

[. . .]

References

American National Standard Institute (1969) *American National Standards Specification for Audiometers,* ANSI, S3.6.

American Standards Association (1951) *American Standard Specification for Audiometers for General Diagnostic Purposes,* Z24.5, New York, American Standards Association.

Beasley, W.C. (1940) 'Characteristics and Distribution of Impaired Hearing in the Population of the United States', *Journal of the Acoustical Society of America, 12.*

Beasley, W.C. (1957) 'What is Zero Hearing Loss?', in Davis, H. and Usher, J.R. (eds) *Journal of Speech and Hearing Disorders, 22.*

British Standards Institution (1954) *The Normal Threshold of Hearing For Pure Tones by Earphone Listening,* BS 2497, London, British Standards Institution.

Bunch, C.C. (1943) *Clinical Audiometry,* St Louis, MO, C.V. Mosby.

Dadson, R.S. and King, J.H. (1952) 'A Determination of the Normal Threshold of Hearing and its Relation to the Standardization of Audiometers', *Journal of Laryngology and Otology, 66.*

Davis, H. (1970) 'Audiometry: Pure Tone and Simple Speech Tests', in Davis, H. and Silverman, S.R. (eds) *Hearing and Deafness,* (3rd edn) New York, Holt, Rinehart and Winston.

Davis, H., Stevens, S.S., Nichols, R.H. Jr., Hudgins, C.V., Marquis, R.J., Person, G.E. and Ross, D.A. (1947) *Hearing Aids: An Experimental Study of Design Objectives,* Cambridge, MA, Harvard University Press.

Davis, H. and Usher, J.R. (eds) (1957) 'What is Zero Hearing Loss?' *Journal of Speech and Hearing Disorders, 22.*

Glorig, A. (1958) A Report of Two Normal Hearing Studies, *Annals of Otology, Rhinology and Laryngology, 67.*

Glorig, A., Quiggle, R., Wheeler, D.E. and Grings, W. (1956) 'Determination of the Normal Hearing Reference Zero', *Journal of the Acoustical Society of America, 28.*

Harris, J.D. (1954) 'Normal Hearing and its Relation to Audiometry', *The Laryngoscope, 64.*

International Organization for Standardization (1964) *Standard Reference Zero for the Calibration of Pure-Tone Audiometers, ISO Recommendation,* R389, Geneva, 150.

Spoor, A. (1967) 'Presbycusis Values in Relation to Noise Induced Hearing Loss', *International Audiology, 6.*

Steinberg, J.C., Montgomery, H.C. and Gardner, M.B. (1940) 'Results of the World's Fair Hearing Tests', *Journal of the Acoustical Society of America, 12.*

Sunderman, F.W. and Boerner, F. (1950) *Normal Values in Clinical Medicine,* Philadelphia, Saunders.

United States Public Health Services (1938) 'Preliminary Analysis Audiometric Data in Relation to Clinical Histories of Impaired Hearing', *The National Health Survey, Hearing Study Series,* Bulletin No. 2, Washington, DC, US Public Health Service.

Watson, L.A. and Tolan, T. (1949) *Hearing Tests And Hearing Instruments,* Baltimore, MD, Williams and Wilkins.

Wheeler, L.J. and Dickson, E.D.D. (1952) 'The Determination of the Threshold of Hearing', *Journal of Laryngology and Otology, 66.*

4.3 The Hearing Aid as a System

Ivan Tucker and Michael Nolan (1984)

The hearing aid

At the present time there are four main types of hearing aid systems in use with hearing-impaired children. These are:

1 Body worn or pocket aid.
2 Post-auricular or behind the ear aid.
3 Radio hearing aid of the pocket type.
4 Radio hearing aid of personal type which links up with the conventional aid of category (1) or (2) via direct connection or by loop induction.

In addition, an increasing but very small number of children use 'in the ear' or modular aids. Certain groups of hearing-impaired children also have access to amplification systems specific to education. The Group Hearing Aid, which is a hard-wire system, is perhaps the most familiar member of this category.

A system which uses infra-red light is finding more widespread use particularly in special schools for the deaf. The auditory training unit (in effect a 'single module' of a group aid), which finds application particularly with pre-school hearing-impaired children, is not specifically an educational aid, but rather an extension of the child's personal hearing aid, to be used for short sessions such as an interactive play situation with mother, these sessions being aimed at fostering development of the child's linguistic skills.

The role of the hearing aid

All of these amplification systems are designed to improve the auditory experience of the hearing-impaired child. The quality of this hearing experience is of paramount importance, because without effective experiences of the sounds of speech, hearing-impaired children will have little or no chance of developing spoken language. A child's language development proceeds most rapidly in the early years of life. If a child's hearing is such that some or all of the sounds of everyday conversational speech are inaudible, then that child's speech and language will be severely restricted.

[. . .]

A child's ability to make use of his residual hearing depends to some degree on the severity of the hearing loss. It is vitally important to appreciate the potentially devastating effect that hearing-impairment can have on a child's linguistic attainments. While a hearing aid will not restore a child's hearing to normal, it will provide experiences of sound that would be otherwise unheard. It therefore plays a vital role in the child's sensory stimulation and contributes enormously to subsequent linguistic development.

Effective hearing aid management
The effective management of hearing-impaired children requires a comprehensive child-oriented service. Professionals have to deal with a completely different population (having child-specific problems) to that encountered by those working with the adult deaf. It is a fact of life that young hearing aid users rely heavily on their parents, and later, teachers to ensure that their aids are used efficiently. Generally speaking, young children are not able to set their own aids or even fit them. Furthermore, they rarely indicate when a fault arises, even when it results in reduced, distorted or total lack of output. Parents and teachers therefore have the responsibility of ensuring that hearing aids are well maintained and used to maximum effect.

The fundamental point of note at the onset of a management programme is that one is not simply dealing with a handicapped child—one is dealing with a family with a handicap. Families have a very important role to play in the utilization of the child's residual hearing via a hearing aid fitting. They must therefore be carefully counselled, advised and supported, not only early on immediately following the traumatic time of diagnosis, but throughout the child's pre-school years and during the school years where necessary.

Hearing handicap in a young child is often unrecognized by the public at large—that is, until people see the child wearing hearing aids. This concept of 'total child' being child plus hearing aids is one which parents may need time to come to terms with and fully accept. Parental acceptance of the hearing aid and an understanding of the importance of its continued efficient use is without doubt the primary aim of the early habilitative programme. This programme should provide a saturation service for the family, whereby guidance sessions, both in the home and perhaps on occasions at the resource centre, are organized on a regular basis, but with a built-in flexibility of support and help on demand.

Parents initially find it difficult to absorb information so the sessions should be spaced over time and new information only introduced gradually. This will include aspects of hearing aid management and day-to-day fitting procedures. Obviously, in the initial stages following diagnosis the *care* of the aids will be the sole responsibility of the professional, but gradually parents must be encouraged to develop their own hearing aid management skills. The eventual aim should be that the parents are competent hearing aid handlers (*but* not technicians or electronics experts). They should be able to fit aids, routinely check them prior to fitting and be able to spot faults and remedy the commonly occurring ones without recourse to the hearing aid clinic.

Concept of the hearing aid

It is important for everyone concerned with the day-to-day management of hearing-impaired children to conceptualize the hearing aid not from their own 'adult' or 'audiological specialist' viewpoint, but through the eyes of the child. Only in this way is it possible to begin to appreciate those child-specific problems which, if left unchecked, can spell disaster for effective auditory stimulation. Furthermore, such an approach also enables the 'professional advisor', who may have studied hearing aids over many years, to appreciate the difficulty that those 'new' to hearing aids (that is, parents and teachers alike) face in understanding just what kind of device is the hearing aid, how it works, what can go wrong, and what potentially it has to offer to the future of a hearing-impaired child. It is all too easy for familiarity to breed a 'too technically offputting' explanation on what is a vital piece of equipment that must become an integral part of the child.

The hearing aid is best seen as an interactive system, a system comprising a number of building blocks or components; that is, a chain of building blocks. If a single component is weak or faulty, the overall performance of the system will be INEFFICIENT—putting at risk the child's reception of auditory information. It is the job of parents, teachers and professional advisors to maintain this interactive system in as efficient a condition as possible. The aid is only as effective as the weakest link in the chain of building blocks.

Many of the problems influencing the efficient day-to-day use of hearing aids by children relate to the ergonomic design of the hearing aid (Powell, 1975)—the vast majority of hearing aids being designed for the adult user. These design features produce weak spots on the hearing aid, resulting in a risk of inefficient or totally ineffective amplification.

What is a hearing aid?

While hearing aids come in various shapes and sizes they all basically perform the same function—that of providing the hearing-impaired with experiences of sound which would otherwise go unheard. . . . All hearing aids whether pocket, post-auricular or 'in the ear' comprise [a] system of units. The only difference between these 'conventional' systems and other alternatives (e.g., radio hearing aids, group aids, infra-red, etc.) is simply that the alternatives have extra components 'added on', some of these being worn or used by others. This is why such systems are known by the term 'hearing aids not entirely worn on the listener' (IEC, 1979). However . . . they too are equally vulnerable to 'component faults' the majority of which are common to the conventional systems.

[. . .]

References

International Electro-Technical Commission (1979) *Hearing Aid Equip-*

ment Not Entirely Worn on the Listener, International Electrotechnical Commission, IEC 118–3, Geneva.

Powell, C.A. (1975) 'The Ergonomic Design of Hearing Aids for Children', *Proceedings of the Congress on Education of the Deaf,* Tokyo.

4.4 Information Technology: A Breakthrough for Deaf People?

Rob Baker (1987)

Introduction

This paper concerns the advances in technology which have made life easier and more interesting for hearing-impaired people in the last 10 years and also some of the shortcomings of these advances.

The term 'information technology' covers a range of new methods, mainly electronic methods, which have come into use for storing, transmitting and retrieving information. The information usually comes in the form of text, though 'information' can also include sound and pictures (including computer graphics and television pictures). I will concentrate on the development of television subtitling services in the UK, partly because of my personal involvement in this work since 1979, and partly because I believe that television subtitling has led the field in providing access to information for hearing-impaired people.

[. . .]

Research and development in television subtitling— a historical review

In this section I will give a personal view of the history of television subtitling via teletext. First, however, I would like to say something about the role of research. Research can have at least three different functions:

1 Purely academic interest—how many angels can stand on the head of a pin?

2 Procrastination—research projects are sometimes initiated in order to delay dealing with a problem.

3 Facilitation (the opposite of procrastination)—sometimes research can be seen as a way of focusing attention on a problem so that something is done about it—a way of making things happen!

The history of subtitling has involved all three types of research at various times. The work began when the Labour MP Jack Ashley contacted Southampton University in the mid 1970s. He had recently become totally deaf and wanted some means of coping with debates in the House of Commons. Although a skilled lipreader, he found this insufficient for dealing with a large number of speakers in different places and at varying distances, and with varying clarity of speech! What he really wanted was a computer that could automatically receive all the speech and display it simultaneously on a screen in front of him. This was impossible 10 years ago, and it still is. The system that was eventually developed in the Electronics Department at Southampton University was based on a shorthand machine, known as Palantype, which had been used in courts of law in the 1940s and 1950s for keeping a word for word record of court proceedings. A highly trained operator sits at a special keyboard and uses a phonetic code to type in everything that is said. The code enables him or her to type roughly twice as fast as a high-speed audiotypist—and that was what was needed. The codes that the Palantypist types in are 'translated' by a small computer into something approximating English, but with occasional peculiarities in spelling. The peculiarities are partly due to the difficulty of translating phonetics into conventional English spelling (which is far from phonetic), and partly due to inevitable human errors in working at very high speeds under considerable stress. The 'translated' Palantype is relayed to a TV screen in front of Mr Ashley, and with some initial determination on his part, Palantype rapidly enabled him to participate fully in House of Commons proceedings.

Around the same time as the Palantype system was being developed a major breakthrough in television technology was taking place—teletext. Teletext is a means of transmitting information in a hidden code which does not appear on ordinary TV screens. However, by using a special TV set [or video] the teletext signal can be decoded into pages of text and simple graphics, either instead of the normal picture, or superimposed on to it in the form of subtitles. It is said that teletext was originally invented as a technique for adding optional subtitles to ordinary TV programmes. The aim was to provide subtitles which would not intrude on to everyone's TV picture, since there was evidence that the general public did not like subtitles. The subtitles would be there only for those who wanted them. However, although teletext was invented in 1974, the first subtitles did not appear until 6 years later. The main reason for this delay seems to be to do with marketing. In those days a teletext TV cost three times as much as an ordinary colour TV set. In order to make teletext sets cheaper they would need to sell a lot of them. It was considered that teletext should be of interest to the public at large, not just to hearing-impaired people, and it was originally sold as a bit of a gimmick. Teletext could be used to get up-to-date news, sports results, weather forecasts, TV programme details, travel information, horoscopes, recipes, etc.—all interesting enough in themselves, but with all this going on, the marketers lost sight of subtitling. However, some people were not satisfied, notably the late Mr Bill Northwood of the BBC, and Jack Ashley once again.

Jack Ashley contacted Southampton University with the suggestion that Palantype could be used as an efficient method of producing subtitles via the teletext system. Dr Alan Newell of Southampton University approached the broadcasters; the idea was not greeted with much enthusiasm, but eventually the Independent Broadcasting Authority were persuaded to set up a research project at Southampton to look into the whole subject of teletext subtitling. At this time the role of research could properly be seen as procrastination—putting off actually doing subtitling by supporting research into it. However, there were a number of quite good reasons for this:

1   The broadcasters did not have appropriate equipment or suitably trained personnel to begin running a subtitling service.

2   Although Palantype could be read by highly motivated hearing-impaired people with above average English skills, it was doubted whether it would be suitable for broadcasting to a general viewership of hearing-impaired people with a wide range of educational backgrounds.

3   The conventional method of preparing subtitles in advance, as in foreign language films, was considered to be too time-consuming and expensive for the full range of TV programmes. In those days it took at least 40 hours to subtitle one hour of television.

4   Nothing was known at the time about hearing-impaired viewers' requirements—their viewing preferences, or the styles of subtitling that would be appropriate for various types of TV programmes.

The attitude taken by the broadcasters was that they should aim to set the highest possible standards of subtitling from the beginning, and they were not prepared to proceed until a great deal more was known. The research team at Southampton was given three jobs to do:

(i)   to look into ways of improving the Palantype system, and to examine alternatives, especially for sub-titling live TV programmes;

(ii)   to design special-purpose subtitling equipment which would reduce the time required for preparing conventional subtitles by at least 50 per cent;

(iii)   to investigate hearing-impaired viewers' subtitling needs and preferences, with a view to establishing a code of practice.

My main interest, when I was appointed as research fellow on the project in 1979, was in item (iii), and I must admit that at that time it was mainly an academic interest. I had previously done research into the psychology of the reading process, and here was a new and interesting area of reading research. I was quickly persuaded that reading a subtitled TV picture was a very different matter from reading a page from a book. The main differences were that, in reading subtitles:

(a)   the speed of reading is not under the reader's control. Subtitles appear and then disappear, whether you're ready or not; and

(b)   the reader is being asked to do two different things at once, i.e. read and watch television pictures.

It was clear that so little was known about this, the only way to make quick progress was to jump in at the deep end, to go out and meet hearing-impaired people as soon as possible and show them lots of subtitles. So I organized a programme of visits to hard-of-hearing clubs and social clubs for the deaf, demonstrated different methods of subtitling on all sorts of television programmes, and asked people for their reactions and their preferences. The issues under investigation included the layout and position of subtitles on the screen, the uses of coloured subtitling, treatment of sound effects, and the extent of script editing required to allow the viewer sufficient reading time.

Hearing-impaired people gave me clear information on these and many other issues, and very quickly my academic interest turned into research type 3—using research to inform people about possibilities, and to make things happen. Having seen what subtitling was all about, hearing-impaired people themselves began to make loud and clear demands for a proper subtitling service. I became convinced that good quality subtitling was possible provided that the broadcasters continued to listen to the views of hearing-impaired people. Ceefax's special information pages for hearing-impaired people 'No Need to Shout' and Oracle's 'Earshot' could be used to canvas people's opinions of the quality of subtitling. Within a year the first experimental subtitles appeared on Ceefax and Oracle.

Meanwhile engineers at Southampton worked to produce better subtitling equipment, incorporating the subtitling guidelines which were beginning to emerge from the research in deaf and hard of hearing clubs. The equipment is now in use at Oracle and enables subtitlers to do at least twice as much subtitling per working hour as they could in 1980. The output of subtitles from both BBC and ITV has risen from about half an hour a week in early 1980 to about 20 hours a week on each network in 1987, representing a firm commitment to the service. So far so good.

Problem areas

Psychological disadvantages of teletext

Cost and take-up In 1978 a teletext receiver cost nearly £1,000. Nowadays the difference between a teletext set and an ordinary colour TV set is about £50. Nevertheless, many hearing-impaired people feel that they are being asked to pay more money simply to get access to the same TV programmes that hearing people watch. This perception is unlikely to change until teletext is included as a standard feature of all TV sets.

A more serious problem in the current economic climate, is that many people, deaf and hearing, simply cannot afford colour TV sets and colour TV licences. In some cases people are reverting to black and white television. Black and white TV sets with teletext are not on the market.

No one knows what proportion of teletext sets owners are hearing-impaired, or what proportion of hearing-impaired people have teletext sets. One unfortunate effect of this is that the subtitlers at Ceefax and Oracle feel cut off from their viewers, and feel a great need for feedback from them. Hearing-impaired viewers, having got used to subtitles, are likely to have very different expectations from the service than they did when I completed my research in 1983. Now that teletext subtitling has come of age, it is time for proper audience research, which only the broadcasters are in a position to carry out adequately.

Teletext is invisible   In recent years there have been great changes in the attitudes of hearing people towards the needs of hearing-impaired people. Television has played a major part in this, with programmes like the BBC's 'See Hear' and a number of other special series reaching mass audiences well beyond the deaf community. The role of the Deaf Broadcasting Campaign has been highly significant in making deaf people visible to the general public through such programmes. However teletext subtitles are invisible to those who do not choose to watch them. Is this a bad thing?

A recent survey carried out by the Nottingham and Nottinghamshire Society for the Deaf has come up with some fascinating results (Doyle, 1986). The views of 253 ordinary hearing adults in the Nottingham area were sampled, and it was found that 82 per cent of them had watched Ceefax or Oracle subtitles. The reasons for this would themselves be worthy of research. Furthermore it was found that, contrary to earlier research, 78 per cent of these people did not find that subtitles interfered with their viewing pleasure. This may in itself reflect a major shift in public opinion. It may also reflect different ways of asking questions, reminiscent of recent discussions about income tax cuts. When asked, 'Would you prefer tax cuts or more public spending?', people would tend to favour tax cuts. However, if the question is, 'Would you prefer tax cuts or better provision of health, housing, and education services?' a different reply is forthcoming. Similarly, if the question is, 'Subtitles or no subtitles?', most hearing people are likely to say, 'No, thanks'. But if it is made clear that the purpose of subtitles is to allow hearing-impaired people to enjoy television in the same way as everybody else, a more favourable response can be expected.[1]

[. . .]

Technical shortcomings

Subtitling live television programmes   For 7 years some of the best minds in broadcasting engineering have been trying to get to grips with this. The first problem is that there is no automatic method for transcribing real live speech word for word. Even if there was, it would not be satisfactory for some live programmes, such as the news, because it would result in subtitling that was too fast for the majority of viewers to read.[2]

There have been two main approaches to subtitling live programmes with varying degrees of success. The first is to use a shorthand machine, such as Palantype. This can give a word for word transcription of speech rates up to about 200 words per minute (a few news correspondents speak at up to 220 words per minute, so there will still be problems with them.) However, many viewers will have difficulty reading the transcription at the rate it is presented. The BBC have used Palantype on several major public occasions (Royal Wedding, Wimbledon finals, etc.). The BBC have not been happy with the quality of the transcription—on one famous occasion a viewer wrote in to complain about the 'Welsh language' subtitles on his screen! In addition there have been difficulties in getting sufficiently skilled Palantype operators to run the system on a regular basis.

ITV Oracle have adopted a different approach. This involves using a conventional audiotypist, but with a lot of advance preparation. It should be said that for most live programmes a great deal of information is available in script form before the programme begins, and so some subtitles can be prepared in advance. When covering public events the greater part of what is likely to happen can be predicted fairly accurately (e.g. the TV commentator filling in background to the history of the event during lulls in the action, texts of hymns and prayers and Order of Service for weddings, etc.) and so a subtitle file can be prepared during the research stages of the programme. These pre-prepared subtitles are then sent out 'live' at the correct points in the programme. A truly live facility is still needed for instance when the unpredictable takes place. At a recent live-subtitled event the Queen was several minutes late, the commentator improvised, and the subtitler had to work as fast as possible to give a summarized rendering of what was said. The first problem with this approach is that the subtitler must summarize very heavily in order to have time to type, and this can lead to misinterpretations. Furthermore the subtitler also needs time to think before he or she can begin typing, and this can mean that when the subtitles eventually arrive, they appear over a completely inappropriate picture. A classic instance of this was during the coverage of the Prince of Wales' wedding in 1981. The TV pictures showed a beautiful stately home where the couple were to stay immediately after the wedding. A subtitle was composed:

> This is where the Royal couple will spend
> the first few days of their honeymoon.

By the time the subtitle actually appeared, the TV camera had moved inside the house and was showing a beautiful four-poster bed!!

For reasons like this neither the BBC nor ITV have been eager to risk subtitling live news and current affairs programmes, feeling that their reputations for accuracy are too much in jeopardy. Although as much as two thirds of a newscaster's speech is fully scripted and available an hour before transmission, there can be sudden last minute additions, changes in stories or in the order of stories. Moreover, the film and video reports from correspondents, interviews and outside broadcasts, which nowadays make up as much as 50 per cent of a news bulletin, are not scripted at all. It is worth pointing out, however, that live subtitles on news programmes in the USA, using a system similar to Palantype, have been seen for the last 2 or 3 years. The only reason I can think of for this difference in broadcasters' attitudes is that the news in the USA is considered to be just another aspect of show biz!!

[. . .]

This brief examination of current developments should indicate some of the areas of potential growth and also some of the limitations. Technology may develop quickly but it also has to be delivered to the user. The developments may not be effective if the users are not first consulted.

[Notes

1   The Government have announced that the new Channel 3 and 5 licencees will be required to subtitle at least half of all their programmes within 5 years of the start of their franchises in 1993. Deaf people had lobbied intensively on this issue and 150,000 signatures were collected on a petition presented to MPs.

2   Since 1988, however, ITN News at Ten and Channel Four News have been subtitled live.]

Reference

Doyle, M. (1986) *Television Viewers' Attitudes Towards Programme Comprehension Aids for Hearing Impaired People,* Nottingham and Nottinghamshire Society for the Deaf.

Section 5
Educational Perspectives: Learning to Communicate or Communicating to Learn?

Within the education system, special provision is made for the education of deaf children and adolescents. In the educational context in the UK the term 'deaf' is increasingly being replaced by 'hearing-impaired'. This terminology suggests a deficit model in which emphasis is placed on the remediation of a perceived disability and the normalization of deaf children with the aim of making them as much like hearing children as possible.

Audiological criteria are used in determining which children will come under the auspices of special educational services. The British Association of Teachers of the Deaf (BATOD) paper describes the audiological definitions in current use. It advocates an audiological characterization rather than an account of functional hearing loss and provides a powerful labelling device for professionals working with deaf children. This approach, which subdivides children into pre-defined labelled categories, may be contrasted with the cultural definitions of deafness discussed earlier in relation to membership of the Deaf community in which audiological criteria are perceived as irrelevant. It also implies more stability of hearing loss over time than may in fact be found in practice.

As deaf children in the UK came to participate in compulsory education after 1893, communication became a very obvious concern for educationalists. The problem arose of how deaf children were to access a curriculum devised and delivered by hearing people. The obvious solution seemed to be to promote oral language as the medium of instruction. Throughout the history of deaf education, however, there have always been people who have recognized and valued sign language as the natural language of deaf people and advocated its use in education. The long-standing debate between oralists, advocating spoken language, and manualists, advocating sign language, is a recurrent theme in deaf education.

The Milan conference of 1880 is often cited as a watershed in this debate. The final resolution of the conference decreed that 'the oral method ought to be preferred to that of signs for the education and instruction of the deaf and dumb'. Markides and Lane provide different perspectives on the Milan conference. Implicit in Markides' paper is the idea of deafness as pathology and an emphasis on the normalization of deaf people through the acquisition of spoken language. Lane, on the other hand, sees Deaf people as a cultural minority group and views the conference as an example of the oppression of Deaf people and their language.

Controversy continues to surround the choice of communication methods to be used in the education of deaf children. The construction of deafness as a disability to be overcome through amplification and the acquisition of spoken language, to enable deaf people to participate fully in a hearing society, continues to be most forcefully seen in approaches emphasizing oral language development. We have chosen Lynas, Huntington and Tucker as a recent statement of this perspective.

Initially, Total Communication developed as a reaction to pure oralism, and viewed gestures—finger spelling and/or sign language—as valuable in facilitating communication. Its aim continued to be, however, the subsequent development of oral language. The implicit model of deafness as deficit remained, with its attendant emphasis on the acquisition of the language of the dominant culture, so that deaf people could be assimilated into the hearing world. The philosophy of Total Communication, with its emphasis on communication rather than language is, however, compatible with a range of teaching methods including the bilingual option mentioned below.

As deaf people have become increasingly conscious of their own community and culture, they have become more actively involved in educational debate. This, combined with the linguistic recognition of sign language (see Section 6) and views of Britain as a multi-lingual society, has led to the development and implementation in some areas of a bilingual approach, and the recognition of British Sign Language (BSL) as the first language of deaf children, as described by Llwellyn Jones. The bilingual model of deaf education, with its emphasis on BSL, reflects a construction of deafness which views Deaf people as a cultural linguistic minority group.

While the oral/manual controversy continues to provide the background for much educational debate, attempts have been made to remove discussion of educational principles and practice from this area and to focus on interactive styles rather than mode of communication. A leading proponent of this approach is Wood who, with his colleagues, has analysed the outcomes of various teaching styles (see Article 5.8 by Wood, Wood, Griffiths and Howarth). Although the extract used here is based on work in oral schools, more recently Wood's group has used the same methodology to look at teachers in schools using Sign Supported English, with very similar results (Wood, Wood and Kingsmill, in preparation).

As implied above, attitudes towards oral and/or sign language use in the education of deaf children imply differing perceptions of deafness which may be seen to be reflected in the current debate about integration. Schools for deaf children have been viewed as necessary to the development and continuance of a Deaf culture since they provide a meeting ground for deaf children and an opportunity for deaf children to develop sign language (see Ladd, 1990, for example). Some advocates of a cultural view of deafness, therefore, are opposed to integration with its apparent emphasis on the assimilation of deaf children to the hearing world, since they view this as an approach which reinforces a deficit model of deafness. Lynas epitomizes such an approach to integration as assimilation, although a close reading of her own findings demonstrates that the situation is more complex than she suggests. Booth, on the other hand, radically challenges this normalizing notion of integration.

Commitment to a cultural definition of deafness may lead to a view of integration commensurate with the idea of a pluralistic society. Deaf children could be taught in a mainstream setting, but access to the curriculum would be provided in their first language, sign language, and they would learn English as a second language, so that integration would involve a bilingual approach aimed at children's eventual participation in a multicultural society (see Article 5.7 by Llwellyn-Jones).

Gregory and Bishop's paper looks at integration from the perspective of deaf children placed individually in mainstream settings. They indicate that discussion of integration should be concerned not only with whether children have access to the full range of the curriculum (which these children did not) but also with how children themelves construct their experiences. They suggest that the children they studied developed coping strategies which were counter-productive to the long-term goals of education, whether that goal be assimilation or cultural diversity.

References

Ladd, P. (1990) 'Making Plans for Nigel: The Erosion of Identity by Mainstreaming', in Taylor, G. and Bishop, J. (eds) *Being Deaf: The Experience of Deafness*, London, Pinter Publishers.

Wood, D., Wood, H. and Kingsmill, M. (in preparation), *Signed English in the Classroom*.

5.1 Audiological Descriptors

British Association of Teachers of the Deaf (1981, amended 1985)

The National Executive Council (NEC) has agreed on descriptors for the following audiological terms:

Average hearing loss
Prelingual hearing loss
Slightly hearing-impaired
Moderately hearing-impaired
Severely hearing-impaired
Profoundly hearing-impaired

These descriptors are given below.

The NEC also wishes to standardize the forms used to plot the results of pure tone and speech audiometry. [. . .]

Average hearing loss

There seem to be a number of ways by which a child's average (or overall) hearing loss is calculated. The method which is adopted will yield different results, and this can cause confusion when comparing the hearing losses of both individuals and of groups of children unless the full audiograms are given. This is seldom practicable, and there is a need to be able to use a global figure in spite of the disadvantages inherent in global figures. For the sake of standardization, therefore, the NEC has decided that the method of calculating average hearing loss given below should be adopted by our Association. Members are asked to use this method when quoting average losses for children. The editions of this Journal [in which this article was originally published] will also ask contributors to use this method of calculation where hearing losses are quoted in articles.

Method of calculation

The average hearing loss for a child should be calculated in the following way. The loss in dB (HL) at the five frequencies 250Hz, 500Hz, 1kHz, 2kHz, and 4kHz should be averaged for each ear. The ear which shows the smaller loss (i.e. the better ear) is then taken as the child's *average hearing loss*. If there is no response at any of the five frequencies, then for the purposes of the calculation a numerical value is given to that no response (NR). The actual value used will be 130 dBHL.

Example—JOHN

Frequency	250Hz	500Hz	1kHz	2kHz	4kHz
Left ear	80	90	100	NR	110
Right ear	60	80	90	110	NR

The average loss in John's left ear is
$$\frac{80 + 90 + 100 + 130 + 110}{5} = \frac{510}{5} = 102 \text{ dBHL}$$

and in his right ear
$$\frac{60 + 80 + 90 + 110 + 130}{5} = \frac{470}{5} = 94 \text{ dBHL}$$

John's *average hearing loss* therefore is 94 dBHL.

Descriptors relating to levels of hearing loss in children
It is clear that the statutory descriptors of the terms deaf and partially
hearing, that is:

Deaf children 'Pupils with impaired hearing who require education by
methods suitable for pupils with little or no naturally acquired speech or
language' (HMSO, 1962)

and

Partially-hearing children 'Pupils with impaired hearing whose development of speech and language even if retarded is following a normal pattern
and who require for their education special arrangements or facilities
though not necessarily all the educational methods used for deaf pupils'
(HMSO, 1962)

no longer serve the needs of the profession as a whole. The inadequacy of
these descriptors is highlighted by the increasing use of terms such as
educationally deaf, educationally partially hearing, audiologically deaf,
audiologically partially hearing. Though these terms are usually used in an
attempt to clarify a child's hearing status, it often adds to the confusion in
that a child may be educationally deaf, but audiologically partially hearing,
or educationally partially hearing but audiologically deaf, etc. There is a
need therefore to move to simpler descriptors.
    These new descriptors should be based on two factors:

1   The age of the child when hearing impairment occurred.
2   The average hearing loss for pure tones, as calculated using the method
described above.

The first factor, age at onset, is clearly important since a child who has acquired language before a hearing loss occurs presents a different problem to the child who has a prelingual loss. The next question that has to be decided is after what age should a loss be considered post-lingual? Due to the considerable variation that exists between children, this presents a difficulty. However, to achieve a suitable definition an age has to be stated, and the NEC believes that this age should be 18 months. A hearing loss that occurs after this age should not be considered to be prelingual. A prelingual loss is therefore defined as:

A permanent hearing loss which occurs before the age of 18 months.

The second factor, the degree of hearing loss, is somewhat easier to resolve. It is simply a question of agreeing on suitable terms to describe the varying levels of hearing loss. The NEC **RECOMMENDS** that the terms DEAF and PARTIALLY-HEARING should no longer be used to describe the hearing status of hearing-impaired children. In their place the following terminology and descriptors should be used:

1 **Slightly hearing-impaired:** Children whose average hearing loss, regardless of age at onset, does not exceed 40 dBHL.
2 **Moderately hearing-impaired:** Children whose average hearing loss, regardless of age at onset, is from 41 dB to 70 dBHL.
3 **Severely hearing-impaired:** Children whose average hearing loss is from 71 dBHL to 95 dBHL, and those with a greater loss who acquired their hearing-impairment after the age of 18 months.
4 **Profoundly hearing-impaired:** Children who were born with, or who acquired before the age of 18 months, an average hearing loss of 96 dBHL or greater.

Summary
Average hearing loss: The average of five frequencies (250Hz to 4kHz).

Prelingual loss: Onset before 18 months.

Slightly hearing-impaired: Up to 40 dBHL.

Moderately hearing-impaired: 41 dBHL to 70 dBHL.

Severely hearing-impaired: Losses 71 dBHL to 95 dBHL and post-lingual losses greater than 95 dBHL.

Profoundly hearing-impaired: A prelingual loss exceeding 95 dBHL.

NB: The terms 'deaf' and 'partially-hearing' should not be used to refer to children.

[. . .]

Reference

HMSO (1962) 'Handicapped Pupils and Special Schools Amending Regulations 1962', *Statutory Instrument No. 2073*, London, HMSO.

5.2 The Teaching of Speech: Historical Developments

Andreas Markides (1983)

[. . .]

Nineteenth century

Flight from speech teaching

. . . The first half of the nineteenth century saw the establishment of asylums and institutions for the deaf and dumb in urban areas of the United Kingdom, such as Edinburgh, Aberdeen, Glasgow, Birmingham, Manchester, Liverpool, Doncaster, Brighton, Exeter, Bristol, Aberystwyth. This expansion came about mainly as a result of the endeavours of humanitarians who considered it their religious duty to provide 'places of refuge from a cruel and unsympathetic world' where the handicapped, the destitute and of course the poor should be taught to live upright and industrious lives in the position it had pleased God to place them!

The method of instruction followed in these 'schools' for the deaf was exclusively manual and the protagonist for this was Louis du Puget, a Swiss who was an ardent supporter of the methods of Abbé de l'Epée. He was appointed to the headship of the General Institution for the Instruction of the Deaf and Dumbe Children in Birmingham in 1825.

It is true that during this period there were one or two isolated attempts to teach speech but they were without success. For example, John Anderson, during his headship of the Glasgow institution, devised a model of the human speech mechanism which could be used to demonstrate the different positions required to articulate different sounds. This, however, was of no practical use and it was on show mainly to impress visitors. Also Arnold in the 1840s, whilst a young teacher in the deaf institution in Liverpool (Arnold, 1888), reported that a certain amount of articulatory work (speech teaching) was attempted but without any success.

[. . .]

Teaching of speech revived

The first signs of the revival of teaching speech to deaf children in the United Kingdom appeared in the early 1860s when Gerrit van Asch arrived at Manchester as tutor for the deaf-mute daughter of a wealthy Jewish merchant. A year or two later (1862), van Asch opened a private school for deaf children in London. The method of instruction in his school was oral, based on the 'German system'. In the same year, another private school for deaf children was opened in London by Susannah Hull. According to Hodgson (1953) her methods were purely oral.

In 1866 the Jewish school, under the patronage of Baroness Mayer de Rothschild, decided to adopt the oral method of education and for this purpose another Dutch national from the Rotterdam school for the deaf came over to help. The man in question was the young William van Praagh—a teacher totally committed to oralism. His oral methods proved so successful that in 1871 an Association for the Oral Instruction of the Deaf and Dumb was formed. Its aims were to publicize the oral system and to 'nationalise the oral instruction of the deaf by lipreading and articulate speech, to the rigid exclusion of the finger-alphabet and all artificial signs' and 'to train qualified teachers on this system and to maintain a normal school for instructing deaf and dumb children' (Arnold, 1888). The school and training college were opened in Fitzroy Square, London in June 1872.

By the middle of the 1870s the change in favour of teaching speech to deaf children was gathering momentum. In 1876 James Howard, the headmaster of the Yorkshire Institution for the Deaf at Doncaster, arranged for the Abbé Balestra from Italy (a convert to the 'German system') to come and instruct himself and his staff in the principles of oralism. A year later, in 1877, a conference of headmasters of institutions for the deaf was held in London. This conference, spearheaded by Richard Elliott of Margate and James Howard of Doncaster, resolved that reforms in institutions for the deaf were necessary. The next year James Watson resigned his headship at the Old Kent Road school rather than be part of the newly proposed changes.

Apart from Elliott another person was emerging to prominence at this time. He was Rev. Thomas Arnold, a successful oral teacher of the deaf and a prolific writer. Arnold's publications influenced generations of teachers of the deaf. In particular his book *A Method of Teaching the Deaf and Dumb Speech, Lip-reading, and Language* which first appeared in 1881 was adopted by the College of Teachers of the Deaf and was reprinted, with slight amendments, as recently as 1954 under the title *Arnold on the Education of the Deaf. A Manual for Teachers*.

Another influential person during this period was St John Ackers MP who had a deaf daughter. In his desire to provide for his daughter the best possible education, he visited schools for the deaf both in continental Europe and in the USA. He returned to England a firm believer in the 'German system' and he set about influencing people and events with the zeal of a missionary. He founded the 'Society for the Training of Teachers of the Deaf and the Diffusion of the German System in the United Kingdom'. In 1878 he opened a private college for training teachers of the deaf at Ealing. He publicized widely the aim of the society; he organized meetings, read papers and published pamphlets. He participated in the Royal Commission on the Condition of the Blind, and Deaf and Dumb etc. (1889) which recommended the 'pure oral method' in the education of the deaf.

The big manual 'schools' for the deaf, both in England and in continental Europe, especially in France and Italy, came under increasing public scrutiny. Their work, the living conditions of the children, their academic achievements, the calibre and training of their teachers and above all their methods of instruction were examined and found wanting. Change was demanded and change was achieved, especially following the International Congress for the Deaf, held at Milan in 1880. This congress passed the following resolutions:

> . . . considering the incontestable superiority of speech over signs in restoring the deaf-mute to society and in giving him a more perfect knowledge of the language, the Congress declares that the oral method ought to be preferred to that of signs for the education and instruction of the deaf and dumb . . . and considering that the simultaneous use of speech and signs has the disadvantage of injuring speech, lip-reading and precision of ideas, declare that the pure oral method ought to be preferred . . . and considering that a great number of the deaf and dumb are not receiving the benefit of instruction recommends that Governments should take the necessary steps that all the deaf and dumb may be educated.
> (Buxton, 1880)

Following these recommendations the official French delegate expressed his complete conversion from the manual to the oral system. So did the Italians. The English, including St John Ackers, his wife and Susannah Hull, were jubilant; the American delegation was dejected. Soon the wind of change in favour of oralism became a hurricane. In 1893 in England an Act of Parliament made the education of deaf children compulsory between the ages of 7 and 16 years. Local school boards started establishing day schools for the deaf and almost all of these schools were oral from the very beginning. Residential institutions for the deaf, in order to benefit from state financial assistance, started organizing speech lessons for selected groups of deaf children.

[. . .]

References

Arnold, T. (1888) *Education of Deaf Mutes*, London, Werthimer Lea.

Buxton, D. (1880) *Speech for the Deaf*, Essays, Proceedings and Resolutions of the International Congress on the Education of the Deaf.

Hodgson, K.W. (1953) *The Deaf and Their Problems*, London, Watts.

Royal Commission on the Blind, The Deaf and Dumb and Others of the United Kingdom Report (1889), London, HMSO.

5.3 Why the Deaf Are Angry

Harlan Lane (1984)

[. . .]

Long after many other nations accepted education as a fundamental right of all its citizens, hearing and deaf, deaf education remained in Great Britain a matter of private charity rather than public responsibility. Late in the last century, however, the Crown created a Commission to consider these issues. At first it was charged with investigating the education of the blind and feebleminded but an influential barrister, member of Parliament, and father of a deaf girl, St John Ackers, managed to have himself appointed to the Commission and to have its scope enlarged. Ackers wanted his daughter to speak, although she had become deaf at only a few months of age, and he hired a teacher from the United States. 'I would call upon all interested in the success of the [oral] system', Ackers wrote, 'to unite together resolutely to refuse admission into their schools of any who can converse by signs'. The Chairman of the Commission had recently opened a new wing of the Manchester school for the deaf with the claim that, 'If only the education of children were begun at an early age, in 99 cases out of 100 the deaf and dumb could be taught to speak by the oral system'. No one on the Commission was deaf, nor an expert on teaching the deaf. In short, the combining of deaf issues with those of the blind and feebleminded which guaranteed a medical model, and the make-up of the Commission, left little doubt that it would recommend oralism for the deaf.

One of the leading witnesses before the Commission was Edward Minor Gallaudet, son of Thomas Gallaudet, the Protestant minister who, with Laurent Clerc, created the network of residential schools in the United States. The leader of his profession in America, and son of a deaf woman, Edward Minor Gallaudet believed that sign language was the irreplaceable vehicle of educating the deaf, and that speech and speechreading were valuable supplementary skills when they could be acquired. Opposing him was one of the most famous British subjects alive: a professional teacher of speech and inventor of the telephone, Alexander Graham Bell. Bell was the leading figure in the attack on the Deaf community in the United States. Bell sought to banish the sign language; to scatter the deaf and discourage their socializing, organizing, publishing and marriage; to have deaf children educated in and use exclusively the majority language. To this cause he devoted his great prestige, personal fortune, and tireless efforts; thus he became 'the most fearful enemy of the American deaf, past and present', to quote the President of the National Association of the Deaf.

The report of the Commission was called a victory by both sides. It concluded: 'All children should be, for the first year at least, instructed in the oral system; those who cannot profit should then be taught manually'. The adult deaf may, of course, have disagreed with putting signs in second place, using the language only with those who fail speech, but the report explained that signs tend to isolate the deaf with the result that they 'are not at all competent witnesses as to which is the best system; those that have lived in cages all their lives are so much attached to the cage that they have no desire to fly outside. The children themselves may prefer the sign system as more natural to them and the parents of poor [deaf] children are sometimes indifferent and careless'.

The most flagrant and destructive disregard of the views of the deaf in history is to be found, however, in the international congresses, organized by hearing teachers of the deaf, that finally sealed the unhappy fate of the deaf in Europe and America to the present day. It all began at the French Exposition of 1878, when a meeting of hearing instructors of the deaf was hastily convened. Only fifty-four persons attended, half of them instructors, and all but two of these from France. No deaf people were allowed to attend, although a majority of the instructors of the deaf in France were themselves deaf. Nevertheless, the hearing group grandiosely proclaimed themselves the 'First International Congress on the Education and Welfare of the Deaf', affirmed that only oral instruction could fully restore the deaf to society, and chose Milan as the site of the second congress to be held in 1880.

In fact, the Milan meeting was a brief rally conducted by opponents of manual language. At the congress, which lasted some twenty-four hours, three or four oralists reassured the rest of the rightness of their actions in the face of troubling difficulties. Nevertheless, the meeting at Milan was the single most critical event in driving the languages of the deaf beneath the surface; it is the single most important cause—more important than hearing loss—of the limited educational achievement of the modern deaf man and woman.

Writing from Milan, a British teacher raved, 'The victory for the cause of pure speech was gained before [the] congress began'. The headmaster at the Royal School for Deaf Children reported that the congress 'was mainly a partisan gathering. The machinery to register its decrees on the lines desired by its promoters had evidently been prepared beforehand and to me it seemed that the main feature was enthusiasm [for] "orale pure" rather than calm deliberation on the advantages and disadvantages of methods'. The location chosen, the make-up of the organizing committee, the congress schedule and demonstrations, the composition of the membership, the officers of the meeting—all elements were artfully arranged to produce the desired effect.

The Italians made up more than half the 164 delegates, and there were fifty-six from France; the committed delegates from these two countries were seven-eighths of the membership. Of the eight British delegates, six were brought by St John Ackers.

Apart from the Ackers group, the British delegation included Rev.

Thomas Arnold, author of a monumental oralist history of deaf education. Arnold was shortly to become the intellectual leader of his profession in Britain. He told the congress, 'Articulate language is superior to sign, because it is the method employed by nature. Modern science teaches us that what is natural ends up with the upper hand'; and, 'No doubt signs are often animated and picturesque but they are absolutely inadequate for abstraction'; and much more of the same.

The officers of the Milan congress—like the location and membership—were chosen to ensure the oralist outcome. The organizers selected Guilio Tarra, a rabid oralist, as the president by acclamation. Tarra preached to the congress:

> Let us have no illusions, to teach speech successfully we must have courage and with a resolute blow cut cleanly between speech and sign . . . Who would dare say that these disconnected and crude signs that mechanically reproduce objects and actions are the elements of a language? Oral speech is the sole power that can rekindle the light God breathed into man when, giving him a soul in a corporeal body, he gave him also a means of understanding, of conceiving, and of expressing himself . . . While, on the one hand, mimic signs are not sufficient to express the fullness of thought, on the other they intensify and glorify fantasy and all the faculties of the sense of imagination . . . The fantastic language of signs magnifies the senses and inflames the passions, whereas speech elevates the mind much more naturally, with calm, prudence and truth and avoids the danger of exaggerating the sentiment expressed and provoking harmful mental impressions . . .

When a deaf-mute confesses an unjust act in sign, Tarra explained, the sensations accompanying the act are revived. For example, when the deaf person confesses in sign language that he has been angry, the detestable passion returns to the sinner, which certainly does not aid his moral reform. In speech on the other hand, the penitent deaf-mute reflects on the evil he has committed and there is nothing to excite the passion again. Tarra ended by defying anyone to define in sign the soul, faith, hope, charity, justice, virtue, the angels, God . . . He concluded: 'No shape, no image, no design can reproduce these ideas. Speech alone, divine itself, is the right way to speak of divine matters'.

All but the Americans voted for a resolution sanctifying the dominant oral language and dismissing the sign language whatever the nation:

> 1   The congress, considering the unarguable superiority of speech over signs, for restoring deaf-mutes to social life and for giving them greater facility in language, declares that the method of articulation should be used instead of the method of signs in the education of the deaf and dumb.
>
> 2   Considering that the simultaneous use of signs and speech has the disadvantage of injuring speech, lipreading and precision of ideas, the congress declares that the pure oral method should be used.

In the closing moments of the congress, a delegate from the French government cried from the podium, *'Vive la parole!'* This has been the slogan of hearing educators of the deaf down to the present time. But an American deaf leader has written: '1880 was the year that saw the birth of the infamous Milan resolution that paved the way for foisting upon the deaf everywhere a loathed method; hypocritical in its claims, unnatural in its application, mind-deadening and soul-killing in its ultimate results'.

5.4 The Deaf School Child

Reuben Conrad (1979)

We include here three short extracts from Conrad's seminal study in which he considered all deaf young people of school leaving age, 15 to 16½ years of age, in England and Wales in the mid 1970s (1974–1976). The study is detailed, and we can only include some of the main findings here.

The study, which reported low attainments of deaf young people on a number of measures, has been influential in much of the discussion concerning the education of deaf children, since its publication in 1979. These results are not unique to England and Wales, similar findings are reported in studies throughout Western Europe and North America. Such results also illustrate why language and communication method has been such a pervasive theme in any discussion of the education of deaf children.

[. . .]

[Reading]
The median reading age, when the entire school population is considered is 9:0. The combined values covering the two age-groups 15 and 16 years reported by DiFrancesca (1972) for 17,000 children in the USA, yields a grade level of 3.15; that is, a median reading age of 9:2. In spite, therefore, of the use of different reading tests and different procedures for collecting data, there is remarkable concordance. In practical terms a useful way of taking an overall view of the reading ability of these children is the presentation in Figure 1. Partly because there seems to be a genuine discontinuity at about a hearing loss of 85 dB, and partly to maintain adequate numbers, reading ability is shown in the form of cumulative frequencies for those children with a hearing loss up to 85 dB and separately for those above this value. The figure then shows the percentage of children reaching different levels of reading age in months. Since, with the test used, zero reading comprehension is represented by a reading age of 7:0, the lowest detectable ability shows as a value greater than this. It will be seen that of the deafer section of the population almost 50 per cent have no reading comprehension at all—they are totally illiterate. With the same test, this would be the case for hearing children only at the chronological age of 7 years. For the less deaf children, some 25 per cent are without any reading comprehension. It is worth noting performance at the other end of the range as well. Here we can see that some 8 per cent of the less-deaf children have a reading ability commensurate with their chronological age—a value which reduces to five such children out of 205 when deafness is greater than 85 dB.

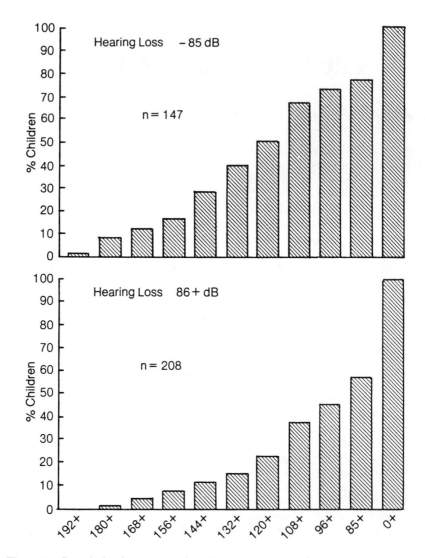

Figure 1 Cumulative frequences of reading age in months (after Conrad, 1977a)

[. . .]

[Lip-reading]
Think of the case of hearing people listening to speech in normal conditions. With unimpaired hearing, we must assume that they can understand everything that they linguistically know. That is, if they do not understand a spoken statement, neither would they were it written.

Partially hearing children, whose hearing is imperfect but far from gravely impaired, may be expected not to do so well. We now count the proportion of children with hearing losses up to 65 dB who can in fact understand through speech almost everything—let us say 95 per cent or more—of what they can understand in print. We find 93 per cent of such children. This means that nearly all of these partially-hearing children comprehend the language they know through speech, more or less as well as do hearing people. Evidently vision can effectively substitute if necessary for their mild hearing impairment.

Now, however, consider the case of children whose hearing loss is beyond 95 dB—those very deaf—and ask the same question: what proportion have speech comprehension at the level of their linguistic knowledge (95 per cent or more)? Here we find no more than 16 per cent. For the vast majority there is a gap, of varying size, between what they can understand and what they know. While all hearing children and 93 per cent of slightly deaf children can understand (through speech) whatever they know, only 16 per cent of profoundly deaf children can. This provides a dramatic idea of the deficit incurred when most of known spoken information has to be derived visually.

The second suggestion involves a direct comparison with hearing children. Essentially what is being evaluated here is the effect of some 10 years of training and practice at lip reading by deaf children. We took a group of seventy-five hearing children aged 15–16 years from a state school. White noise was passed through headphones to a degree where no speech sounds at all could be perceived. In this condition they were in fact more 'deaf' than probably all of our deaf population, since their 'deafness' was literally total. They were given one practice run through the Donaldson test followed by a test run. We omitted the print-reading version because three tests would have begun to strain patience. We gave the latter test to forty-three different hearing children from the same school. Otherwise the test conditions were identical to those used with deaf children. For comparison, we used all of the deaf children with a hearing loss greater than 95 dB who were in schools for the deaf. An earlier article (Conrad, 1977a, b) reporting this aspect of the study compared the hearing group with a subsample of deaf children selected to be free from additional handicap and with an intelligence distribution fitted to that assumed for the hearing children. The results were so close to those for the entire profoundly-deaf group that it seems simpler to present them now for the more complete population.

Table 1 shows the outcome of this comparison. The speech comprehension scores for the two groups are, coincidentally, identical. It is difficult to assess the auditory benefit derived by the deaf children from whatever residual hearing was available to them. In varying degree, some element of the prosodic features of speech are likely to have provided a little information. But at the very least we cannot say that they lip-read better than untrained and inexperienced hearing children.

Table 1   Speech comprehension by deaf and noise-masked hearing children

	Speech comprehension (max. = 38)	Print-reading (max. = 38)
	Mean	Mean
Deaf	25.3	32.0
	$N = 150$	
Hearing	25.3	36.7
	$N = 75$	$N = 43$

[. . .]

Speech rating, speech intelligibility and deafness

How easy would it be then for people unfamiliar with deaf children to understand what they say? The simplest evaluation can be seen in the proportions of children allocated to the five rating descriptions by their own teachers:

Wholly intelligible	14%
Fairly easy to understand	20%
About half understood	18%
Very hard to understand	25%
Effectively unintelligible	23%

(Children in Special Schools only: $N = 331$)

Evidently there would be little difficulty in holding a conversation with about one-third of these children. But it would be extremely difficult to do so with nearly half of them.

[. . .]

References

Conrad, R. (1977a) 'The Reading Ability of Deaf School-leavers', *British Journal of Educational Psychology, 47,* pp. 138–48.

Conrad, R. (1977b) 'Lip-reading by Deaf and Hearing Children', *British Journal of Educational Psychology, 47,* pp. 60–65.

DiFrancesca, S. (1972) *Academic Achievement Test Results of a National Testing Program for Hearing Impaired Students*, United States, Spring 1971. Series D, Number 9. Washington, DC, Gallaudet College, Office of Demographic Studies.

5.5 A Critical Examination of Different Approaches to Communication in the Education of Deaf Children

Wendy Lynas, Alan Huntington and Ivan Tucker (not dated—published 1988)

[. . .]

The case for oralism

Oralists support the idea that attempts should be made to *overcome* the barrier to communication caused by deafness by exploiting the use of residual hearing to the maximum rather than by *circumventing* the problems of deafness and communication by, for example, substituting sign language for speech.

Oralists accept that in the past conditions were not so favourable as they are today to the oral success of the profoundly deaf child. As a consequence of such things as late diagnosis, inadequate hearing aids, an absence of pre-school services, teaching based on 'incorrect' assumptions of the way in which children develop language, some deaf young people left school not only unable to speak intelligibly or to understand the speech of others, but also without having achieved basic literacy (Conrad, 1979).

Oralists claim, however, that more recently sufficient evidence has accumulated (e.g. Clark, 1978; Oxford Polytechnic 1980; Aplin, Hostler and Tucker, 1985) to justify and sustain considerable optimism over the capability of even very deaf children to develop a fluency of spoken language which allows them to live comfortably and efficiently in hearing society. Oralists claim that the prospects have never been better for the very deaf child. As a result of recent advances—namely, the development of technologically sophisticated high powered hearing aids; an improved understanding of the process of language acquisition; more extensive parent guidance services and better educational practice—even very deaf children, that is those with profound hearing losses[1], can be enabled to produce and understand spoken language.

Oralists generally do not deny that sign language in many situations provides an effective means of communication. They question, however, the capacity of sign language to perform all the educational functions that can be achieved by a conventional language, such as, for example, English. Sign language is used by a restricted number of people in a restricted range of social contexts. English, on the other hand, is used by an enormously wide range of people in a great many different contexts. English over time has thus developed a much broader range of expressive functions than sign language could possibly have done. The vocabulary of British Sign Language (BSL), for example, is several times smaller than that of English.

Oralists argue that if deaf children are to develop spoken language effectively, it is important that their residual hearing is exploited to the full from the earliest age. This does not mean that visual clues are insignificant. Where hearing impairment exists, the auditory sense will be supported by visual communication, such as facial expression, lip movements and normal gesturing. Oralists believe, however, that the deaf child should not be directed to the extra visual information that would be provided by a separate and distinct visual means of communication such as sign language. The signs of sign language do not have a direct relationship to the sounds of spoken language and, therefore, do not reinforce the elements of spoken language. In fact, oralists maintain that a young deaf child, if persistently exposed to the visual communication of sign language, will not learn to make best use of his residual hearing. Too much attention paid to visual input, it is argued, impedes the auditory development of deaf children and this may foreclose the possibility for some deaf children of ever achieving satisfactory levels of oral language and intelligible speech. This matter is particularly serious in relation to profoundly deaf children who need *every possible* opportunity to make use of and develop residual hearing in order to learn to talk and understand the talk of others. Thus most oralists share the belief that the early and continued use of sign language interferes with the deaf child's ability to make progress with spoken language.

Oralists claim that deaf individuals without the ability to communicate orally are condemned to feel lonely and isolated in the hearing world. It is true that they can participate in the deaf community and deaf subculture for some of the time, for example, by attending Deaf Clubs and meeting deaf friends, but as deaf people form such a tiny minority within society as a whole, and do not live in exclusive deaf neighbourhoods or work in deaf offices and deaf factories, they are surrounded for most of the time by normally hearing people. The deaf individual whose only significant social contacts are formed within the deaf group thus, arguably, leads a restricted life.

If a deaf person wishes to participate in the signing deaf subculture then an oral approach in education does not preclude this, but learning to sign from an early age, it is argued, precludes for some the possibility of ever learning to talk. Sign language, on the other hand, it is suggested, can be learnt as a second language at any age and once a young child or young person has a good foundation of oral language, learning sign will not detract from his or her ability to continue acquiring spoken language. It may well be the case for some deaf young people, acquiring the ability to sign offers them a sense of pride and satisfaction at being able to communicate in 'their own special language', but oralists insist that educators have a *moral* responsibility to enable deaf children to acquire the *dominant* language of our society as a first priority. Only an oral approach allows the life objectives of the deaf person to be as wide as those of all other people. Oralists refer to the testimony of oral deaf adults (Ogden, 1979; Lynas, 1986) who indicate that, whilst they encounter numerous obstacles in normally hearing society, they feel their lives to be significantly expanded through participation in the hearing world.

[. . .]

The development of oral language in the young deaf child

Oralists contend that even severely and profoundly deaf children can develop oral language sati[s]factorily but that in order to do so maximum use must be made of the deaf child's residual hearing. For this to occur it is important that deafness is diagnosed early and that the young deaf child is fitted with appropriate hearing aids. So, we need to consider the question of early diagnosis and to know how effective hearing aids are because the oralists' case depends entirely on their use.

Early diagnosis and fitting of hearing aids

Very precise measurements of hearing loss in very young infants and children are not at the moment possible, though technological advances are increasing the possibility of accurate and reliable audiological assessments of even young babies (Hostler, 1987). There is every reason, therefore, to be optimistic about current and future possibilities for the detection of severe hearing impairments at an early age. If deafness is diagnosed early and hearing aids fitted, this affords the opportunity of exploiting residual hearing and developing auditory acuity during the first few months and even weeks of the deaf child's life. What is emphasized by oralists is that even if there is no measurable hearing at the young infant stage it is most unlikely that the child will have *no* residual hearing. The overwhelming majority of even profoundly deaf children have some usable hearing, and it is important, therefore, oralists say, that they are fitted with powerful hearing aids as early as possible. It is quite commonly found that children who make no response to sound at diagnosis will show some auditory acuity at a later stage after stimulation by hearing aids.

Research by Tucker (1986) provides firm evidence on this foregoing point. In a two-year detailed longitudinal study nine young profoundly deaf children were investigated, commencing from the time of diagnosis. A considerable amount of data was collected on these children: regular and detailed observations were made of their interaction with their mothers; their linguistic and communication progress was carefully monitored throughout the study. Five of the nine children on initial audiological testing made 'no response' to sound at any frequency but by the end of the period of study *all* the children were found to have measurable hearing which, with the help of powerful hearing aids, they were using to develop oral communication skills. Thus, whilst initial testing indicated 'no response' in some children, none was 'totally' deaf or without usable residual hearing.[2]

The development of auditory acuity in profoundly deaf children is without doubt, oralists claim, accelerated by the continuous *efficient* use of hearing aids and this will facilitate spoken language acquisition. Provisions under the National Health Service and pre-school educational services should ensure that no deaf child in Britain need be without effective and properly maintained hearing aids. Furthermore, it can certainly be argued, say the oralists, that the general quality and capability of hearing aids has improved in recent years because of advances in technology so that deaf children can now benefit from greater amplification over a wide range of frequencies.[3] Thus many deaf children are today quite literally hearing sounds that 10 years or so ago they would not have been able to hear and this has an important bearing on the prospects for the development of speech.

[. . .]

Summary and conclusions

Our examination of the communication options available for use with deaf children confirms our conviction that for the majority, the overwhelming majority of deaf children, the oral-auditory approach offers the best chance of developing language and providing a means of communication. Through an oral-auditory approach, therefore, we believe the deaf child is offered the most satisfactory preparation for life in the wider society. We contend on the basis of the evidence we have examined that 'total communication' in any of its forms has been found to be seriously wanting. Whilst the idea of using all sensory modalities to develop language in children with impaired hearing has 'commonsense' appeal, the practice of presenting and receiving two different symbol systems of language simultaneously seems impossible to achieve. That the barriers to providing effective total communication are insurmountable is supported by the research findings we have reviewed which indicate that the use of total communication approaches in the education of deaf children depresses rather than raises educational and linguistic standards.

The achievement of bilingualism in deaf children, that is competence in oral language and in sign language, may be possible where the deaf child is brought up by deaf signing parents *and* is also given the opportunity to mix with normally hearing people. However, it is rare for deaf children to grow up in such circumstances and, as we have seen, normally hearing parents generally do not achieve sufficient fluency in sign language to provide their deaf children with an adequate sign language environment. Furthermore, research evidence indicates that deaf children born of deaf parents make greater linguistic progress if their parents use speech rather than signing as the predominant means of communication.

Generally, given that for most deaf children total communication is an impossible goal because an impossible practice, the alternatives seem to lie between selecting a pure oral-auditory *or* a sign-only approach to communication. If one believes that the main purpose of deaf education is to prepare the deaf individual for a life of exclusive participation in the deaf signing community then the choice of a sign-only approach is justified. However, we do not envisage that normally hearing people will in large numbers be prepared to learn 'the language of the deaf' in order to communicate in sign language with deaf people. If, on the other hand, one believes that the central goal of deaf education is to enable the deaf individual to participate in the wider community of hearing-speaking people, then one must surely reject the sign-only option as a vehicle of education. We would, of course, not deny the right of the deaf individual to learn sign language in order to communicate with deaf signing people. We contend, however, that unless an oral-auditory approach is used in the education of deaf children, there is a serious risk that the deaf individual will have *no choice* but to form relationships of significance within the deaf-signing community.

[. . .]

Notes

1 A profound hearing loss has been defined (BATOD, 1981) as an average loss in the better ear exceeding 95 dB. It is worth pointing out here that total deafness in children is extremely rare.

2 The mean hearing loss established after the study period was 100.67 dB in the better ear.

3 Modern hearing aids can amplify sound to a level of around 135 dB over most of the speech frequencies.

References

Aplin, Y., Hostler, M. and Tucker, I. (1985) 'A Longitudinal Study of a Population of Children with Sensori-Neural Hearing Impairments', paper presented at the 1985 *International Congress on Education of the Deaf*, University of Manchester.

BATOD National Executive Committee (1981) 'Audiological Definitions and Forms of Recording Audiometric Information', *Journal of British Association of Teachers of the Deaf, 5* (3).

Clark, M. (1978) 'Preparations of Deaf Children for a Hearing Society', *Journal of British Association of Teachers of the Deaf, 2* (5).

Conrad, R. (1979) *The Deaf School Child*, London, Harper and Row.

Hostler, M. (1987) 'Hearing Aid Policy with Babies and Young Children', *Journal of British Association of Teachers of the Deaf, 11* (1).

Lynas, W. (1986) *Integrating the Handicapped into Ordinary Schools: A Study of Hearing Impaired Pupils*, London, Croom Helm.

Ogden, P. (1979) *Experiences and Attitudes of Oral Deaf Adults Regarding Oralism*, unpublished Doctoral Dissertation, University of Illinois.

Oxford Polytechnic (1980) *1980—One hundred Years After Milan*, videotape, Lady Spencer Churchill College, Oxford Polytechnic, Oxford.

Tucker, I. (1986) *Some Aspects of the Verbal and Non-Verbal Interaction of Parents and their Hearing-Impaired Children*, unpublished Doctoral Thesis, University of Manchester.

5.6 Total Communication

Lionel Evans (1982)

[. . .]

During the 1960s, the prevailing attitude towards teaching method became increasingly questioned by educators in the United States. Evidence of the results of the oral approach gave rise to dissatisfaction. Vernon (1971) surveyed studies by Schein and Bushnaq in 1962, Boatner in 1965, and McClure in 1966, which revealed that of the deaf student population, over 30 per cent were illiterate, 60 per cent were at a fifth-grade level or below, and only 5 per cent reached tenth-grade level or better, and these were mostly hard of hearing or adventitiously deafened students. An important study of the actual attainments of deaf students on completion of their schooling provided further evidence. A survey of results of the National Achievements Tests standardization study carried out from the Office of Demographic Studies of Gallaudet College in 1974 (Trybus and Karchmer, 1977) found that in the 20-year-old deaf population (who had passed through primary education in the 1960s) the average student had a reading ability below fifth-grade level, only 10 per cent read at above eighth-grade level.

[. . .]

Gradually there emerged a new attitude. Garretson (1976b) recorded that during the 1960s 'a segment of the profession began to articulate the need to develop a philosophical framework that would recognize the value of manual modes as useful adjuncts to accepted aural/oral approaches' (p. 89). The theoretical interest in manual communication was heightened when such distinguished linguists as Lenneberg (1967, p. 320) and Chomsky (cited in Vernon, 1972) expressed critical views on pure oral communication for all severely deaf children.

Out of this growing concern there developed a more liberal outlook which advocated the use of oral and manual media in combination. This became known as *total communication*. Although the term had an earlier usage, as for instance in a work by Margaret Mead (1964), it has become associated with the liberal communication approach for deaf people. Garretson (1976b) records that the term total communication was used in 1968 by an educator, Dr Roy Holcomb, to describe a flexible approach to communication in teaching deaf children at Santa Ana, California.

The term was quickly taken up, and in 1968 it was adopted by Dr David Denton to describe the philosophy at the Maryland School for the Deaf. Denton (1976) described the approach there as comprising 'the full spectrum of language modes, child-devised gesture, the language of signs, speech reading, fingerspelling, reading, and writing . . . the development of residual hearing for the enhancement of speech and speech reading skills'.

The importance of fingerspelling and signing, to supplement the inadequacy of lipreading, has been emphasized. Vernon (1972) explained total communication as 'a constructive coping with the reality of the limitations of lipreading . . . the deaf child is taught and is given the opportunity to communicate through a system no more ambiguous to him than the spoken word to the hearing child' (p. 531).

The obligation of both hearing and deaf people to adjust their skills to meet the needs of the particular situation was stressed in a description of total communication as a concept that:

> . . . involves the use of all means of communication with deaf people and by deaf people. It requires that a hearing person use his speech, signs, fingerspelling, and English syntax. It holds the deaf person to these same requirements. It also requires that every effort is made by the deaf person to use residual hearing.
> (Merrill, 1973)

The concept of a multimedia approach to communciation gained further acceptance, so that in an international seminar held at London in 1975, total communication was said, by Brill (1976), to involve:

> . . . the use of any and all modes of communication. This includes the use of a sign language system, fingerspelling, speech, speech reading, amplification, gestures, pantomime, drawing and writing . . . expressive modes can be used simultaneously such as speech, one of the forms of manual communication, and amplification. The individual . . . may receive through only one of the modes or by two or more modes simultaneously.
> (Brill, 1976, p. 80)

[. . .]

By 1976, interest in total communciation had reached such a level as to warrant an official definition. The Conference of Executives of American Schools for the Deaf at the Forty-Eighth Meeting held at Rochester, New York, agreed upon a definition of total communication as:

> . . . a philosophy incorporating the appropriate aural, manual, and oral modes of communication in order to ensure effective communication with and among hearing impaired persons.
> (Garretson, 1976a, p. 300)

This hallmark of official recognition reinforced the widely understood concept of total communication as an eclectic attitude towards the selective use of appropriate media to suit the needs of the situation. Subsequent developments in educational practice emphasized this interpretation of total communication as a philosophical attitude towards the acceptance of oral and manual media, rather than a methodological prescription as to how they should be used.

This outlook was exemplified in the description developed for the Pre-College Programs at Gallaudet College, which held that:

> . . . total communication is not a method, but rather a philosophy of approaching any given communication situation . . . It is a recognition that not all modes of communication are effective for individuals in all situations . . . a commitment to a selection of those modes or combination of modes which will be most effective with individual children.
> (Cokely, 1979, pp. 9–10)

Parallel changes in Britain

The trend in the United States was paralleled by developments in Britain, where concern for the level of educational attainment of hearing impaired children led to similar changes in attitude and practice. During the 1950s, most of the formative influences on education of the deaf had been centred on a pure oral philosophy. Teachers were trained to use oral methods only; the communciation research was concerned mainly with use of residual hearing, lipreading and speech intelligibility; and the early guidance to parents emphasized the role of speech and lipreading. It is not surprising that, against this background of influence, the majority of British schools for the deaf aspired, at least officially, to use pure oral methods of teaching. The opening of many partially hearing units meant that by the mid-1960s the majority of children receiving full-time special educational treatment because of their impaired hearing were placed in ordinary schools. It was expected that when properly assessed, partially hearing children should be capable of making satisfactory progress in speech and language by oral teaching. With the continuing trend towards integration of hearing-impaired children in ordinary schools, the special schools became preoccupied with the needs of the more severely handicapped, and this brought into question the suitability of pure oral teaching for all deaf children.

In 1964, an important committee of inquiry was set up by the British Department of Education and Science under the chairmanship of a distinguished educator, Professor Michael Lewis, to consider the possible place of fingerspelling and signing in the education of deaf children. The report of the committee (Department of Education and Science, 1968) strongly endorsed a place for oral communication and urged improvements in the conditions for oral teaching. But it also recommended that research should be carried out to determine whether 'the introduction of manual media of communication would lead to improvement in the education of deaf children' and to evaluate the 'effects of combining oral and manual media' (p. 106). The publication of this report, popularly known as the 'Lewis Report', opened the way for scientific study of communication in British schools in the 1970s, including evaluation of the results of oral teaching and the introduction of combined teaching methods.

[. . .]

In 1976, the Royal National Institute for the Deaf published the proceedings of an important international seminar on methods of communication currently used in the education of deaf children. Twenty participants from Great Britain, Ireland, Holland, the United States and Canada presented papers. Of those experienced in education, psychology, psychiatry, or social work, some advocated the continuation of a predominately pure oral approach (Braybrook; Lowell; Reeves; Watson), but others proposed, or discussed evidence for, the use of combined oral and manual media for some deaf children (Brill; Craig; Davis; Denmark; Evans; Freeman; Meadow; Montgomery; Reed; Stuckless; Verney; Vernon). In a summary of these papers, Conrad (1976) commented on 'the difficulty of assessing exactly what oralism has been able to achieve'. He pointed out that in contrast to 'a very substantial body of research [into the use of combined media, there is] a curious, dramatic, and . . . unfortunate imbalance in documentation [with lack of] a single published account which sets out the outcome, the achievements, and the shortcomings of good oral education' (p. 148).

[. . .]

By the late 1970s, a number of British schools for the deaf had introduced combined methods of teaching or formally adopted the term total communication for their teaching approach. These include some of the older schools with past experience of manual methods, such as the Royal School for Deaf Children at Margate, the Royal West of England School for the Deaf at Doncaster, as well as some more recently opened schools, such as Heathlands School for the Deaf at St Alban's, and Beverley School for the Deaf at Cleveland. In the south of England, the widening interest led to the setting up of a working party to develop practical guidelines for the most effective ways of combining lipreading, speech, residual hearing, signing and fingerspelling into teaching method (Robson, 1980). In Scotland, there has been research into the effectiveness of signing and fingerspelling (Montgomery, 1966, 1968; Montgomery and Lines, 1976), and the term total communication has been widely applied for the combined teaching methods in Scottish schools. The support for total communication from professionals in fields allied to education included strong advocacy for the use of sign language. Verney (1976), a social worker, believed that 'the manual component of total communication should be a standardized and systematized version of the sign language already in use by deaf adults' (p. 71). Denmark (1976), a psychiatrist, also maintained that total communication should include 'the sign language as used by deaf people in this country' (p. 77).

[. . .]

References

Brill, R.G. (1976) in Henderson, P. (ed.) *Methods of Communication Currently Used in the Education of Deaf Children*, London, Royal National Institute for the Deaf, Ch. 14.

Cokely, D. (1979) *Pre-College Programs: Guidelines for Manual Communication*, Washington, DC, Gallaudet College.

Conrad, R. (1976) in Henderson, P. (ed.) *Methods of Communication Currently Used in the Education of Deaf Children*, London, Royal National Institute for the Deaf, Ch. 21.

Denmark, J. (1976) in Henderson, P. (ed.) *Methods of Communication Currently Used in the Education of Deaf Children*, London, Royal National Institute for the Deaf, Ch. 13.

Denton, D.M. (1976) 'Remarks in Support of a System of Total Communication for Deaf Children', *Communication Symposium*, Maryland School for the Deaf, Frederick.

Department of Education and Science (1968) *The Education of Deaf Children: the Possible Place of Finger Spelling and Signing*, London, HMSO.

Garretson, M.D. (1976a) Committee Report Defining Total Communication Proceedings of the Forty-Eighth Meeting of the *Conference of Executives of American Schools for the Deaf*, Rochester, New York.

Garretson, M.D. (1976b) 'Total Communication', in Frisina, R. (ed.) *A Bicentennial Monograph on Hearing Impairment*, Trends in the USA, Volta Review, 78.

Lennenberg, E.H. (1967) *Biological Foundations of Language*, New York, John Wiley and Sons.

Mead, M. (1964) 'Vicissitudes of the Study of the Total Communication Process', in Sebeck, T.A. (ed.) *Approaches to Semiotics*, The Hague, Mouton.

Merrill, E.C. (1973), President, Gallaudet College, Washington, DC (personal communication).

Montgomery, G.W.G. (1966) 'The relationship of Oral Skills to Manual Communication in Profoundly Deaf Adolescents', *American Annals of the Deaf, 111*.

Montgomery, G.W.G. (1968) 'A Factorial Study of Communication and Ability in Deaf School Leavers', *British Journal of Educational Psychology, 38*, (3).

Montgomery, G.W.G. and Lines, A. (1976) 'Comparison of Several Single and Combined Methods of Communicating with Deaf Children', paper presented at *Seminar on Visual Communication*, held at Northern Counties School for the Deaf, Newcastle upon Tyne.

Robson, P. (1980) Inspector of Special Education, Inner London Education Authority (personal communication).

Trybus, R.J. and Karchmer, M.A. (1977) 'School Achievement, Scores of Hearing Impaired Children: National Data on Achievements Status and Growth Patterns', *American Annals of the Deaf, 122.*

Verney, A. (1976) 'Planning for a Preferred Future', in Henderson, P. (ed.) *Methods of Communication Currently used in the Education of Deaf Children*, London, Royal National Institute for the Deaf.

Vernon, M. (1971) 'Psychological Evaluation of the Severely Handicapped Deaf Adult', in Stewart, L. (ed.) *Towards More Effective Rehabilitation Services for the Severely Handicapped Deaf Adult*, Hot Springs, Arkansas Rehabilitation Research and Training Center.

Vernon, M. (1972) 'Mind Over Mouth: a Rationale for Total Communication', *Volta Review, 74.*

5.7 Bilingualism and the Education of Deaf Children

Miranda Llwellyn-Jones (1988)

[. . .]

In this paper I would like to discuss the relevance of bilingualism to the education of deaf children. Bilingualism is a well-established concept when applied to hearing speakers on a world-wide scale yet in this country the response to the issue has been piecemeal in terms of the education of hearing children from a variety of linguistic and cultural backgrounds. For the purpose of this paper bilingualism should be understood in the following ways. Pupils who operate in two or more languages to whatever degree of competence should be regarded as bilingual.

> The bilingual child is one who is learning and using two languages (of which one is mother tongue) irrespective of level of achievement in the languages at any given point in time.
> (Fitouri, 1983)

The emphasis on the functional aspects of language is important as it highlights the significance of communication. Within the term bilingualism one can envisage a range of communication skills according to the range of situations which the communicator faces. Not only are there the discrete languages being used but also a range of registers and styles for that individual. Language use does not necessarily imply full literacy. The notion of mother-tongue, literally the language learned on the mother's knee, relevant to many bilingual hearing people, is problematic in our field but I will discuss this further, later. Bilingualism does not require one to be fluent in both or all languages; indeed the balance of fluency will vary not only in one individual but also over time. When one uses the term 'first language' one must beware of restricting it to the relative temporal earliness of its acquisition. 'First' may come to mean dominant, preferred, or most frequently used even when that language has been acquired relatively late.

Attitudes to bilingualism have changed from negative to positive in recent years as the research evidence has demonstrated the advantages inherent in being bilingual. No longer is bilingualism seen as being 'a problem'. Despite the claims being made for bilingualism, however, the impact on education is limited. As long ago as 1975 the Bullock report said:

> . . . no child should be expected to cast off the language and culture of home as he crosses the school threshold, to live and act as though school and home represented two totally separate and different cultures which have to be kept apart.

> . . . the school should adopt a positive attitude to the pupils' bilingualism and whenever possible, help to maintain and deepen their knowledge of their mother tongue.
> (Bullock, 1975)

However, the more recently published Swann report, despite recognizing linguistic diversity as a positive asset, said:

> . . . we cannot support arguments put forward for the introduction of programmes of bilingual education in maintained schools.
> (Swann, 1985)

> we believe that essential to equality of opportunity, to academic success and more broadly to participation on equal terms as a full member of society, is a good command of English and that first priority in language learning by all pupils must therefore be given to the learning of English.

The education system in this country has not, on the whole, forwarded the maintenance and use of ethnic minority languages, marginalizing bilingualism and shifting responsibility away from schools.

In another report, Rampton described three patterns of teachers' attitudes in relation to the dialects spoken by some West Indian children: deficient, that is the language was inadequate for learning and required changing; dialect interference, that is the different structures make learning English difficult; repertoire, that is increasing the awareness of the child to the different language forms. The third positive attitude does not require the child to change his/her language, and contrasts with many present practices:

> whereby the school's failure to understand or capitalise on the linguistic concepts such a child brings to the classroom often results in the over-representation of black children in groups perceived as having problems.
> (Khan, 1987)

> If teachers of English as a second language do not use or refer to the pupil's mother tongue as an aid to learning, then this may signal a low evaluation of the minority languages.
> (Linguistic Minority Project, 1985)

The background to the issue of bilingualism in education as a whole is bound up with the historical relationship between English speakers and the speakers of community languages such as Urdu, Punjabi and Creole. Users of English exerted political and cultural dominance over the colonies; South Asian and Afro-Caribbean languages are thus accorded low status.

Linguistic minorities lacking fluency in the use of the dominant language are relatively powerless. The language of the majority is used in institutions and policies by decision-makers on behalf of the minority. The link between language, culture and the community is inextricable.

> . . . learning a language which may be used more than the mother-tongue, may pose a threat to self-concept and cultural identity which then interferes with the learning of the other languages.
> (Khan, 1987)

The role of native users in education is undervalued. There are a few community language teachers but they are not widespread. The curriculum may not reflect the linguistic and cultural diversity of the children. English may be taught on a withdrawal basis in units or language centres, practices which many people regard as an example of institutional racism. Testing procedures for second language learners may not take into account first language skills and result in inappropriate assessments of the children. It is in these issues that we can see parallels with deaf education and this is to be developed later. The fact that there is so much literature on bilingualism from which we can draw and that there is growing pressure from community language users for bilingualism to be taken seriously have helped to raise the level of awareness of the concept generally. To what extent has deaf education been affected?

Should profoundly deaf children be educated bilingually?

[. . .]

Given the current confused situation in education concerning bilinguals, it may be a mixed blessing to regard the deaf as a linguistic and social minority. However, without such a realization, real beneficial changes in deaf education are unlikely to occur.

Bilingualism in relation to the deaf refers to the use of sign language and English with a repertoire of communication systems in between. Deaf people can be considered as functional bilinguals in English and BSL even though we may question their levels of facility in both. Sign language, recognized as a language in its own right, often represents the primary language for deaf children, easiest acquired, preferred to use, and the basis of cognitive growth. To quote Conrad in 1979:

> Sign language can provide an easily learned mother-tongue, which may serve not only a communicative function but, much more important, it may preserve and develop the crucial organization for language upon which second-language learning must be based.
> (Conrad, 1979)

Even in 90–95 per cent of profoundly deaf children born to hearing parents, where Sign is not strictly speaking the mother-tongue, this is seen to be the case. No one denies the critical importance of English skills to deaf children: where there is disagreement is in how these should be developed: that is, within a monolingual or bilingual approach.

[. . .]

Attitudes

Bilingualism involves a positive attitude towards deaf people and sign language; it involves a move from monolingualism to multilingualism; from normalization to a respect for linguistic minorities and their identity; from a deficiency or interference model to a repertoire approach to language and communication skills. It demands increasing *deaf awareness* in the general public. Sign language is recognized as the language of many deaf people and English as the *target* or second language. Sign language is not solely the means of acquiring English. Negative attitudes towards BSL and the subsequent enforced use of English in education have lead to the same kinds of underachievement that have marked other minority individuals.

Attitudes of the hearing majority influence how deaf people regard themselves. There is a widespread feeling among deaf people that they are held back educationally as a result of teacher pressure to learn in English, little if any creditability being awarded to BSL use in education.

Status, power and control

Bilingualism allows users of sign language to exert control and to have status. English is no longer the powerful language nor users of it in a dominant position. Hearing users of English may indeed find themselves in an inferior position, the minority. Deaf children make decisions, have some say in their education. There is a shift in the balance of power in the classroom and elsewhere.

Institutions and policies

These begin to represent the interests of deaf people. Local authorities respond to deaf communities' demands for a say in the education of deaf children. Deaf people are involved in decision-making and in preparing policies. Changes from the *top-down* by enlightened policy-makers are balanced by those from the *bottom-up*, those at the chalk-face as it were.

Language, culture and community

Deaf children are more affected by negative attitudes than other minority groups as they are rarely brought up in an environment where their language is used by the rest of the community and family. Deaf people do not have the ethnic roots to fall back on and so have been even more at risk. Bilingualism fosters the links between sign language, deaf culture and the deaf community. The deaf are a handicapped group and also a linguistic minority, whose culture, and in a wider sense their whole way of life, is based on sign language. This is why sign language is of central importance when it comes to deaf people's equal participation, cultural identity and self respect:

> Sign language is the only language deaf people can learn in a natural way, without schooling, the same way as hearing children learn their surrounding's language: in association with persons who use this language.

Sign language should therefore be accepted as deaf people's first language. The language is an important part of a person's identity. If the society accepts sign language, it also accepts the deaf person as a human being.
(Working Programme for the Northern Council of the Deaf, 1987)

It gives children access to the deaf community and the opportunity to, as adults, find a place in hearing and deaf society.

Deaf adults are the link between the children and the deaf community.

The role of native users

Deaf adults can represent linguistic and role models for the children. They function as mother-tongue speakers, sharing the children's preferred method of communication and their identity:

> Sign Language is the deaf chld's first language, and to learn this, the child needs sufficient natural sign-linguistic interaction with the surroundings. The deaf child needs people within its surroundings who sign to the child as well as to each other. The deaf child needs contact with deaf adults and also with other deaf children.
> (Working Programme for the Northern Council of the Deaf, 1987)

Bilingualism involves hearing and deaf people working together as a team. This is often very threatening to hearing teachers, so deaf adults themselves need to be aware of these feelings.

As a profession we teachers of the deaf have jealously guarded our qualification, yet what more appropriate qualification can be found than being deaf?

The curriculum

Through sign language the deaf child gets knowledge and advice, learns values and standards, develops socially and emotionally, and learns how to express feelings. Through sign language, the cultural traditions of both deaf and hearing people can be brought to the deaf child.

Can sign language be used across the curriculum? Can we teach geography, history, science through a language other than English? Why not; if the children are to have true access to the curriculum this must be based on their understanding of the content. The support offered to deaf children must have a linguistic basis. Sign language interpretation may be required for some children. Integration is intended to give the children a better, broader education alongside their hearing peers. For this to be meaningful, language support has to be clearly defined in a bilingual way: for example, immediate understanding through sign language interpretation and written back-up in English. The curriculum has to be multicultural: there are many deaf children from ethnic minorities and white deaf children have to be prepared for a multicultural society.

[. . .]

References

Bullock Report (1975) *A Language for Life*, London, HMSO.

Conrad, R. (1979) *The Deaf School Child*, London, Harper and Row.

Fitouri, A. (1983) 'Working with Young Bilingual Children', *Early Child Development and Care, 10,* pp. 283–92.

Khan, S. (1987) *Towards a Policy for Bilingualism*, Leeds, Community Relations Council.

Linguistic Minorities Project (1985) *The Other Languages of England*, London, Routledge and Kegan Paul.

Roaf, C. (1987) 'The Special Need for Human Rights (Second Opinion)', *Times Educational Supplement*, 18 September 1987.

Working Programme for the Northern Council of the Deaf (1987) Bergen, The Deaf Publishing Company.

5.8 Teaching and Talking with Deaf Children

David Wood, Heather Wood, Amanda Griffiths and Ian Howarth (1986)

[. . .]

Teaching and conversing

When we began to consider ways of trying to describe the structure of conversation, we were working both in schools for deaf children and in nursery schools and playgroups for preschool hearing children. Most of the teachers in both these settings considered talking to and with children an important part of their work. The general climate of opinion in early childhood education includes a stress on the importance of communication and language in helping children to become competent individuals and effective learners. In recent years, research into the processes of language development and the study of individual differences in children's acquisition and use of language have reached almost epidemic proportions (e.g. Tough, 1977; Blank, Rose and Berlin, 1978; Wells, 1979; Tizard and Hughes, 1984; to mention a few). The emphasis on the importance of langauge in education is commonplace in many countries.

Working in twenty-four different preschool settings for hearing children and in six schools for the deaf over a period of a year or so, we were struck both by marked similarities between and revealing differences across the various settings. In some classrooms, children seemed relatively active, loquacious and responsive. They talked a good deal, asked questions and contributed to discussions. In others, children seemed rather reticent and unforthcoming. They spoke little and often in short phrases or even monosyllables. Although the deaf children were considerably older than the hearing preschoolers, they were, as one might expect, far less verbal. Most of the deaf children in our studies had better-ear hearing losses of at least 80 dB, but we were still struck by marked variations in the language of deaf children with similar hearing losses but in different classrooms. We accepted that, in part, such variations might reflect 'intrinsic' differences between children but we also felt that they were influenced by the ways in which teachers communicated with them.

The basic idea behind the system we eventually devised to try to capture the essence of differences and similarities across settings suggested itself when one of us was listening to a conversation between a teacher and a group of children from outside the room in which they were talking. Although not able to see the participants, he was struck by the fact that each time the teacher talked, there was little doubt about what sort of response the children were likely to make next. Anticipating how the teacher would react after the children had spoken was a little more uncertain, but still usually possible. The structure of the interaction was so predictable, we felt, because the teacher's different verbal 'moves' towards the children exerted so much *control* over the children's part in 'conversation'. Unless they were to ignore her or strike up a topic of conversation outside the one she had initiated—which, as we shall see, children are unlikely to do—then their pattern of response was usually preordained.

This led us to the notion of 'control' in conversation. Subsequently, we were to find (as one usually does in research) that several other students of classroom discourse had come up with very similiar ideas (e.g. French and MacLure, 1981; Dillon, 1982). In fact, a number of quite detailed and elaborate systems exist for describing and analysing such discourse. Our aim, however, unlike that of most researchers in this area, was not to develop a comprehensive, linguistically sophisticated analysis of discourse. Rather, we wanted to find a way of describing the interactions that would explain why children seemed more or less active and loquacious in different interactions. The main categories of the system we developed are shown in Table 1 . . .

Table 1   Levels of control in conversation

Level of control	Examples
1 Enforced repetitions	Say 'I have one at home'.
2 Two-choice questions	Did you have a good time? Did you go with Jim or Pete?
3 Wh-type questions	What happened? Where did she go? Tell me about Sunday.
4 Personal contributions, comments, statements	That must have been awful! They call it a zoom lens. I love the lakes in Scotland.
5 Phatics	Oh lovely! Super! I see. Hmm.

Imagine overhearing a conversation in which each of these different 'moves' occurs in turn. The person or people *listening* to these moves are being co-operative and compliant, attempting to meet the 'force' of any requirements laid down by the current speaker. After the first, most controlling move (an enforced repetition) the response of our compliant listener is fully predetermined. Within the limits of his receptive and expressive language ability, what he says next is fixed. The next move, 'two-choice' questions, specify at least one word that the listener should respond with. Should he so wish, he can meet the 'force' of this move with a single word (which, as we shall see, children usually do). The next category, 'Wh-type questions' also dictates the nature of the ensuing response. If the listener understands the move, the 'semantic focus' of his response (e.g. where—a place or location; when—a time; who—a person) is predetermined. The current speaker still controls the direction and content of the conversation.

After a 'contribution', however, the listener is left with a number of alternatives. He may simply acknowledge what is said in some way (perhaps saying nothing, just nodding), he might ask a question, continue with the theme or make a contribution of his own. The speaker tacitly offers the listener a chance to take over the control and direction of the subsequent conversation. The final category, 'phatics', includes any move that fills a 'turn' without offering any substance or direction to the *content* of discourse (unless, of course, it involves irony, sarcasm or some other 'hidden' meaning). It may signify reception and comprehension of what is said, but leaves the next person to speak with control of the conversational floor. If *he* then responds with a phatic move of his own, this may be a signal that the current focus or topic of conversation has been exhausted (e.g. John: 'I went home then'; Mary: 'Oh really'; John: 'Yup'), in which case someone may introduce another topic, ask a question or they may part conversational company.

In the study of children in nursery schools and playgroups already mentioned, we found that preschool hearing children acted like compliant listeners most of the time when in conversation with the teacher. In other words, they responded to different types of teacher moves in the manner described above. This led us to some very specific measures of child *initiative* in conversation that we need to consider before discussing conversations with deaf children. What does it mean to be 'active and forthcoming' in a conversation? Well, for us, it involves the following ingredients. An active participant will sometimes take *control* of the interaction by asking questions. They will also *contribute* readily and frequently after a contribution or phatic from their partner. They will extend the theme being discussed and occasionally introduce new topics of talk. Finally, when they answer questions addressed to them (particularly two-choice ones) they will characteristically not do so with a single word but will go on to add further information (i.e. make a 'double move' by answering *and* contributing to the topic).

As we shall see, whether or not children are active and forthcoming in conversation depends mainly upon the ways in which teachers manage the interaction. What about older deaf children? Do they understand enough of what is going on even to be 'compliant' listeners?

When we first posed this question (see Wood *et al.*, 1982) we were unsure of the answer we would get. For deaf chldren to be influenced by different structures of conversation in the same way as hearing children, they must be 'aware' of the basic force of different moves from the teacher. They would have to be able to discriminate questions from statements and phatics, for example. They would also have to be able and ready to follow the less controlling moves from the teacher (e.g. contributions) by saying something themselves. If they do not readily take initiative in conversation (by saying something or asking questions after a contribution or phatic) then it may be the case that teaachers have to *question* deaf children in order to encourage them to play any role in conversation at all. We were not sure what the answer would be.

In fact, we found that deaf children's patterns of response to different teacher 'moves' were almost identical to those of hearing children. They did, as one might expect, tend to confuse different 'Wh-questions' more frequently; otherwise, their reactions were the same.

Having established this level of competence in children, the next question we asked was whether different teaching styles had similar effects on the two groups of children. Did the way the teacher controlled the conversation influence how much children said and how much initiative they showed? It did.

Teacher power, child initiative and loquacity

The conversation that we analysed were based on audiotaped (hearing groups) and videotaped (deaf groups) interactions between teachers and children in their own classrooms. With the deaf groups, these involved 'news sessions' in which teacher and children talked about what had happened, say, over the weekend at home. Having transcribed the interactions 'verbatim' we classified teachers' and children's turns into the move categories shown in Table 1 . . .

The principle measure of teaching style, 'teacher power', is simply the proportion of each teacher's conversational turns that end in a controlling move (questions and enforced or requested repetitions). A second measure (more sensitive with preschool children) also includes all 'tag' moves since young children tend to respond to these as two-choice questions. A teacher who asks questions and/or demands repetitions frequently at the expense of other moves, thus gains a 'high power ratio'; one who asks relatively few gains a low ratio.

We measure children's responses in two main ways. One is an assessment of how much 'initiative' they show, the other estimates how talkative or loquacious they are. The most general measure of child initiative takes into account a number of features of children's talk. How often does a child not only answer a question but go on to elaborate on his answer by making an unsolicited contribution? How likely is he to make a contribution after the teacher has made either a contribution or has simply acknowledged what he has already said? How often does he ask questions?

Broadly speaking, what we find is that this measure of child initiative in conversation is related *negatively* to teacher power. Consequently, teachers who ask the most questions are least likely to gain elaborated answers from children, receive spontaneous contributions or be asked questions by them. Thus, children become increasingly passive as a teacher increases control via questioning.

Another way of examining the child's involvement in the conversation is to see how *much* he says. On average the deaf children in our studies produce responses of between two and three words (or word-like sounds) in length, but how much they say in each turn depends upon what the teacher has just said. They offer short reponses after two-choice questions (they only elaborate on them about 25 per cent of the time) and relatively long ones after contributions and phatics. Thus, where controlling moves are frequent, children's turns tend to be short. In sessions where teacher control starts high and stays high, children become progressively less likely to show any signs of verbal initiative and their responses become more and more terse. Thus, if we want to understand why some children say a lot in conversation and others very little, it is not enough to consider the relative talkativeness or linguistic competence of the children. What they say and how much they talk is also strongly influenced by the conversational style of the teacher.

Teaching style also influences the readiness with which children talk to (and hence listen to) each other. When teacher control is high, children seldom address comments or questions to their peers. However, when control is low, children are most likely not only to contribute comments and questions to the teacher but also to converse with each other. Thus, the whole 'tenor' of a group conversation is directly influenced by very specific, and very simple, features of teaching style. In the next chapter, we offer some examples of conversations to illustrate these general principles.

If a teacher wants to get children talking and showing initiative, she should be prepared not only to question but also to inform, react, listen and acknowledge. Rather than directing the conversation by questions or trying to use it to 'improve' language (we shall return to this topic later) she needs to become more contingent upon and accepting of what the children have to offer. Of course, if the goal is *not* to get children showing initiative and being talkative, all this goes by the board.

[. . .]

What do teachers use conversations for?
Teachers of the deaf are specially trained to 'teach' or, perhaps, to help children acquire language. How do they go about it? There are, as we shall see, 'special' features of teachers' talk to deaf children. Are these a product of training and of benefit to the child? Perhaps the differences we found are a reflection of the expertise of teachers. Before addressing these possibilities, however, we need to outline the system of analysis we developed to explore such differences (Table 2).

Repair
When a conversation is running smoothly, most of the 'moves' made by speakers will be 'substantive' in nature. Contributions that develop, elaborate and extend the topic at hand and questions designed to solicit additional information or elaboration will usually be serving *substantive* functions. The listener, meanwhile, when not asking questions designed to solicit substantive replies, will be showing non-verbal and verbal signs of attention, interest and understanding. If the conversationalists are achiev-

ing mutual understanding, then 'continuity' moves from the current listener (such as 'Mm', 'Really!', 'You don't say!') help to fulfil their obligations to the speaker.

Table 2   The function of teacher moves

Function	Examples
Substantive	Tell me about your dog. What happened on Sunday? I like cream cakes too.
Continuity	How nice. Oh, it was red, was it? Yes, I see
Repair	What? Say that again. Say 'I have one at home'. I don't understand. Wait a minute, you saw a *train* or a *crane*?

Occasionally, however, the listener may be distracted or not hear what is said. Or they may lose the thread of conversation, finding something ambiguous or unintelligible. In these circumstances, the listener is likely to take control over the interaction, 'stop' the flow of conversation and try to 'repair' the breakdown in understanding. They may do so by asking a repairing question 'Did you just say . . . ?', a repairing phatic (e.g. 'Sorry?', 'Pardon?') or with a repairing contribution such as 'I didn't understand what you just said'.

When we examined a series of conversations involving teachers with hearing children and compared these to classroom conversations with deaf children, we found, perhaps unsurprisingly, that the greatest difference between the two lay in the incidence of 'repair'. However, less obviously, most of the repairing moves came from the teachers and not the children. Although the children involved were very deaf, they seldom exercised 'listener control'. Either they were understanding everything said to them (which seems rather doubtful) or they did not know 'how' to seek clarification; or the asymmetry of power between teachers and children inhibited them from taking control of the conversation. [. . .] the latter explanation is most likely to be the case.

A lot of teacher repair with deaf children arose as a 'natural' product of unintelligible speech and ambiguous utterances from children. Other repair sequences, however, seemed more 'pedagogically' inspired to help children 'improve' their utterances. When we measured the frequency of repair by teachers of hearing children in classroom talk, we found between 6 and 10 per cent of their moves were repairing. Although repair of deaf children by their teachers was most frequent, we found very marked individual differences between teachers of the deaf in their readiness to repair children's utterances. For example, one teacher with a group of children with average hearing losses of 83 dB displayed 14 per cent repair. Another teacher, whose group had average losses of 87 dB, made 68 per cent repairing moves. Whilst some teachers seized almost every opportunity to clear up ambiguity or to check the meaning of an unintelligible utterance, others did not. Also, some teachers made more frequent demands for 'enforced repetitions' which, by their nature, always go 'backwards' and serve a repairing function.

Enforced repetitions are extremely rare in interactions between hearing children and teachers. They may occur occasionally in play (e.g. the teacher says to a child 'Say goodbye to Uncle Fred for me'), in 'lessons in etiquette' (e.g 'Say please') or in teaching songs or nursery rhymes. Some teachers of the deaf (though by no means all) use such moves relatively frequently when talking to deaf children. One teacher, in our initial study, employed them in 43 per cent of her turns. For example, one child having said 'Yesday—Mother Day', his teacher responded with 'Say, "Yesterday was Mother's Day"'. We presume that the purpose or function underlying such tactics is to 'teach language', but syntactically motivated repair is uncommon in the speech addressed to hearing children. As Roger Brown (1977) observes somewhat wryly, we often repair children's meaning but almost never their grammar, yet they grow up to tell lies (violate meaning) but with a capacity to speak in well-formed utterances!

Our notion of 'repair' thus covers two main activities: the deliberate modelling or teaching of 'better English' and also natural reactions to the handicap. In all cases, however, it is a hallmark of repair that it goes 'backwards' into previous conversational territory rather than moving it, or permitting it to move, on.

[. . .]

Causes and effects: who does what to whom?

Teaching styles, which we have described in terms of power and function, are highly correlated with a number of features of children's responsiveness and productivity in conversation. Certain aspects of teaching style, we have argued, stem from implicit or explicit theories about how language should be 'taught'. Others are responses to the *nature* of the handicap and the way in which it is likely to distort the structure of interactions by evoking *natural* but often counter-productive responses from the hearing adult. The fact that teachers vary substantially in the way they control conversations and in their levels of tolerance for ambiguity in children's language suggests that high power and frequent control are not, however, *inevitable* outcomes of conversations with deaf children.

[. . .]

References

Blank, M., Rose, S.A. and Berlin, L.J. (1978) *The Language of Learning:*

The Pre-School Years, New York, Grune and Stratton.

Brown, R. (1977), Introduction to Snow, C.E. and Ferguson, C.A., *Talking to Children, Language, Input and Acquisition*, Cambridge, Cambridge University Press.

Dillon, J.T. (1982) 'The Effect of Questions in Education and Other Enterprises', *Journal of Curriculum Studies, 14*.

French, P. and MacLure, M. (1981) 'Teacher's Questions: Pupil's Answers. An Investigation of Questions and Answers in the Infant Classroom', *First Language, 2* (1).

Tizard, B. and Hughes, M. (1984) *Young Children Learning: Talking and Thinking at Home and at School*, London, Fontana.

Tough, J. (1977) *The Development of Meaning*, London, Allen and Unwin.

Wells, G. (1979) 'Variation in Child Language', in Fletcher, P. and Gorman, M. (eds) *Language Acquisition,* Cambridge, Cambridge University Press.

Wood, D.J., Wood, H.A., Griffiths, A.J., Howarth, S.P. and Howarth, C.I. (1982) 'The Structure of Conversation with 6 to 10 year-old Deaf Children', *Journal of Child Psychology and Psychiatry, 23*.

5.9 Integrating the Handicapped into Ordinary Schools

Wendy Lynas (1986)

[. . .]

Investigation into the perceptions of and perspectives on an integrated education of hearing-impaired pupils and young people who were attending, or who had attended, ordinary schools, was . . . a central concern and feature of my research. Interviews with deaf pupils and deaf young adults revealed a mixture of views concerning themelves in relation to the normally hearing and to others who were deaf. Their views reflected both a desire to be as 'normal' as possible; that is, to talk normally, and to be part of the normally hearing group, and to a greater or lesser degree a sense of special identity as a deaf person. At one end of the spectrum of perspectives were hearing-impaired pupils and young people who had a weak sense of their deaf status and who felt to all intents and purposes 'normal'. These interviewees believed themselves to be assimilated into normally hearing society. At the other end of the spectrum were hearing-impaired individuals who had a strong sense of the difference between themselves and those with normal hearing and who, whilst participating on several levels in the hearing-speaking world, generally preferred the company of other deaf people. In many of the hearing-impaired pupils and young adults a simultaneous sense of being both 'normal' *and* 'deaf' could be detected.

All the hearing-impaired pupils and young people subscribed to the principle of normalization in that they all believed the major goal in deaf education should be teaching deaf children to talk. They believed that the ordinary school, in providing a normal spoken language environment, offered them as deaf pupils the best available means of acquiring the ability to talk normally. This view was held by deaf pupils and young people who used sign language together with those who eschewed any form of manual communication. Thus, virtually all the hearing-impaired pupils and young people who had views on the matter stated a preference for an education in an ordinary rather than in a special school. This does not, however, necessarily mean that they found life easy or always pleasant in the ordinary school.

Many hearing-impaired pupils and former pupils acknowledged that there were sometimes problems and even painful experiences in the ordinary school, such as difficulties in following ordinary class lessons, inconvenient and sometimes distressing noise, occasional experiences of being made fun of or victimized by certain of their normally hearing peers. None the less, despite day-to-day problems in and out of the classroom there was considerable agreement that the ordinary school provided the best 'preparation for life' in the adult hearing-speaking world. There seemed to be a universal desire among the deaf interviewees to acquire the behavioural norms of their normally hearing peers in order for them to be able to adapt to, and be accepted in, a hearing-speaking society. None questioned that they would need to conform to the expectations of the normally hearing if they were to cope with life as adults in a hearing-speaking world. The views of the hearing-impaired pupils and young people I interviewed are quite likely to be typical of deaf young people in the country as a whole as they were not specially selected, but I cannot with complete confidence make such a claim. In order to ascertain whether or not the opinions cited are representative of British deaf chldren and young people generally, it would be necessary to interview a much larger sample of deaf pupils and young people and one which included a proportion who were attending, or who had attended, special schools for all or most of their school lives.

That the research findings indicate a desire on the part of hearing-impaired pupils and young people to talk normally and become socialized into the ways of the normally hearing will undoubtedly be much welcomed by those teachers of the deaf who believe their chief responsibility is to teach deaf children to talk. However, there was evidence that some hearing-impaired pupils displayed on some occasions what might be seen as too strong a desire 'to be normal', or at least too strong a desire *to be perceived* 'as normal'. This was made apparent when deaf pupils tried to conceal their handicap and disattend to or deny the existence of the many problems associated with the handicap of deafness. Attitudes and behaviours reflecting a 'denial of handicap' were most apparent in relation to receiving special attention from teachers in the ordinary classroom.

Negative attitudes towards special attention from class teachers reflect the kind of feelings which perhaps any pupil might have in not wanting to be 'in the limelight', or to be seen by others as the 'teacher's pet'. Special attention was also unwelcome in the opinion of some deaf pupils and young people, though not all of them, because they felt it exposed their handicap and made them feel unacceptably different from other pupils. Some hearing-impaired interviewees admitted that they would 'pretend to understand' rather than admit that they were having difficulties in following lessons or rather than ask for help from teachers.

Oversubscribing to the idea of being 'normal' or affecting appearing to be 'normal' rather than acknowledging 'abnormality' is likely to be counter-productive for the deaf pupil. The long-term effect of strategies designed to deceive the teacher into believing that they were coping adequately and following the lessons, when the converse is true, might well be to increase the gap between hearing-impaired pupils' educational attainments and those achieved by normally hearing pupils.

An inspection of the public examination attainments at 16 years of age of the hearing-impaired young people who featured in the study did indeed reveal that the deaf pupils' attainments were below national norms of attainment for all pupils. This finding reinforces the well established belief that if deaf pupils are to have equal opportunity to develop their educational potential then they require positive discrimination. On the other hand, my research has demonstrated that offering positive discrimination to deaf pupils in ordinary classes can be a problem. It may be a problem for class teachers in relation to the scarcity of resources such as time and expertise; it may be a problem for normally hearing pupils in that they are likely to feel resentment if deaf classmates are given what they see to be unfair 'favouritism'; and, very importantly, it may be a problem for hearing-impaired pupils who might not want attention drawn to their special problems and special status.[1]

In addition to ensuring that class teachers have adequate resources to enable them to offer special help to the deaf pupil, and in addition to ensuring that normally hearing pupils are made aware of the special problems caused by a hearing handicap and the consequent special educational attention that deaf pupils so often need, it is also likely to be necessary to counsel hearing-impaired pupils themselves to come to terms with special attention. This is so that they do not feel ashamed or embarrassed about their handicap, and are not afraid to ask for help when experiencing difficulties in following lessons. Deaf pupils should be encouraged not to feel humiliated if a teacher offers extra help or checks their understanding. Indeed, some hearing-impaired pupils in ordinary schools may need to be firmly advised that pretending that their problems in main school classes do not exist might offer short-term relief but is likely in the long run to exacerbate rather than lessen the effects of their handicap.

Consideration might also be given to other additional forms of compensatory education for the hearing-impaired. One compensation might be simply to inform the hearing-impaired pupil and his parents that greater than average efforts are required at home and in school in order to enlarge his educational opportunity and help to overcome the effects of a hearing handicap. The deaf child, if possible with the help of his parents, might be encouraged to do extra school work, or extra reading and language work at home. Another form of positive discrimination would be to extend the period of compulsory education for severely and profoundly deaf pupils.

Generally, then, my research findings indicate that, however much a deaf pupil appreciates and values the 'normalizing' environment of the ordinary school and however much parents and educators support the goal of normalization in the education of the deaf, normalization will not just 'happen' simply by placing a hearing-impaired pupil in an ordinary school. Appropriate positive discrimination is clearly necessary if deaf pupils are to fulfil their expressed desire to talk normally and be capable of adapting to the demands and expectations of hearing speaking society. When a consideration is being made concerning the kinds of special help and extra support that might be offered to deaf pupils in ordinary schools it is crucially important that such help and support is given in a way that is made acceptable to the consumer of the service; namely, the deaf pupil himself.

[. . .]

That the hearing impaired featuring in the research held different viewpoints, and adopted different stances in respect of their relationships with others in society, suggests that they were not subject to a single source of influence. Their attitude and behaviour were almost certainly affected by parents and teachers of the deaf. But there was no evidence that I could detect to suggest that those who chose to identify primarily with the normally hearing had been 'indoctrinated' to espouse 'normality', or compelled to cast off their deaf identity. Likewise, there were no grounds for believing that those who chose to attend Deaf Clubs and use sign language had been told that they must preserve their special identity and participate in deaf culture. Whether or not those deaf pupils and young people, particularly those with profound hearing losses, who strove to be part of the normally hearing world, and who disliked the idea of communicating through sign language had 'false consciousness', or whether, indeed, they were acting in their own best interest is a matter of value judgement. The responses of the hearing-impaired people, no matter what their attitude towards coping with their handicap, did not, however, support the allegation that the ordinary school forced:

> . . . the deaf individual into a situation in which he must try to deny his deafness, imitate a hearing person and pretend he enjoys it.
> (Merrill, 1979)

No hearing-impaired pupil or young person observed or interviewed found it impossible to interact at some level with those who had normal hearing and the majority had regular and frequent social contact with others who were not deaf. Variations among them in their perceptions about themselves in relation to others and variations in their social orientation were manifest mainly in terms of the *degree* of assimilation into handicapped society. Those who believed that they were full members of normally hearing society felt themselves to be 'normal'. Others, who oriented to hearing-speaking society but had maintained contact with other deaf people mainly for mutual support and understanding felt more or less 'normalized'. Even the minority who formed their closest associations from among the deaf group were not part of a close-knit deaf community and no one expressed a wish to belong to any such group.

Some knew sign language and frequently or occasionally used visual/ manual communication when interacting with other deaf people. A few deaf young people believed it would be beneficial if deaf children were taught sign language as part of their school education. Such a belief did not, however, detract from the conviction of all the hearing impaired that the acquisition of spoken English was and should be the major goal of their education and of their personal aspiration.

Many of the deaf people interviewed not only felt that they had no need to know sign language but rejected the idea of using sign, mainly on the grounds that to do so would tend to make them too closely identified with what they saw as a rather exclusive and separate deaf world. The hearing-impaired pupils and young people who could not sign did not feel a sense of deprivation at not being able to use their so-called 'biologically preferred mode' of communication.

Generally, though, the findings of this aspect of my investigation suggest that, whilst most deaf pupils and young people do not want to be part of a distinctive and exclusive deaf subculture, with its own special language, nearly half felt a need for association and friendship with others who were similarly handicapped. It is significant, I believe, that most of the hearing-impaired pupils and young people who had been individually integrated into their local school, and who did not have the opportunity at school to meet other deaf pupils, expressed some regret at not knowing someone of similar age with a similar handicap. Thus, whilst placing a deaf pupil individually in his local school might be considered to be serving his best interests in terms, of say, extending opportunities for increasing his academic or linguistic attainments, such placement can mean a restriction of opportunity in terms of being able to have companionship with other deaf people. Being able to talk about problems shared in common with other deaf people can be very important to the deaf individual's sense of well-being. Enthusiasm for assimilation and normalization should not blind educators from acknowledging that a severe sensori-neural hearing loss represents a permanent and serious handicap for a deaf individual. Education cannot cure deafness; it can only alleviate its worst effects. Thus it may well be necessary for educators to take special measures to enable individually integrated deaf pupils to form contacts with others who are deaf, if they so wish. Education, most people would agree, is concerned with extending opportunities and enlarging choices for individuals and not restricting them. Furthermore, my research indicates that educators, who, we may assume, want to help the deaf individual gain independence and overcome his handicap to the maximum extent possible, might devote more attention to advising deaf pupils of the many special services available for deaf people to make use of because many of the deaf participating in my research were unaware of the range of facilities, services and aids designed to make life easier for someone with a hearing handicap.

Finally, I would propose that in order to help deaf pupils eventually to become more self-sufficient, independent adults, such pupils should be consulted about their education more often than is currently the case. My research findings indicate that an education in an ordinary school is popular with hearing-impaired pupils and young people. This does not mean, as we have seen, that there are no problems associated with an integrated education for the hearing impaired, nor that matters could not be improved so that deaf pupils receive a more effective education in an ordinary school. It would, I suggest, be wrong to assume that teachers of the deaf in this country, who almost invariably have normal hearing, always know what is best for the deaf pupil. Consulting and counselling deaf pupils about the education they are receiving in ordinary schools may not only lead to improvements in their education but also give deaf pupils the experience of having some say in, and influence over, their own destiny. This is particularly important in relation to the current criticisms voiced by 'anti-integrationists' such as Merrill (1979) and McCay Vernon (1981) that too little account is taken of the 'voice of the deaf' when planning educational provision for the hearing impaired.

Note

1   The increasingly popular practice of providing support teachers, usually teachers of the deaf, to assist hearing-impaired pupils in ordinary classes relieves class teachers of the extra work such pupils are likely to entail. But, support teachers cannot be in ordinary classes all the time and class teachers have, therefore, to take some responsibility for the education of the deaf pupil despite the demands which doing so might entail. Furthermore, though the presence of a special teacher in the classroom might benefit the class teacher, it is potentially very stigmatizing for the deaf pupil receiving assistance.

References

Merrill, E.C. (1979) 'A Deaf Presence in Education', supplement to *British Deaf News*, August 1979, Carlisle.

McCay Vernon (1981) 'Public Law and Private Distress' in Montgomery, G. (ed.) *The Integration and Disintegration of the Deaf in Society*, Edinburgh, Scottish Workshop Publications.

5.10 Challenging Conceptions of Integration

Tony Booth (1988)

[. . .]

The normalization of the deaf; the denial of prejudice[1]

For some authors . . . the recognition that people with disabilities may be prey to devaluations finds no place. In her book *Integrating the Handicapped into Ordinary Schools: A Study of Hearing-Impaired Pupils* (Lynas, 1986), Wendy Lynas applies the concept of normalization, in its narrowest form, with clear approval. She makes no reference to any other discussion of the principle and assumes that its definition is straightforward, 'making the hearing-impaired as like or as similar as possible to his[2] hearing peers' (p. 63). This involves 'attempting to eliminate as far as possible those differences that distinguish him from "normals" such as poor speech, lack of comprehension, limited language and consequent low academic attainments' (p. 63).

The purpose of normalization is seen not only as giving deaf and partially deaf young people access to the hearing world but also as making them acceptable to it. The key issue here is signing:

> According to the 'normalization' paradigm of integration a deaf child who could talk would be more acceptable than one who could communicate only by means of sign language. One might suggest that the more normal the speech and language, the more acceptable the hearing-impaired child would become.
> (Lynas, 1986, p. 63)

It might seem from this quotation that it is not signing, *per se*, that Lynas sees as unacceptable to the hearing world but only an inability to talk. Yet she is unable to see that implication. She is locked by her ideological position here into one side of the oral/signing dispute. She leaves a hidden implication that an ability to sign precludes an ability to speak and decode spoken English. Nowhere does she mention the bilingual approach to the education of the deaf which has received much attention in recent years as it has for other minority groups (see Brennan, 1987).

For Lynas, 'normalization' is identified with a process of 'assimilation' of young deaf people into the hearing world. Yet, perhaps as a consequence of sequestering herself from the mainstream of educational debate, she indicates no awareness of the critique of the assimilation philosophy within multicultural let alone anti-racist education. She portrays such a process as part of a natural order whereby minority groups conform to the rules of a majority. The acceptance of the minority depends on their willingness to make themselves acceptable:

> Unless there was prejudice against the deaf, in which case little or no acceptance would be possible, it would be likely that the willingness of the majority group to accept would be dependent, to a significant extent, upon the willingness and the ability of the minority group to adapt.
> (Lynas, 1986, p. 63)

Putting pressure on minorities or powerless groups to run their lives according to the rules of the majority or those in power is, of course, just what others interpret as discrimination. But the idea that prejudice against the deaf does exist is dismissed as a fringe view:

> McGrath (1981) even goes so far as to suggest that in a hearing-dominated society the deaf group, because they are unhearing, are oppressed and stigmatized just as other groups are also accorded inferior social status for being 'unrich' or 'unwhite'.
> (Lynas, 1986, p. 67)

There is an echo of Wolfensberger's stricture here, that 'we practice gross discrimination . . . and then we deny it'. Lynas is only willing to give conscious acknowledgment to the existence of prejudice against people with disabilities if it occurred in the past: 'From Ancient Times *right up to the Victorian Age*, handicapped people had characteristically been accorded extremely low status' (p. 2, my emphasis).

When the mind hears

Yet in this book, as elsewhere in the field of deaf education as one reads or listens to some of the comments of those involved in the education of the deaf, one feels one has entered a time warp: 'Most educators in Britain', Lynas tells us, 'regard both assimilation and normalization as proper goals in deaf education'. The idea that a deaf person is not *'essentially "abnormal"'* is set up as an alternative to the mainstream of thought (p. 66, my emphasis). Now Wendy Lynas, like anyone else who has been around the world of deaf educators even for a relatively brief period, must have encountered the profound prejudice that exists against sign language and deaf people that is voiced by some educators of the deaf. But the fact that in her writing she shows no awareness of it suggests to me that there are processes of denial and repression in operation. One might predict that this effort to distort reality would lead to contradiction and I believe that her text as a whole reveals precisely that.

When I first became involved in the area it came as quite a shock that prejudice was voiced with less restraint than against any other group within the education system. Thus, while I was gathering material for a TV programme on the politics of deaf education in 1985, one teacher of the deaf referred to the adult deaf community as the 'deaffies' and to one deaf man who had the temerity to challenge her as 'some deaf Jamie'. Another spoke of the use of sign language as akin to 'barking at print for hearing children'; having the surface trappings of a real skill but without the involvement of comprehension. This same teacher of a postgraduate course in deaf education began a lecture to postgraduate students by telling them how the eating of baked potatoes by a group of deaf people in the lounge at a conference she had attended confirmed the relative inability of deaf people to acquire social skills. Another suggested that signing challenged God's physiological acumen: 'If he had meant us to sign, the functions of language would not have been organized in the left hemisphere of the brain'. Another educator, an ex-head teacher of a school for the deaf, went even further. He moved from a discussion of the medieval doubt of the presence of a soul in the deaf to a sudden espousal of his own present views:

> If you look at a Minister signing the Lords Prayer it can look beautifully expressive—but what does that waggling of hands mean to the deaf? No-one knows what they are thinking about. We were not intended to learn the language of signs . . . Faith can only come through hearing . . . isn't it a fact that faith was transmitted orally?

These examples were gathered over a relatively brief period and similar examples must be common knowledge to teachers of the deaf and others involved in deaf education. They have a long history which has been comprehensively portrayed by Harlan Lane in his book *When the Mind Hears* (Lane, 1984). The lecture he gave, based on this book, at the International Congress on the Deaf, Manchester, 1985, stands out for me as a remarkable piece of academic theatre. He recited orally the catalogue of prejudices and mistaken beliefs about the inadequacies of sign language as a linguistic system over the last hundred years whilst these were simultaneously and dramatically disproved by their translation into American Sign Language, British Sign Language and Swedish Sign Language.

[. . .]

Revealing contradictions

Now I do not intend to prove in this paper that arguments against the use of sign language are primarily based on prejudice. That job has been eloquently performed by Harlan Lane as well as the thousands of deaf people through history who in their ordinary spontaneous interchanges show how signing can provide unfettered expression for their thoughts and emotions. But what I can indicate is how one author in her uncritical inheritance of a position based on domination and control unthinkingly reproduces a series of profound prejudices and fails to subject her own data to a proper analysis.

She is certainly led to some strange conclusions. She claims that her findings 'will undoubtedly be much welcomed by those teachers of the deaf who believe their chief responsibility is to teach deaf children to talk'. She also argued that there was a conviction among all the young people with 'hearing impairment' whom she interviewed that 'the acquisition of spoken English was and should be the major goal of their education and of their personal aspiration' (p. 251).

I heard a similar sentiment expressed in a joke told to me by an Irishman and I think it is worth risking a repeat of it here:

> A politician was addressing a large crowd and hoping to impress them with his patriotic principles. He puffed out his chest, adopted a stern expression and began:
> 'I was born an Englishman, I have been brought up to be an Englishman and, when the time comes, I shall die an Englishman. . . '
>
> As he paused, there was just time for a member of the audience to call out: 'Jesus, have you no ambition?'

The idea that educators of the deaf and young deaf people themselves should lower their educational sights to such an extent that acquiring spoken English is their major educational ambition is absurd. Yet such a view is reproduced by educators as conventional wisdom.[3] If it is successful, education provides a source of enjoyment, a discovery of interests, a knowledge of cultures and the means to continue to develop and control one's own life. The learning of languages may be part of such a process and can be assessed in relation to it but cannot replace it. In their emphasis on acquiring spoken language for the deaf, educators misrepresent the function of language. They portray it as serving only a public function, permitting interchange between the hearing and the deaf. But language is used on our own as a means of thought, as a vehicle of fantasy and a framework for converting wishes and desires into projects and plans of action.

What has been going on in the education of the young deaf people in Wendy Lynas' study if they limit their aspirations for education in the way she suggests? She argues that: 'there was no evidence that I could detect to suggest that those who chose to identify primarily with the normally hearing had been "indoctrinated" to espouse "normality", or compelled to cast off their deaf identity' (p. 251).

My immediate reaction to that comment is to think that Lynas must inhabit a different world to me. In my world everyone seems to be subjected to 'indoctrination' to espouse 'normality'. Lynas' own evidence might lead her to question her conclusion if she had not started out with the assumption that indoctrination to espouse an amorphous normality was a natural and legitimate goal:

> There seemed to be a universal desire among those interviewed to adopt the behavioural norms of the normally hearing in order to be able to adapt to, and be accepted by, hearing–speaking society. These young people . . . wanted to talk as normally as possible, understand the speech of normally hearing people, achieve as near normal as possible academic standards and become socialized into the ways of normally hearing society . . . They hoped that by being in a normally hearing school, some 'normality' would rub off on them. (Lynas, 1986, p. 169)

For her to detect an overpressure to appear normal Lynas would have to find some striking evidence. She says that despite wanting to appear normal in every respect this does not mean these young people were 'ashamed or embarrassed about being deaf' (p. 169). Yet interestingly enough Lynas' own evidence straightforwardly includes such sentiments. She reports it and fails to see it and when she sees it, she then denies it. What is going on here? Thus on pages 179–192 she records the strategies deaf pupils use for coping in ordinary classes and many of these involve hiding their difficulties and are 'undoubtedly motivated by a desire to conceal their handicap' (p. 180). Thus they hide their hearing aids (p. 181), pretend they understand lessons when they don't (p. 182) or copy other pupils work (pp. 183–184). Sometimes the belief that hearing pupils had privileged access to the right thing to do belied a deaf pupil's own abilities. A teacher reported of one child, Christine:

> She can paint well, but she always, but always, does what Gail (normally hearing) does. If Gail does a butterfly, then Christine does a butterfly; if Gail does a snowstorm, then we get a snowstorm from Christine.
> (Lynas, 1986, p. 187)

She leaves her contradictory assertions unacknowledged and unexamined. At the conclusion to the book she is able to report: 'there was evidence that some hearing-impaired pupils displayed on some occasions what might be seen as too strong a desire "to be normal", or at least too strong a desire *to be perceived* "as normal"' (Lynas, 1986, p. 247).

That some pupils should try to hide their disability was met with surprise by some teachers, as one put it: 'I don't know why they try to hide their aids; everyone knows they're deaf' (p. 181). Whilst some pupils attempt to *pretend* to others that their deafness makes no difference, some fall into the trap of believing it themselves.

> These deaf young people did not, on the whole, see their hearing impairment as an insurmountable barrier to their participation in normally hearing society. They therefore did not believe that the acquisition of sign language should be a priority in their education.
> (Lynas, 1986, p. 238)

Their belief that their deafness is not an 'insurmountable barrier' is to be encouraged because it leads them to play down the importance of sign language in their education. But their lack of awareness of their relatively poor attainment is at the same time to be deplored:

> Many, though not all, hearing-impaired pupils in ordinary schools, do not have a strong sense of their academic 'abnormality' . . . it would seem that if hearing-impaired pupils were made more aware of their difference from others in relation to the attainment of academic success, they might be better motivated to aim for higher standards, work harder, and thus achieve more 'normality' in the long run.
> (Lynas, 1986, p. 209)

Here we have the end result of the 'normalization' philosophy. It is propounded by deaf educators but when it is absorbed by young deaf people they are taken to task for succumbing to personal failings. Pupils, like Alison who say 'I hate it if people know I'm deaf' (p. 234) can then receive the stricture: 'Oversubscribing to the idea of being "normal" or affecting appearing to be "normal" rather than acknowledging "abnormality" is likely to be counter productive for the deaf pupil' (Lynas, 1986, p. 248).

Now for part of one page, at least, Wendy Lynas is well aware of what constitutes the barrier to achievement for many young deaf people:

> . . . a severe and profound hearing loss represents a serious barrier to the educational development and normalization of a deaf pupil and is hence a barrier to his ultimate full assimilation into normally hearing society.
> (Lynas, 1986, p. 240)

The trouble then, acknowledged here, is that young deaf people have difficulty with an education carried out through spoken English because they are deaf. They cannot become hearing and cannot be passed off by others or themselves as if they were hearing. The problem is not that young deaf people cannot acknowledge that they are deaf but that this constitutes a problem for many hearing educators. For to acknowledge that they are deaf means to not only accept that they may need and wish to communicate in sign language but also that a denial of access to sign language represents a severe form of prejudice. But this is a prejudice to be hidden from oralist educators of the deaf by themselves and for those pupils they educate.

A close reading of Lynas' text provides evidence for the counter hypothesis to her own. Young deaf people may be encouraged to espouse a commitment to a 'normality' which is against their own interests. Where this leads them to curtail their freedom and dominate their educational aspirations with the acquisition of spoken English then it is clearly indoctrination. It is hardly surprising that many deaf people have reacted vehemently against this view of integration within deaf education which provides ideological support for their subjugation. It is a tribute to the power of mechanisms of defence that some educators of the deaf can insulate themselves so effectively against the contradictions of their position.

[. . .]

Acknowledgement

I would like to thank Len Barton for his comments on an earlier version of this chapter.

Notes

1 There has been a growing awareness in recent years that some

expressions can contribute to the disadvantage of people with disabilities (see Merry, 1981, p. 29). I tend to avoid terms where a person's identity appears to be depicted by a disability such as 'an epileptic', or 'the disabled'. However, some people with disabilities use the latter term, themselves, to convey a sense of solidarity and a positive identity. In the case of 'the deaf' I use this term in my own writing because of my acceptance of the arguments from deaf people for an overwhelming need to reclaim their deafness as a positive contribution to their lives.

2 Wendy Lynas used this sexist language throughout her text, written in 1986. Wolfensberger's 1972 text as well as the quote from Binet and Simon 1914 use male pronouns at a time when the ideological climate on such matters was less accessible to question, though looking back now, some passages look ridiculous. Wolfensberger writes: 'In the next chapter we will review how ideologies have forged man's patterns of response to devalued groups of fellow men (Wolfensberger, 1972, p. 10). Did I really head a chapter I wrote in 1975 *Nature and Change in Man* (Booth, 1975, p. 130)? Some authors writing currently are digging in their heels on such usage. I have analysed the effect that such a determined lack of self-consciousness can have on the way gender roles are ascribed in a review of Cole's *Residential Special Education* (Cole, 1986; Booth, 1987).

3 Two examples come to mind immediately but there are many others. Hegarty and Pocklington (1982) report that 'developing pupils' ability to communicate, preferably in an oral way' is the 'central goal' of 'deaf education' (p. 158). Cole (1986) referring to the education of the deaf tells us that 'language development must be the central facet of their educational programme' (p. 85).

References

Binet, A. and Simon, T. (1914) *Mentally Defective Children*, London, Edward Arnold.

Booth, T. (1975) *Growing up in Society*, London, Methuen.

Booth, T. (1987) 'Backwards into the Future; Residential Special Education', in *Disability, Handicap and Society, 2*(2), pp. 187–92.

Brennan, M. (1987) 'British Sign Language: The Language of the Deaf Community', in Booth, T. and Swann, W. (eds) *Including Pupils with Disabilities*, Milton Keynes, Open University Press.

Cole, T. (1986) *Residential Special Education*, Milton Keynes, Open University Press.

Hegarty, S. and Pocklington, P. (1982) *Integration in Action*, Windsor, NFER-Nelson.

Lane, H. (1984) *When the Mind Hears*, New York, Random House.

Lynas, W. (1986) *Integrating the Handicapped into Ordinary Schools: A Study of Hearing-Impaired Pupils,* London, Croom Helm.

McGrath, G. (1981) 'Language Competency in the Evaluation of Integration: A View from Australia', in Montgomery, G. (ed.) *The Integration and Disintegration of the Deaf in Society,* Edinburgh, Scottish Workshop Publications.

Merry (1981) in Campling, J. (ed.) *Images of Ourselves: Women with Disabilities Talking,* London, Routledge and Kegan Paul.

Wolfensberger, W. (1972) *The Principle of Normalization in Human Services,* Toronto, National Institute on Mental Retardation.

5.11 The Mainstreaming of Primary Age Deaf Children

Susan Gregory and Juliet Bishop (1989)

Introduction

The findings presented here come from a study of twelve children, each with a significant hearing loss, individually placed in mainstream schools. Data were collected when the children were 5½ and again when they were 6½ years of age in a one-to-one situation with the teacher, and in a group situation.

[. . .]

Access to the curriculum

At first sight it seemed that the deaf children were participating. We analysed the group situation to see whether the teacher interacted as much with the deaf child as the hearing children. In terms of the number of comments that the teacher made to the deaf child it was clear that he or she did. In fact there were more comments addressed to the deaf child and this difference was statistically significant. (All the statistics are based on comparison with the 'target' children when both children were 6½ years of age.) Thus deaf children were not excluded in the group situation, in terms of the number of teacher child interactions.

It may, of course, be that this result is not typical of the normal classroom interaction in that the teacher knows we are recording the deaf child and thus makes a special effort with respect to him or her. However, another possible explanation is that the deaf child has difficulty in understanding the teacher, and the teacher in understanding the deaf child, and thus more questions and comments from the teacher are necessary in order to clarify the communication.

Let us consider the following example with Katherine Ashdown . . . The teacher is talking about when they were newborn babies in hospital. According to the conventions of maternity hospitals they would have been known as baby + surname. The teacher goes around the class saying to each one, 'What would you have been called—baby . . . ?' Each replied baby + their own surname. None of them had any problem with this except Katherine, who after many attempts by the teacher, is still unable to answer and has finally to be told.

Teacher: What would you have been called Katherine?
Katherine: I don't know.
Teacher: What's your second name?
Katherine: ??? (indecipherable utterance)
Teacher: Baby Ash . . . ?
Katherine: Ash
Teacher: What's your second name? What comes after Katherine?
Katherine: (no response)
Teacher: Baby who?
Katherine: Ash
Teacher: Ash De. Come on.
Katherine: Ash De
Teacher: I'll give you Ash De. Ash who? What's your second name?
Katherine: Ash De?
Another child: Down
Katherine: Ash De
Teacher: Ashdown isn't it? So you would have been 'Baby Ashdown'.
Katherine: (laughs)
(Group session—6½ years)

Thus a lengthy dialogue involving eight attempts by the teacher to get the appropriate response was necessary, whereas each individual hearing child replied straight away. It seems then, that the teacher talked more to the deaf child than to each individual hearing child, because this was necessary to achieve understanding.

[. . .]

The maintenance of classroom interaction

Child's strategies
Of more consequence, however, than the limitations on the communications with the deaf child, are the strategies used by both teachers and deaf children to maintain and sustain interaction. These strategies, while facilitating the situation in the short term, are often counter-productive in respect of long-term educational goals.

One simple strategy used by the child is that of nodding in response to the questions that are asked.

Teacher: To go to the Christmas parties in? Did you? So you could have a nice pretty dress.
Deaf Child: (nods)
Teacher: Isn't that lovely? Did your mummy make it for you?
Deaf Child: (nods)
Teacher: Or did she buy it?
Deaf Child: (shakes head)
Teacher: She made it?
Deaf Child: (nods)

Teacher: Did she? Has she got a sewing machine?
Child: (nods)
(Individual session—5½ years)

The teacher often facilitates the child's responses by indicating by facial expression or tone of voice which particular nod or shake of the head is required. This is even more apparent in the next example.

Teacher: What did you do? Did you stay in bed all day?
Deaf Child: (nods yes)
Teacher: In bed all day?
Deaf Child: (nods yes)
Teacher: You didn't stay in bed all day, did you? (She shakes her head)
Deaf Child: No.
(Individual session—5½ years)

One child had worked the nodding strategy to a fine art in that he could nod his head (indicating yes) while saying 'no'.

Another strategy was to use contextual clues—thus, for example, if the teacher is pointing at something the child would respond by naming it.

[. . .]

A further strategy is to repeat the last thing that has been said, as the following examples, all taken from a lesson about telling the time, illustrate . . .

Teacher: Three o'clock. Now what's that? (points)
Hearing child: Five past three.
Teacher: Five past three. Five past three.
Deaf Child: Three.

Teacher: Twenty-five to . . . (?)
Hearing child: Four.
Teacher: Twenty-five to four.
Deaf Child: Five to four.
Teacher: No. Twenty-five to four.
(Group session—6½ years)

This conversational move also occurs in hearing children, but at a much younger age, usually reaching a peak at 2 years 6 months and fading away quickly after that. Moreover, in hearing children the repetitions are almost always appropriate within the wider context of the conversation (Ochs Keenan, 1977).

A further strategy observed in several of the children is that of giving the name of a colour in response to a question, as the following excerpts taken from conversations with two different deaf children illustrate.

Teacher: Oh, you've got a skipping rope, have you?
Deaf Child: (nods) Yes.
Teacher: Can you skip?

Deaf Child: Yes.
Teacher: What can you skip? How can you skip?
Deaf Child: White and brown.
Teacher: Mm?
Deaf Child: White and brown.
Teacher: White and brown colour . . . Oh, is the skipping rope white
  and brown?
Deaf Child: Yes.
(Individual session—6½ years)

[. . .]

Teacher: Do you know what vegetables he grows?
Deaf Child: Pink.
Teacher: Peas?
Deaf Child: (nods)
Teacher: Do you keep saying 'pink'?
Deaf Child: (nods) then (shakes head)
Teacher: No, well don't keep saying 'pink'. That's a colour, isn't it?
  Now, what sort of vegetables does he grow?
Deaf Child: White.
Teacher: Pardon?
Deaf Child: White.
(Individual session—5½ years)

It may be a comment on our methods of teaching deaf children that they
have learnt that naming colours is often a good way of maintaining
interaction. Colour naming is certainly a feature of early work with deaf
children, and in the transcripts there were many examples of teachers
asking about colour, and in those cases such answers would be appropriate.

All of these strategies clearly are effective in the short term and they
are in fact often only detectable when they fail to work. It is possible that
for much of the time the techniques are being used successfully and are not
apparent. Thus much of what actually passes for good dialogue with deaf
children is not based on a mutual understanding but on the ability the child
develops to satisfy, albeit superficially, the social requirement of the
situation.

Teacher strategies

The teachers too have strategies for maintaining the semblance of good
classroom interaction. In the above examples of children's strategies the
teacher's part was not insignificant in maintaining the interaction, by using
gesture, or indicating by facial expression the form of reply required. It
seems likely the teacher often framed the question so that to repeat the last
few words would be an appropriate reply. Also, as has been indicated,
requests for colour names were common enough to lead to over
generalization of this response.

As already mentioned earlier, teachers would use one or two words to make some sense of what the child was saying—which became apparent if other members of the class requested clarification.

Teacher: Where are you going for your holidays, Harriet?
Deaf Child: ??????
Teacher: To where?
Deaf Child: I going to? for my holidays
Teacher: Are you? I wonder if there are any lighthouses there?
Hearing child: What did she say?
Teacher: I don't know.
Deaf Child: I don't know.
(Group session—5½ years)

Incidentally, the last comment is yet another example of a deaf child repeating the last thing that they had heard.

The teachers would also minimize the breakdown in communication by assimilating the deaf child's comments into the dialogue as a minor misunderstanding, and then continuing with the main topic.

Teacher: What did mummy wear yesterday? Do you remember?
Deaf Child: Sweets and lollipop.
Teacher: Mummy ate sweets. I said, 'what did she wear'?
(Individual session—5½ years)

Alternatively, the teacher could put words into the child's mouth and use the child's elicited nods as confirmation. This would facilitate the conversation which could then proceed.

[. . .]

Another teacher's strategy was to construe the child as teasing him or her. Rather than attributing the child's inappropriate response to misunderstanding it was seen as an attempt to tease.

Teacher: And what else did you eat yesterday besides your egg and bacon and tomatoes?
Deaf Child: Sausages.
Teacher: Sausages as well? I see. What did you have for your tea?
Deaf Child: Lunch.
Teacher: You're teasing me, aren't you?
Deaf Child: (shakes head)
Teacher: Yes, you are, you're teasing me, aren't you?
Deaf Child: (nods)
(Individual session—5½ years)

This was not an isolated occurence, and in fact the teachers claimed the child was teasing in three of the twelve sessions recorded at this age.

Analysis
Why then do teachers and pupils collude with each other in maintaining the

semblance of classroom interaction, when for neither party is the communication itself based on mutual understanding. This will be the most speculative part of the paper as it is one area we have only just begun to consider in detail.

One way of thinking about this centres around Goffman's idea of 'passing'—the notion that stigmatized individuals pass for normal to the extent they are able to gain acceptance for themselves, rather than having a role forced upon them related to their stigma. He says 'because of the great rewards in being considered normal, almost all persons who are in a position to pass will do so on some occasions by instinct' (Goffman, 1968, p. 95).

He gives the example of a deaf person who had developed an elaborate technique to cope with dinner parties. She would either '(1) sit next to someone with a strong voice, (2) choke, cough or get hiccups, if someone asked a direct question, (3) take hold of the conversation herself, ask someone to tell a story she had already heard, ask questions the answers to which she already knew' (Warfield, quoted in Goffman, 1968, pp. 127–8).

Many of these techniques are reminiscent of those described in this paper, which are utilized by young deaf children. It seems unlikely that they were deliberately trying to 'pass' or be seen as hearing children. However, many of the deaf children had clearly developed techniques which reduced the ways in which they could be seen as different. It may well be better to understand their behaviour as resistance to being singled out and treated differently rather than as actively trying to 'pass' as normal.

A further line of thought on the development of teachers and pupils' strategies looks at the classroom system as a whole. Teachers have a responsibility to the whole class and at a simple level this comes over in their having to balance the needs of the deaf child with that of the class as a whole. Most teachers found, right from the start, that they were having to do extra work because of the deaf children in their classes.

> Every night I go home and think will . . . (child's name) be able to do this or have I got to think of some alternative? You have got to find time really, you have got to treat him as an individual. I mean, when you have chatted to the whole class about a robin or something, then you have to go over it all with . . . (child's name).

This, of course presented a dilemma for the teachers because their class sizes were not reduced to take account of the deaf child's presence. Many teachers expressed concern about the other children in the class.

> I think he is going to need more extra help—the teacher has to ask herself what time you can spend with . . . (child's name) when there are 29 other children in the class.

One way of coping with this on a day-to-day basis would be to maintain the semblance of communication as far as possible, rather than disrupting the flow of classroom interaction.

However, at a more complex level, classroom discourse is embedded within a context, which takes for granted a basic ability to communicate and is concerned with formulating appropriate styles of interaction for the various acts of learning. The classroom is a particular environment, providing a specific context in which educational discourse is developed. As Bruner (1968) has said, 'I have come increasingly to recognize that most learning in most settings is a communual activity, a sharing of the culture' (p. 127).

The work of the teacher is not just to impart information but to develop and maintain a context appropriate to education. This requires the establishment of certain conventions of classroom behaviour. As Edward and Mercer (1987) point out in their detailed analysis of classroom interaction in the mainstream school.

> An important part of the contextual basis of classroom discourse is the body of rules which define educational activities and which are required for successful participation in educational discourse. (. . .) These rules are problematic for both teachers and pupils, for reasons which stem from the fact they normally remain implicit. They form part of the 'hidden agenda' of school work which is rarely, if ever available for scrutiny and discussion by teachers and pupils together.
> (Edwards and Mercer, 1987, p. 162)

In order to develop and maintain the educational context, the teacher may have to take for granted that there is a mutual understanding of the language that is used. To pause and clarify the language we may well be inconsistent with the development of ideas through conversation which is part of the classroom task with children at this age. Misunderstandings, rather than requiring attention to the comprehensibility of the language, necessitate eleboration in educational terms. Thus the teacher has to collude with the child to maintain a sense of good communication in order that the work of the classroom proceed. Hearing children nod when they do not understand, or respond affirmatively to questions that seem to require such an answer, without really understanding the questions. It may well be that in these cases, continuing with the dialogue may be productive as the topic may be clarified as the conversation proceeds. The teacher can assume the hearing child will catch up because they will gain information from the next part of the lesson. While this is appropriate with hearing children, with deaf children it is problematic, for the deaf child is unlikely to pick up the meaning later in the lesson and catch up. Thus such strategies when used by the deaf child are counter-productive in terms of the long-term goals of education.

[. . .]

References

Bruner, J. (1968) *Actual Minds, Possible Worlds,* London, Harvard University Press.

Edwards, D. and Mercer, N. (1987) *Common Knowledge,* London, Methuen.

Goffman, E. (1968) *Stigma,* London, Penguin.

Ochs Keenan, E. (1977) 'Making it Last: Repetition in Children's Discourse', in Ervin Tripp S. and Mitchell Kernan C. (eds) *Child Discourse,* London, Academic Press.

Section 6
The Linguistic Perspective:
The Status of Sign Language

It is only relatively recently that sign language has been accorded the status of a language. Following Stokoe's pioneering work in the USA, Brennan was the first person to introduce the term 'British Sign Language' (BSL) and her paper in this book indicates some of the linguistic parameters of BSL. Volterra offers further validation of its linguistic standing. She focuses on sign language acquisition in young children and provides insights into the nature of sign language and early language development. Woll places current BSL in a historical context and indicates the dynamic development of language. In doing so she counters a frequent assertion that sign language is merely mime and essentially iconic. An example of such criticism is given in the paper by van Uden whose arguments are countered by Stokoe.

In their studies of language, linguists often rely on native users as informants. Working within this tradition, Brennan, Stokoe, Volterra and Woll have all obtained their primary data from Deaf people themselves. Thus, within the linguistic perspective deafness is not constructed as essentially problematic or disabling, but Deaf people are seen as a minority group who share a specific language. Prior to its recognition as a language, BSL was often viewed by hearing people as an elaborated system of mime and gesture, parasitic on English. With the recognition of sign language as a language in its own right, the role of teaching and assessment, which was formerly undertaken by hearing people and focused largely on signs used in English word order, has been increasingly assessed by Deaf people, as indicated by Simpson and Denmark. The use of video in assessing Deaf students represents a move away from conventional forms of assessment derived from the hearing world to an exploration of methods more appropriate to Deaf culture.

By validating the status of sign language, linguists have enhanced the status of its users. The construction of Deaf people as a cultural group, rather than a disability group, is legitimated by the assimilation of the study of their language into professional linguistic discourse.

6.1 British Sign Language: The Language of the Deaf Community

Mary Brennan (1987)

[. . .]

British Sign Language (BSL)

It does not come as any surprise to hearing people to learn that Deaf people communicate by means of a sign language. However, most of us have not thought very deeply about what kind of a communication system this might be. There is, for example, a widely held misconception that there is a single, universal sign language, comprehensible to deaf people throughout the world. When hearing people are informed that Sweden has its own sign language, America another, Britain another and so on, they often ask, in some bewilderment, why this should be so. Thus, despite accepting without question that there are numerous different spoken languages in the world, hearing people are usually surprised at the variety of sign languages. This is possibly because they have not fully recognized that sign languages are genuinely comparable to other human languages.

BSL is a *visual–gestural* language and both elements of that description are crucial to an understanding of this communication system. It is a language which is perceived by the eye and it therefore exploits forms of patterning which are easily visible. It is produced in the form of gestures which occur in space and in order to understand BSL fully we need to understand something about the specific forms these gestures take and the use which is made of the so-called signing space.

The words of BSL

We can begin to understand the nature of linguistic gesture if we look firstly at the individual sign; that is, the unit which corresponds most directly to the spoken word. The notion of *linguistic gesture* is important here. We can all use gestures to communicate if necessary. Indeed, most of us use gesture as an accompaniment to speech. Some gestures have communicative significance, but they rarely have specific meanings. Others may take on generalized meanings such as the thumbs up sign, the victory V sign and the alternative V sign with its obscene connotations. The gestures have one thing in common with the linguistic gestures of BSL: they can be described very precisely.

In Figure 1, you can see some examples of individual signs of BSL. The hands in each sign have different configurations. In NAME the handshape used has the index and middle finger extended from the closed fist; in CHEAT the hand is closed into a fist and the thumb is extended; in BIRD the thumb and index finger are held parallel to each other and in FAR both index finger and thumb are extended but held at right angles to each other. The gestural words of BSL are made up of separate elements which combine in different ways to produce the individual signs of the language. One of the types of element involved is that of *handshape*.

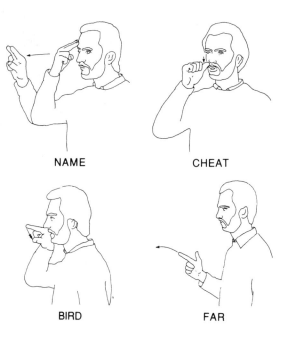

Figure 1

Another significant kind of element is the *position* of the hand in relation to the body. NAME is made at the forehead; CHEAT on the cheek; BIRD at the mouth and FAR in what is known as neutral space: the area directly in front of the body.

A third element of individual sign structure is *movement*. In NAME the fingers touch the forehead and then twist outwards away from the signer's body; in CHEAT the hand moves downward while the thumb contacts the cheek; in BIRD the index finger and thumb make a repeated closing and opening action and in FAR the hand moves in an arc away from the body.

The same realizations of these elements of handshape, position and movement keep recurring, just as the sound elements which make up English words, the phonemes of the language, occur again and again. In much the same way that a relatively small number of significant sounds allows us to create thousands of English words, a relatively small number of handshapes, positions and movements allows us to produce thousands of BSL signs.

As in English, quite tiny differences in form can bring about a change of meaning. The difference between a voiced sound and a voiceless sound in pairs such as [b] and [p] or [t] and [d] is phonetically very slight, but it allows us to make important distinctions in meaning. We do not find it strange that such a slight difference in sound accounts for contrasts in meaning like 'bear' and 'pear' or 'bull' and 'pull'. This is because we are so familiar with the system of contrasts which operates in our own language. In BSL, relatively small differences such as whether the thumb is extended or the fingers are bent can be crucial in distinguishing meanings.

By finding 'minimal pairs' of signs, it is possible to discover which changes in handshape, position and movement are meaningful and which are either conditioned by the context or merely idiosyncratic (Brennan, Colville and Lawson, 1984). For example, the difference between the closed fist and the closed fist with thumb extended is linguistically meaningful. The contrasting signs YOUR (with closed fist) and RIGHT (with closed fist and extended thumb) as shown in Figure 2 demonstrate

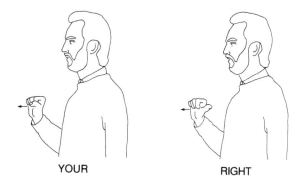

YOUR   RIGHT

Figure 2

the significance of this contrast. It has not been possible to discover a comparable minimal pair to distinguish the flat hand held with thumb parallel to the fingers and the flat hand with thumb extended (Figure 3). Therefore this difference cannot be regarded as 'phonemic'.

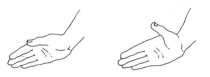

Figure 3   'Non-phonemic' contrast

A close analysis of BSL signs has also revealed other parameters which are significant. Probably the most important of these is what is termed 'orientation'. For example, the only difference between the signs BROTHER and PISTON ENGINE (Figure 4) is the orientation of the palms of the hands and the fingers, otherwise the two signs have the same handshape, position and movement.

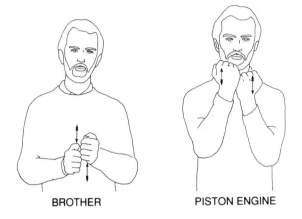

BROTHER   PISTON ENGINE

Figure 4

In a spoken language like English, the primary type of patterning is the sequential combination of units; in BSL the form of patterning is primarily simultaneous. This use of simultaneous patterning operates right across the language, whether we are talking of word structure or grammatical structure. At word level, it simply means that at whatever point we choose to examine the sign, we can describe it in terms of the parameters established above. However, signs do have some sequential structure as well. Recent studies in America suggest it is possible to recognize sign equivalents of syllables (Liddell, 1984). Whether this is the case or not, the interaction of simultaneous and sequential patterning has much to offer in terms of clues towards a greater understanding of human languages in general. This issue is discussed further below in relation to grammatical structure in BSL.

Pictorial signs   Are signs merely pictures in space? The account given so far of individual sign structure focuses on the seemingly arbitrary structural elements which combine together to form BSL signs. So if signs are pictorial, then they are very different from the somewhat idiosyncratic pictures that hearing individuals tend to create if they are asked to present meanings through gesture. Moreover, it is a simple matter of observation to discover that hearing people who do not know sign lanaguage usually have no idea at all what signers are conversing about. This is not really surprising: hearing people do not expect to be able to understand a conversation in Mandarin Chinese or Polish if they do not already know these languages. Nevertheless, there is something in the intuition that most of us have that gestural language is potentially able to show greater links between form and meaning than spoken languages.

The extent to which sign languages show a link between form and meaning is one of the most controversial issues in sign language studies today. There are many more links between form and meaning in BSL vocabulary than can be discerned, say, in English. However, these links are not all of the same type. Some signs of BSL can be regarded as *iconic-pictorial*. They provide some kind of picture in space of what they represent. The signs TREE and HOUSE are typical examples (Figure 5). We can see these signs as almost like stylized drawings or images. Often iconic signs represent an object by showing us only part of that object: the sign ELEPHANT in effect depicts the trunk of the animal, while one of the signs for DOG depicts the legs in the 'begging' position. While BSL structure mirrors the real life aspects of these items, the structure of the signs is highly controlled and stylized. The mime artist may use similar devices, but BSL signs are tighter in structure than mimes. They tend to be more compressed, both spatially and temporally, than equivalent mimes. Moreover, they also use handshapes, positions and movements which may be used completely arbitrarily in other signs.

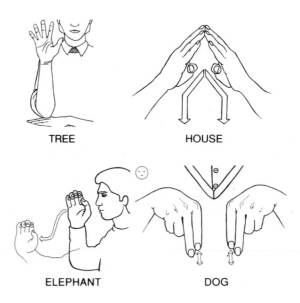

TREE   HOUSE

ELEPHANT   DOG

Figure 5

Some signs are related to their meanings by *conventional* associations of meaning, rather than by inherent links. In BSL, the closed fist handshape with thumb extended is generally associated with meanings which are connected with notions of 'goodness'; the handshape in which the little finger is extended from the closed fist is linked with 'badness'. Thus the thumb up version is used in GOOD and PRAISE, while the little finger version is used in BAD and CRITICIZE (Figure 6). Of course, there is nothing intrinsically bad about the little finger; it is purely a matter of

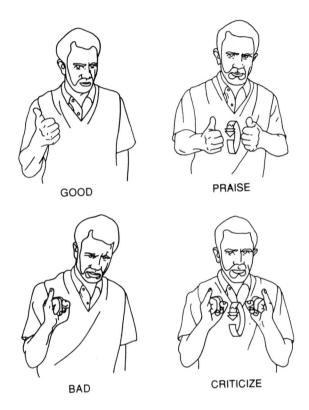

Figure 6

convention that this association is made in BSL. In American Sign Language (ASL) such a convention does not operate: the ASL sign for IDEA and IMAGINE make use of the little finger handshape. A similar form in BSL has the meaning SUSPICIOUS (Figure 7).

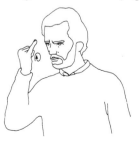

Figure 7 SUSPICIOUS (BSL) or IMAGINE (ASL)

Some signs have what might be thought of as a *metaphorical* link with their meanings. Metaphor is just as pervasive in sign language as it is in spoken language. Thus one of the signs for DOUBTFUL involves the right flat hand making a repeated side to side movement on top of the left hand, while the sign for DEFINITE uses the same handshape, but this time the right hand makes a firm downward movement to contact the left hand. The side to side movement of DOUBTFUL seems to provide a visual metaphor of uncertainty, while the firmness and simplicity of the movement in DEFINITE also seems to echo its meaning (Figure 8).

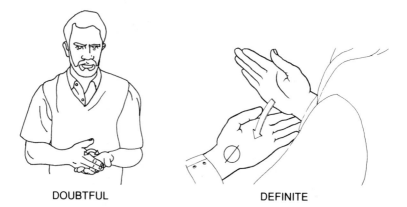

DOUBTFUL   DEFINITE

Figure 8

Many signs of BSL are completely *arbitrary*, as are the majority of words in English. It is difficult to find any explanation of the form of the sign meaning CAN (verb) in BSL (Figure 9). With English, we tend not to look for explanations, simply because we do not expect there to be any links between form and meaning. In BSL, there is a greater chance that such links will be present. The signs of BSL often do have built-in clues to

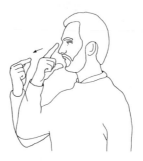

Figure 9   CAN

their meanings, but this is not always the case. Moreover, it is possible to describe BSL signs in a purely structural way, just as we can in English.

Expanding BSL vocabulary   Just as English has ways of expanding its vocabulary to meet new needs, so does BSL. One of the most productive ways is by means of compounding. Many compounds are formed simply by combining sequentially two separate words of the language to create a new word with a new meaning. THINK and GRASP combine together to form the new compound UNDERSTAND; SAY plus TALK produces RUMOUR (Figure 10).

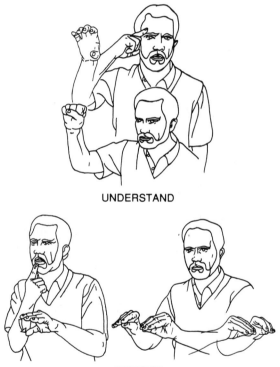

UNDERSTAND

RUMOUR

Figure 10

However, BSL is able to do something which is much more difficult, although just about possible to imagine, in spoken language. BSL can combine two separate meaningful signs together *simultaneously* rather than sequentially. This is because we have two hands and can therefore express one sign with one hand and another sign with the other hand. The telephone device for deaf people known as 'Vistel' which makes use of a keyboard, an electronic print-out and a telephone is represented in BSL by means of a simultaneous compound. The left hand uses the handshape normally used in the sign TELEPHONE, but instead of being placed at the ear, the hand is placed in front of the body. The right hand, fully open with fingers spread, is placed under the left hand and the right hand makes a side to side movement with fingers flickering (as in typing). Thus with one hand the signer represents the telephone receiver, which during telephone communication of this kind is fitted to a location on top of the keyboard, and at exactly the same time, represents the action of typing with the other hand. Similar examples of simultaneous compound signs include PERSON plus LEGS, giving us JUMP DOWN ONE'S THROAT, and PERSON plus SCISSORS, producing BARBER (Figure 11). The presence of *simultaneous compounds* in BSL stresses the way in which the language exploits its medium to full advantage.

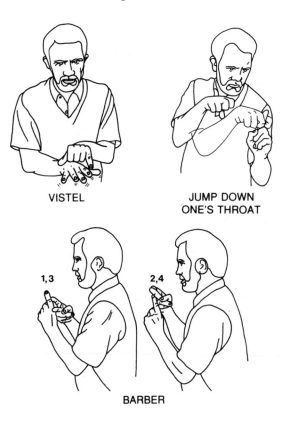

VISTEL

JUMP DOWN
ONE'S THROAT

BARBER

Figure 11

The grammar of BSL

It would take rather more than a few pages, or indeed a few books, to describe the grammatical structure of BSL. Like any other natural human language, BSL has a highly complex and efficient grammatical system.

Here it is only possible to give a hint of the nature of BSL grammatical structure. In order to give a sense of the rather specialized use made of spatial–gestural features, the focus will be on those aspects of structure which are not quite so familiar to English speakers. Every grammatical device or feature so far found in BSL has some equivalent in some spoken language of the world, albeit expressed in a different medium.

Non-manual features   So far I have concentrated almost entirely on the *manual* signs of BSL, but there are other equally important non-manual elements. Such elements can include movements of the head, eyes, mouth, cheeks, shoulders and trunk.

Very often we are dealing with the simultaneous articulation of several non-manual gestures. In some cases, a combination of specific features expresses one particular linguistic function; in other cases, each feature expresses a different function. Yes–no questions in BSL are expressed by means of non-manual features. Typically, the eyebrows are raised and the head and shoulders are pushed forward. These non-manual features combine to express the linguistic function of questioning. The mouth pattern in which the lips are pushed forward as in the production of the sibilant sound 'sh' is used in BSL to express the meaning of existence. It can be used either as an inherent element of the so-called 'existence' signs (Figure 12) or it can be added to a range of signs for emphasis. In the latter case, it would normally be translated by 'really' as in 'Yes, he is really

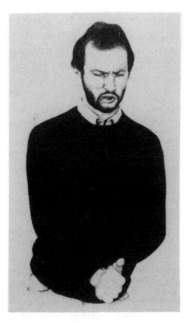

Figure 12   'sh' + existence verb

dead' (Figure 13). It is quite possible to produce a question form, using the non-manual features mentioned earlier in the paragraph, at the same time as expressing the notion of existence through the lip-pattern. An English form such as 'Is he really dead?,' would be expressed by such a combination of non-manual features. When we realize that several further types of non-manual feature could operate simultaneously and that the hands themselves can be conveying separate bits of meaning, then we begin to get some idea of the power and complexity of BSL structure.

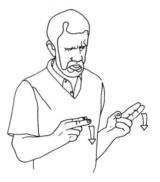

Figure 13   'sh' in 'Yes, he is really dead'

Non-manual modifications make use of some of the same non-manual elements and can be used across a wide range of signs. Their function is often comparable to the function of adverbials in English. Thus the addition of the non-manual feature 'tongue protrusion' (usually referred to as 'th') adds meanings connected with boredom, unpleasantness and weariness. The addition of the non-manual feature 'puffed cheeks' shows intensity and is often translatable by 'very' or 'really' (Figure 13). Again the simultaneous use of such modifications allows the signer to pack a great deal of information into a very short space of time.

Non-manual features also indicate questions, negatives, topic-comment structures, conditional clauses, sentence boundary markers, and turn-taking markers. Research on some of these areas is still at an early stage and there is little doubt that, despite our increasing awareness of the role of non-manual features in BSL, we may, as yet, be underestimating their role in the language.

Manual modifications (inflections)   The study of manual modifications in American Sign Language has led the American linguists Edward Klima and Ursula Bellugi to compare ASL with Latin, insofar as both languages are highly inflected (Klima and Bellugi, 1979). BSL also makes use of regular changes in the movement parameter of manual signs which in turn result in systematic changes of meaning.

Directional verbs in BSL illustrate the way in which changes in movement bring about changes in meaning. These verbs make use of modifications to the direction and/or orientation of the sign to provide information concerning the subject and object of the verb. The sign EXPLAIN can be produced so that the movement is made away from the signer, in which case the meaning is 'I explain to you' or towards the signer as in 'You explain to me'. Here the only change of movement is that of direction. In the sign CRITICIZE there is a change in both direction of movement and orientation of the hands. The two closed fist hands with little fingers extended and palms facing each other move away in a circular action for the meaning 'I criticize you': for the meaning 'You criticize me', the palms face towards the signer and the movement is also towards the signer. There are several different categories of directional verbs (Brennan and Colville, 1984). Not all verbs can be modulated in this way. The learner of BSL has to learn the relevant classes of verbs and the specific changes involved just as one has to learn specific conjugations in Latin.

There are several other types of inflectional change associated with BSL verbs. One group allows us to express certain types of temporal meaning. In English, we are very used to the idea that the verb phrase can express *tense*: the verb itself is able to give us some information as to when an event took/takes/will take place. Such information is often supported by other carriers of meaning, particularly adverbials such as 'tomorrow', 'in three hours time', 'in 1066' and so on. In BSL, this kind of information is usually given through adverbials alone.

However, BSL does express what is known as *aspectual* meaning within the verb, something which English does not do to the same extent. *Aspect* is a less familiar grammatical category for speakers of English than tense. It is concerned with what we might think of as a temporal perspective. It allows us to look at the same event from different points of view in respect of time. We can see the event as completed, ongoing, just about to start, just about to finish, happening again and again, happening gradually and so on. Most of these aspectual choices are made in BSL by modifying the verb. It is again the movement parameter which allows us to express these choices. The sign COME can be made with short movements to express the meaning of coming regularly or habitually; a slower, repeated movement would express the idea of the same activity happening again and again and again. To express the meaning 'It gradually became dark', the sign DARK is produced with a slow movement (Figure 14); to express 'It got darker and darker and darker' the movement is made in several short steps. A sign may be held in its starting position to indicate that the action was just about to take place but did not. Again, not all verbs can take the same aspectual inflection. A detailed grammar of the language would specify the categories of verbs and the inflections they may take.

Location   BSL is a spatial language. The signs are made in space and it is possible to exploit this fact grammatically. BSL does this by using the location of signs in space to express relationships among signs. Signs can be localized in space in a number of different ways: by articulating the sign at a particular point in space to the right of the signer, at head height, to the

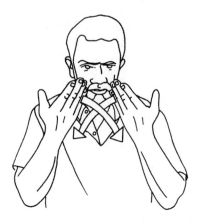

Figure 14   It gradually became dark

left of the signer and so on; by pointing to specific locations, and by using eye gaze to indicate particular locations. The points in space are then made use of in the choice of movement inflections in directional and other categories of verbs.

As well as providing the basis of subject–object relationships, spatial location can also be used to refer to the physical location of objects or people. Meanings such as 'beside', 'in front of', 'under' and so on can be expressed easily by selective use of space. The language also has what may be thought of as a conventionalized set of locations allowing for the expression of pronouns. It is also possible to use space in a metaphorical way to express more abstract relationships. Thus two individuals who are seen as being unequal can be placed so that one is higher than the other in space. BSL exploits such possibilities but in a highly structured manner.

Classifiers   One set of signs which has received much attention in recent years has been the group known as 'classifiers'. There are, in fact, many languages of the world which are described as 'classifier languages'. Perhaps the best known of these is Chinese. Many classifier languages require the use of classifying words in numeral and/or demonstrative expressions. Lyons (1977) quotes Mandarin Chinese 'san ben shu', meaning 'three books', in which the word 'ben' is a classifier for flat object. BSL also has signs which classify objects into categories or groups. Indeed 'flat object' is one of the groups expressed in this way. Other categories include 'round object', 'narrow object', 'long thin object' and so on.

Classifiers play an important role in BSL, although this role is not identical to the use of classifiers in a language such as Chinese. One important function of classifiers in BSL is to act as 'pro-forms', i.e. to stand in place of other signs. If we were describing a journey in a car, we would not constantly repeat the sign CAR, but would replace this sign with what is known as a vehicle classifier. This is made with the flat hand held so that the palm is facing left and the fingers are pointing away. The use of the classifier form allows greater flexibility and allows noun and verb functions to be expressed simultaneously: 'the car went up the hill' will be expressed by a single sign using the vehicle classifier and an appropriate handshape.

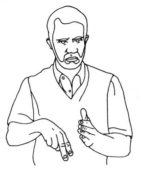

Figure 15   Vehicle classifier + legs classifier 'He stood beside the motorbike'

Classifiers also facilitate the depiction of locative relationships. If we had been talking about a motorbike and then wanted to express the meaning 'He stood beside the motorbike', we could do so by using two classifiers: the flat hand representing the vehicle and the so-called legs classifier (Figure 15). Their position in signing space mirrors their real-life physical relationship. We are able to express all of the information expressed in the English sentence in a single moment of time. The spatial medium and the potential for simultaneity inherent in a gestural language allow this compression of time. The language has adapted to the medium in which it is expressed.

[. . .]

References

Brennan, M. and Colville, M.D. (1984) Final Report to Economic and Social Science Research Council.

Brennan, M., Colville, M.D. and Lawson, L. (1984) *Words in Hand: A Structural Analysis of the Signs of British Sign Language* (2nd edn), Edinburgh, Moray House College/Carlisle, BDA.

Klima, E. and Bellugi, U. (1979) *The Signs of Language*, Cambridge, MA, Harvard University Press.

Liddell, S. (1984) 'Think and Believe: Sequentiality in ASL Signs', *Language, 60* pp. 372–99.

Lyons, J. (1977) *Sematics*, vol. 2, Cambridge, Cambridge University Press.

6.2 Historical and Comparative Aspects of British Sign Language

Bencie Woll (1987)

[. . .]

Background

Most of the literature comparing different sign languages has been concerned with American Sign Language and French Sign Language. It is generally assumed that ASL is historically related to the French Sign Language of the early nineteenth century, researchers seeing evidence of cognate signs in French and American Sign Language. The folk belief among signers in the United States is that French Sign Language was imported into the United States by Laurent Clerc, a deaf teacher of the deaf brought over to Connecticut by Gallaudet to establish the first school for the deaf there. It is quite clear that there has been a strong influence by French Sign Language on ASL, including borrowing of the French one-handed alphabet, and numerous signs which show a French Sign Language origin. However, it is also clear that deaf people in the United States had some sign language in use before French Sign Language was imported, and this language was derived to some degree from British Sign Language (Groce, 1985).

The absence of a simple chain of development from FSL to ASL is supported by a comprehensive study comparing ASL and FSL conducted by Woodward (1978). This was a glottochronological study, using word lists in both languages as the basis for comparison. In glottochronology, developed originally for spoken language comparative research, lists of basic vocabulary are compiled for two languages. Because of the fairly regular rate of change in languages over extended periods of time, the percentage of cognate signs in both languages can be used to give an approximate date at which the languages began to diverge. For example, using this method it is possible to demonstrate that English and German diverged earlier than English and Dutch. In Woodward's study, varying numbers of signs from ASL and FSL (between 77 and 872 pairs) were compared, and using standard glottochronological techniques (Gudschinsky, 1964), he concluded that the approximately 60 per cent rating of cognates found could only be accounted for by viewing ASL as a creole of FSL and some other language or languages, as this figure is far too low for the supposed separation date for ASL and FSL of 1816.

[. . .]

Comparative data analysis

We can also rank individual sign languages in terms of how similar each sign language is to the other sign languages [. . .] On this analysis [of five sign languages] British, Australian and New Zealand sign languages have the highest similarity rankings, with South African and Hong Kong Chinese Sign Languages rated as less similar to each other. This can be explained if British, Australian and New Zealand Sign Languages have been less influenced by other sign languages than Chinese and South African Sign Languages.

A few examples will show that the nature of the similarities in sign language lexicons is unlikely to be due to the presence of coincidentally similar signs. For example, the British sign for BAD is formed by extending the little finger from the closed fist. This handshape also appears in a number of signs with meanings associated with BAD such as ILL, WRONG, DIRTY, etc. All of the sign languages discussed above also produced BAD with the little finger extended. Of the twelve other sign languages discussed in the European comparative study, only Irish Sign Language uses this handshape for BAD. Irish Sign Language, of course, exists in close proximity to British Sign Language, and although believed to be historically unrelated, has borrowed signs to a great extent. The handshape found in BAD in BSL is also mentioned by Bulwer in 1644 as a sign meaning BAD, and thus this sign appears to have been in use in Britain for over 340 years. Many other types are also found only in this group and not in any other sign languages.

There is also historical evidence to support the view that these sign languages are related to each other. All except Chinese Sign Language use the British two-handed alphabet. Although Chinese Sign Language does not, there appears to be some historical vestiges of the use of a two-handed alphabet, as in Shanghai, signed with a fingerspelled 's'. For Australian, New Zealand and South African Sign Languages, there is a known history of deaf signers and teachers of the deaf using sign language in Britain emigrating to those countries. South African and Chinese Sign Languages are the least similar, and these cultures have been influenced by other spoken language groups.

One of the most interesting features arising from the analysis is the discovery of what are likely to be earlier sign forms for which there is no attested BSL version at present, or of signs which have altered along the same principles but with differing results. For example, the Australian sign WOMAN is articulated on the contralateral cheek; the British sign WOMAN is articulated on the ipsilateral cheek; in the earliest version of this sign, the hand passes from one cheek to the other. In the Australian sign HEALTH, the original changing handshape and location of the sign are preserved, while they have disappeared in the British sign.

Old records of signs

Background

Old sources of information about signs were collected for analysis of early sign forms. This was a relatively difficult task, as there exists no central source of information in the form of a bibliography of sign language texts. The main sources providing information about sign language from the nineteenth and early twentieth centuries are a number of small pamphlets which were probably designed for fund-raising, and which began to appear in the 1880s; they consist of sign illustrations (either photographs or drawings) with or without explanatory descriptions of how to produce the signs. One set was drawn and published by Henry Ash (b.1863), who was a deaf draughtsman and designer of wall-paper. Three of his pamphlets dating from the late 1890s to the 1920s have been obtained, all titled 'The Guide to Chirology'. They were advertised in the publication of the British Deaf and Dumb Association, 'The British Deaf Times' . . .

As well as illustrations of signs, the pamphlets contain other information and anecdotes about deaf people, illustrations of the manual alphabet, and illustrations of deaf scenes such as a wedding, a deaf club, and a visit by Queen Victoria to a deaf woman, showing the Queen using fingerspelling.

Another pamphlet was published in Belfast by Francis Maginn, probably early in this century: 'Guide to the Silent Language of the Deaf'. This contains eighty drawings, two alphabets, and a poem about deafness.

A third source of drawings is a pamphlet entitled 'A Pocket Book of Deaf and Dumb Signs', published anonymously in 1895, and which was repeatedly republished in parts in the British Deaf Times, appearing for the last time in 1931. The illustrations are in an apparently random order, but are accompanied by a list of words in English alphabetical order which refer to the illustrations.

The fourth and final source of drawings is from a journal entitled 'Our Monthly Church Messenger to the Deaf and Dumb'. The drawings are 'by a very poor deaf mute', and Henry Ash prepared the block. The signs are described as 'very imperfectly drawn', and while it is clear that a complete set of signs from A to Z was intended, only five blocks were published, from A to G, comprising 120 signs, which are accompanied by brief descriptions.

At the beginning of the twentieth century, photography was first used for sign illustrations, the earliest found being in a brief article in the British Deaf Times in 1904, although there were earlier photographs of signs:

> No maker of signs, to our knowledge, has been so much photographed as the Rev F W G. Gilby. . . . Mr Gilby himself, by force of his position as Superintendent Chaplain of the RADD, is the very first person to whom the journalist or photographer is referred when in the quest of copy or pictures illustrative of the language of gesture.
> (Vol. 1, April, no 5, 1904, p. 97)

Gilby, who was the son of deaf parents, and editor of 'Our Monthly Church Messenger to the Deaf and Dumb' (see above), is shown signing various religious texts, with an accompanying discussion of some features of sign language grammar.

Probably the best-known photographs from this period are found in a pamphlet published by the British Deaf Times, entitled 'Language of the Silent World' (1914). This contains 143 signs, in random arrangement, and a manual alphabet. Until superseded in 1938 by another pamphlet published by the National Institute for the Deaf, this was the most widely available source of information on sign language. The photographs were republished for the final time in 1929.

The final group of photographs discovered were taken at about the same time as the 'Language of the Silent World', and appeared in a similar pamphlet of eighty-four photos, several drawings, anecdotes, etc.

As well as illustrated sources, a number of written descriptions of signs were traced. These include The Deaf and Dumb: their Deprivation and its Consequences; the process of their education with other interesting particulars, by the Rev. Samuel Smith (1864); The Deaf and Dumb: Their Education and Social Position, by W.R. Scott (1870); The Instruction of the Deaf and Dumb, by J. Watson (1809); Education for the People, by Mrs Hippisley Tuckfield (1839); Researches into the Early History of Mankind and the Development of Civilisation, by E. Tylor (1878); and The Sign Language of the Deaf and Dumb, by J.B. Nevins (1895).

[. . .]

References

Groce, N. (1985) *Everybody Here Spoke Sign Language,* Cambridge, MA, Harvard University Press.

Gudschinsky, S. (1964) 'The ABC of Lexicostatistics (grottochronology)', in Hymes, D. (ed.) *Language in Culture and Society*, New York, Harper and Row.

Woodward, J. (1978) 'Historical bases of ASL', in Siple, P. (ed.) *Understanding Language Through Sign Language Research*, New York, Academic Press.

6.3 Sign Languages of Deaf People and Psycholinguistics

A. van Uden (1986)

The lexicology of sign languages
The 'Dictionary of Signs' by Martinus van Beek (Sint Michielsgestel), kept up until 1906, comprises 5,021 signs. The comprehensive American Dictionary (Sternberg, 1981) comprises '5,000 definitions'. It should be noted that by no means all the deaf know these signs, not even when they have been brought up with them.

We are concerned here with *three concepts*: To what extent are signs *iconic*? *esoteric*? and *arbitrary*?

NB Neisser (1967) calls an 'icon': a persistance of visual information as an 'afterimage'. We, however, use the term here in a wider meaning, that is, not purely visual but as a certain resemblance of reality, of feelings, attitudes, reactions, etc. (cf. Griffith *et al.*, 1981).

Iconicity, esoterism and arbitrariness in words
These concepts also apply to words. A word like 'cuckoo' represents the typical sound of a certain bird and can be regarded as iconic in this respect. Or think of a word such as 'gong'. Hoemann (1975) calls this 'meaning transparency', Luftig and others (1983) speak of 'translucency'.

A word like 'fluff' may also have some iconic aspects, more obviously when the meaning of light featherly stuff is known. Or take a word such as 'floppy' disk, used for computers, meaning a very flexible disk. These iconicities are not as clear, however, as those of 'cuckoo' and 'gong'. They 'dawn', become clear, provided the meaning is known. I would call this '*indirect* iconicity', in contrast to the 'direct iconicity' of 'cuckoo' and 'gong'.

The meaning of a word like 'glupy' will not be immediately clear to everyone, since it is not only not directly iconic, but also its meaning may only be known within the circle of people who use this word: consequently it is esoteric (i.e. known only within a certain circle, used only for 'in-group' communication). If, however, we know the meaning: 'a jumping horse', the iconicity dawns. Thus the word is in a way indirectly iconic. Another esoteric word is probably 'heekes'. When someone says this to express his dislike of the skin of the milk in his coffee, the meaning of this word becomes clear through the 'oral mimicry'. It seems a very esoteric, indirectly iconic word.

Very often slang words have typical indirectly iconic aspects, 'deliberately used for picturesqueness' (Sykes, 1976). Poets too use iconic aspects of words and of word groups, for so-called 'phonetic symbolism' or 'oral mimicry'; for instance, this quotation from a poem by Anne Hawkshawe:

'Listen to the kitchen clock' . . . , in contrast to:
'I am a very patient clock, never moved by hope or fear' . .

Most words, however, are purely arbitrary

[. . .]

Iconicity, esoterism and arbitrariness in signs

In spoken languages the iconicity does not occur very often. Esoteric words are exceptional too. By far the greater majority of words are purely arbitrary. This is not the case in sign languages: here the rule is what the exception is in the spoken languages. Research in this area is usually done as follows:

● Testees who do not know any signs at all are shown certain signs and they have to guess what the meaning of these could be.

● With signs which are difficult to identify (their chance of guessing correctly is low), the meaning is given and the testees are asked whether connection with the signs is clear and in what way.

● After that only a few signs remain, where the connection with the meaning is not clear.

This research has been done by means of drawings . . . and also by means of film and/or video recordings. The latter is of course better, because the dynamics of the sign becomes clearer.

[. . .]

Criticism on researches

Quite a large number of researches have been done on the iconicity of different sign languages used by the deaf, particularly American ones[1] . . .

Sternberg (1981) has described the iconic meanings of more than 5,000 signs of the American Sign Language. It is the most extensive dictionary of signs ever published. Hardly any non-iconic sign can be found in this dictionary. The same must be said of other dictionaries as for instance that of French Sign Language (Oléron, 1974; cf. Moody, 1983), of German Sign Language (Starcke and Maisch, 1977), of Dutch Sign Language (van den Hoven and Speth, 1983), of Australian Sign Language (Jeanes, Jeanes, Markin and Reynolds, 1976), etc.

Schlesinger puts it briefly and clearly: 'Iconicity is the single most striking feature of sign language'.

Yet quite a few scientific imperfections are on these researches, the following of which I would like to mention:

● Mainly *hearing* judges have been used, who had to either guess at once what a certain sign could mean, or to indicate on a scale how strongly a certain sign was connected with a certain meaning. It is of course much more important to know, how certain signs live in the minds of the *deaf* sign users. It is typical that quite a few deaf people like to explain to an interested hearing person the meaning or the origin of their signs. This does not always agree with reality, and comprises a lot of 'folk etymology', but this tendency does warn against the opinion, which one often hears, that these iconic meanings are so worn away in the minds of the deaf that they do not (cannot) play a role in their thinking. Unfortunately no thorough research exists on this. The said tendency not only occurs in the directly iconic, but also in the indirectly iconic and even in the so-called arbitrary signs. . . . Hoemann (1978) notes that it is easier to execute the signs, if one knows the iconic backgrounds.

● The meanings of the signs were given in spoken or written words. Do they *per se* reflect the pure meaning of the sign?

● A rather arbitrary number of signs were taken without finding out whether they were a representative sample, whether they belonged to the frequent vocabulary of the average deaf person, whether they were known to all the deaf, or conversely, were fairly unknown, etc.

● Loose signs were given, and not in the flow of a sentence as the deaf use them among themselves. After all in the flow of a sentence, usually expressed with a lot of Body language, the signs can be more iconic than when taken separately. Cuxac and Abbou (1984) found, for French deaf signers, the pantomime 'increasing the iconic features which are already present in French Sign Language' (cf. pp. 76, 87).

In spite of all these imperfections we can sum up the results fairly reliably as follows:

Directly iconic signs　About one third of the signs, in the various kinds of sign-lexicons, are so transparent that everyone who belongs to the culture in which the manual deaf live, can guess the meaning of them (guessing chance more than 50%). We call these signs *directly iconic*, and they are often so clear, with a guessing chance of more than 90 per cent, that they cannot be called esoteric. . . .

Indirectly iconic signs　About half of the signs are not immediately clear, and can be regarded as *esoteric*. But if one knows the meaning, and certainly if the origin of the sign has been explained, the iconicity becomes clear. They are *indirectly iconic*. Often this kind of signs has gone through a process of development, so that at first they were very iconic, sometimes not even esoteric, but are more or less worn, and have lost their direct iconicity in daily use.

Arbitrary signs　About one fifth of the signs can no longer be called iconic, they are more or less arbitrary and thus also esoteric. See Frishberg (1975) about historical changes and arbitrariness. The manual system by Martinus van Beek (1827) comprises a fair amount of these arbitrary signs, for example for 'name', 'to serve', 'man', 'woman', 'parents', 'father', 'mother', 'son', 'daughter', etc., especially, however, for function words or particles such as 'then', 'thus', 'it', 'also', 'still', etc. (However, the latter signs do not originate from prelingually deaf people, but are introduced from the verbal language.)

[. . .]

The sequence of signs: a genuine linguistic syntax?

Introduction
Bonvillian, Nelson and Charrow (1980) say: 'American Sign Language and the sign languages in other countries differ both in the construction of individual signs and in the structure of their sign sentences'. The first assertion is true. There is little evidence, however, for the still unproven second one.

[. . .]

A visual or experiential sequence   As far back as 1908–1911 Wundt tried to compose a certain 'syntax' of deaf signs. His experiments pointed to an experiential sequence of signs, including a sequence of events, of attention and indication, and also to an emotional sequence.
   An example:

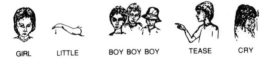

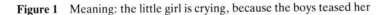

| GIRL | LITTLE | BOY BOY BOY | TEASE | CRY |

Figure 1   Meaning: the little girl is crying, because the boys teased her

   The signed sentence gives a visual sequence of events: first there was a little girl; then the boys were seen; they were teasing; the girl started to cry. The order of 'GIRL LITTLE' is typical too for a sign language. This resembles a sequence of 'topic-comment' or 'given-new' (see below). One first indicates what one is talking about. GIRL, and then how this girl is. The same happens with, for example, a phrase such as 'in the cupboard', which becomes in signs 'CUPBOARD IN'; after all one first has to indicate the cupboard in signs before one can show that something is put into it (cf. Friedman, 1976). Other terms for the same kind of sequences may be 'agent–action–recipient' (see below), in locative sentences 'the immobile precedes the mobile', etc. (cf. Volterra *et al.*, 1984).
   Something similar occurs in ordinary colloquial language, for example (cf. Jansen, 1981, quoted by Van der Toorn, 1982):

'Your brother, where does he live?'
'See the cupboard over there, put the cups into it!'

'The bus, you know the one that goes via Croydon. I could not find it.'
Etc.

An emotional sequence   In our spoken language we can emphasize a word
that is emotionally more loaded, that deserves a special emphasis, at the
start of a sentence, in the middle or at the end. In a sign language one is
inclined to put the emotionally loaded word first. An example:

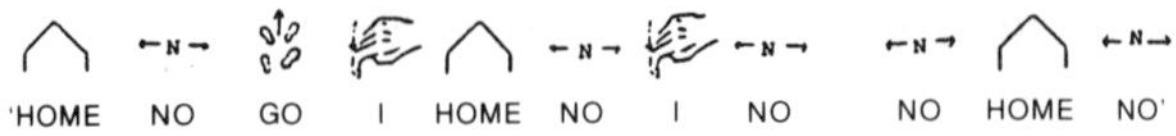

'HOME   NO   GO   I   HOME   NO   I   NO   NO   HOME   NO'

Figure 2   Meaning: I don't feel like going home at all!

Such sequences, however, also occur in spoken language, for example
(Jansen, 1981, quoted by Van der Toorn, 1982):

'You fool, what a fool you are!'
'Forgotten! Of dear, I have left my hat on the train!'
'A flash, thundering, I jumped out of my skin!' . . .

A 'semantic sequence' (Oléron, 1978)   Wundt's findings (see above) are
confirmed in the different textbooks and studies on sign language . . .
Isaac Schlesinger (1981) . . . compared these findings with the word
sequences used by very young, normal, hearing children at the age of about
1½–3 years. He found clear parallels. In a way one may say that such a
young hearing child wrestles as it were with two systems, 'the semantic
sequence' of the words and the more rhythmic groupings of everyday
language. . . . This semantic sequence is used by practically all the deaf,
whatever sign lexica they follow. The same phenomena are found in the
United States, in France, Canada, United Kingdom, Denmark, Sweden,
Germany, Israel, Italy, etc. The term 'natural syntax' was suggested by this
author (van Uden, 1968, 1979–1981), whereby the question remains
whether . . . this can still be called a 'linguistic syntax' in the strict sense of
the word. McIntire (1982) too seriously doubts whether one can apply the
terms 'subject', 'verb' and 'object' to sign languages. . . . One can
especially doubt the presence of 'position-categories' (Paardekoper, 1966),
based on rhythmic groupings of words and phrase structure (cf. van Uden,
1968, 1977). See for several semantic factors determining the order of signs
Volterra *et al.* (in Italian deaf subjects, 1984). . . .
     Consequently, Crystal and Craig (1978) put it coherently and briefly:
'Talking about sign syntax in this way is highly misleading'.
     Happily enough, more and more other than strictly speaking linguistic
terms are becoming more frequently used to describe the typical sequences
of signs: 'topic-comment', and 'given-new' (see above), 'agent-action',
'action-recipient' or 'patient' (= undergoing action, see above), 'recipient-
received', 'experiencer-goal', and similar. These terms have more to do
with the contents of the codes than with purely functional relations.

I find Oléron's term *'semantic sequence'* in this context the best.

The semantic sequence and memory   Is this 'semantic sequence' of signs *a support for the memory*?

Tweney *et al.* (1977) did the following test in order to show that the natural sign language of the deaf uses a real 'syntax'. They departed from what was found in spoken languages; i.e. that more is remembered from normal sentences than from deviating sentences and from unconnected series of words (cf. Clark *et al.*, 1977). Short sentences of four to five signs in natural sign 'syntax' were recorded on video tape and presented to 'fluent manual' deaf. Into each sentence one nonsense-sign or one nonsense-finger spelled word had been inserted. Each time the testee had seen the thus constructed sentence, he had to reproduce the signs and also the nonsense-insertions. These reproductions were compared with those in a different series of presentations with the same nonsense-insertions of mutually unrelated signs in series of unconnected four to five signs, composed from the 125 signs which had been used in the sentences. The result was that both more signs and more insertions were correctly reproduced from the signed real sentences. (No mention is made in the report whether the reproductions also maintained the correct order of signs and insertions.) The researchers conclude that the 'syntax' of the signs is the reason for this favourable result, 'entirely as in spoken languages' . . . Is not this conclusion too rash, however? In our opinion the same result can be explained both by the fullness of content of the sentences presented and by the 'semantic sequence' of these signed sentences, without any 'linguistic syntax'.

[. . .]

Conclusion

Linguistic phonology and functional morphology are not found in signs. A linguistic syntax does not exist either. As a consequence, the following kind of sentence (see, for example, Crystal and Craig, 1978) cannot be expressed in signs, detached from the situation:

> Peter is on a journey with John. Before he left, he said to him that they would meet each other in London at 10.30.'

> 'I asked whether John would help Monique'.

> 'Peter is talking about the friendship between Monique and Carla'.

If a manual deaf wanted to express these signs in Natural sign language, he would first have to dramatize the situation, then break up the whole into small units, every moment checking whether his partner is still following his utterances, explaining the sequence of events in its chronological order, and introducing a lot of Body language and extra-linguistic picturing.

[Note
1   A. van Uden's book is characterized by long strings of references after some assertions. Where these are not related in a specific way to the text, but for general information, we have omitted them, indicated by . . .]

References

Beek, M. van (1827), *Nederlands in Gebaren,* Gemert.

Bonvillian, J.D., Nelson, K.E. and Charrow, V.R. (1980), 'Languages and Language Related Skills in Deaf and Hearing Children', in Stokoe, W.C. (ed.) *Sign and Culture: A Reader for Students of American Sign Language,* Silver Springs, Maryland, Linstok Press, pp. 227–65.

Clark, H.H. and Clark, E.V. (1977) *Psychology and Language. An Introduction to Psycholinguistics,* New York, Harcourt Brace Jovanovich Inc.

Crystal, D. and Craig, E. (1978) 'Contrived Sign Language', in Schlesinger I.M. and Namir, L. (eds) *Sign Language of the Deaf, Psychological, Linguistic and Sociological Perspectives,* New York, Academic Press.

Cuxac, U. and Abbou, M.Th. (1984) 'French Sign Language and Pantomime', in Lancke Ph., Boyes Braem, P. and Lebrany (eds) *Recent Research on European Sign Language,* Lisse, Swets and Zeithinger, pp. 141–8.

Friedman, L.A. (1976), 'The Manifestation of Subject, Object and Topic in the American Sign Language', in Li.Ch.N. (ed.) *Subject and Topic,* New York, Academic Press, pp. 125–48.

Frishberg, N. (1975) 'Arbitrariness and Iconicity, Historical Change in American Sign Language', *Language, 51,* pp, pp. 696–719.

Griffith, P.L., Robinson, J.H. and Panagos, J. (1981) 'Perceptions of Iconicity in American Sign Language by Hearing and Deaf Subjects', *Journal of Speech and Hearing Disorders, 46,* pp. 388–97.

Hoemann, H.W. (1975) 'The Transparency of Meaning of Sign Language Gestures', *Sign Language Studies, 7,* pp. 151–61.

Hoemann, H.W. (1978) *Communication with Deaf People, a Resource Manual for Teachers and Students of American Sign Language,* Baltimore, University Park Press.

Hoven, Zr. M. van den, and Speth, Br. L. (1983) *Icanishe Kinderen,* Van Hoven Zeggen.

Jeanes, D.R., Jeanes, R.C., Marken, C.C. and Reynolds, B.E. (1976) *Aid to Communication with the Deaf,* Board of Management, Victoria School for Deaf Children, Australia.

Luftig, R.L., Page, J.L. and Lloyd, L.L. (1983) 'Ratings of Translucency in Manual Signs as a Predictor of Sign Learnability', *Journal of Child Communication Disorders, 6*, pp. 117–34.

McIntire, M.L. (1982) 'Constituent Order and Location in American Sign Language', *Sign Language Studies, 37*, pp. 345–86.

Moody, B. (1983) *La Langue des Signes, Introduction à l' Histoire et à la Grammaire de le Langue des Signes, entre les Mains des Sourds*, Ellipses, Edition Marketing, Paris.

Neisser, U. (1967) *Cognitive Psychology*, New York, Appleton.

Oléron, P. (1974) *Eléments de Répertoire de Langage Gestuel des Sourds-muets*, Paris, Editions de Centre National de la Recherche Scientifique.

Oléron, P. (1978) *Le Langage Gestuel des Sourds: Syntaxe et Communication*, Paris, Editions du Centre National de la Recherche Scientifique.

Paardekoper, P.C. (1971) *Inleiding Tot de ABN-Syntaxis*, Malmberg, S-Hertogenbosch.

Schlesinger, I.M. (1981) 'Sign Language and Natural Grammar', in Hoffer B.L. and St. Clair R.N. (eds) *Developmental Kinetics. The emerging paradigm*, Baltimore, University Park Press.

Sternberg, M.L. (1981) *American Sign Language. A Comprehensive Dictionary*, New York, Harper and Row.

Sykes, J.B. (1976) *The Concise Oxford Dictionary of Current English*, (6th edn) Oxford, Clarendon Press.

Toorn, M.C. v.d. (1982) Book Review. Jansen, F. Syntaktische Konstrukties un gesproken taal. Tijaschnft voor Nederlandse Taal-en Letter Kinde, *98* pp. 234–9.

Tweney, R.D., Heiman, G.W. and Hoemann, H.W. (1977) 'Psychological Processing of Sign Language: Effects of Visual Disruption on Sign Intelligibility,' *Journal of Experimental Psychology*, general, *106*, pp. 225–68.

Uden, A.M.J. van (1968, 1977) *A World of Language for Deaf Children. Part I, Basic Principles. A Maternal Reflective Method*, Lisse, Swets and Zeilinger, BV.

Uden, A.M.J. van (1979/1981) 'Applied Psycholinguistics and the Teacher of the Hearing-Impaired Child', in Mulholland, A. (ed.) *International Symposium on Deafness: Oral Education Today and Tormorrow*, 1979, Washington, DC, 1981, Alexander Graham Bell Association.

Volterra, V., Laudanna, A., Corazza, S. Radutzky, E. and Natale, F. (1984) 'Italian Sign Language: the Order of Elements in the Declarative Sentence', in Loncke, P., Boyes Braem, P. and Lebrun, Y. (eds) *Recent Research on European Sign Languages*, Lisse, Swets and Zeitlinger, pp. 19–48.

Wundt, D. (1908–1911) *Die Sprache. Völkerspsychologie I und II*, Leipzig.

6.4 Tell Me Where is Grammar Bred?: 'Critical Evaluation' or Another Chorus of 'Come Back to Milano'?

William Stokoe (1987)

In a journal like this [i.e. in which this article first appeared] a review article is expected to scrutinize the matter of the book or books reviewed[1] without much attention to the manner—to ask, in this instance, about sign language and deaf people: What is claimed? What is the evidence and how is it presented? To what degree is the claim sustained? Although a review in this vein could not do justice to van Uden's book, I will begin by addressing these questions, then turn to the larger issue.

What is claimed?
The claim is negative and so it is difficult to prove as are all negatives. It amounts, in fact, to denying that, given a proper definition of 'language', there is any such thing as a sign language. The claim is divided according to the subsystems of linguistics; it denies that the signing of deaf people has a true phonology, a morphology and syntax, and a semology or pragmatics. It will therefore be considered first under these headings.

Of phonology?   Chapter 3, 'A "Phonology" of Sign Languages?', ends thus:

> We cannot subscribe to the following theses of amongst others Bellugi and co-workers (1976): 'These . . . systematic formational properties . . . are like the phonemes of spoken language in general arbitrary in terms of meaning,' . . . 'Deaf people do not encode signs in terms of their iconic representational properties,' . . . 'Iconic aspects of signs . . . are entirely disregarded (by the deaf), etc. [closing ''s missing]

> On the contrary, we think that the elements in the signs are mainly aimed at the depiction (not to be understood purely visual, see above) like bricks for a house, lines for a drawing, notes for music, etc. Their structure is basically determined by the content, not by purely functional relationships. They are basically iconic elements . . .
> (van Uden, 1986, p. 51)

This conclusion is reached by an argument that 'the manual deaf' (van Uden's term throughout for deaf people who have not totally abjured signing and become quasi-hearing through oral education) understand and recall signs because of 'the content, especially the imagery content', of all manual signs (p. 51).

[. . .]

The claim that signs are 'basically iconic' used to depict, not to symbolize, can be refuted by a single instance. The anthropologist Hubert Smith's films of deaf singers in a Yucatec Mayan village in Mexico[2] show a sign language entirely uninfluenced by outside signs or signers. This sign language, known and used by all the villagers (but with more or less proficiency according to their relation to deaf persons), has a systematic way of referring to family members. The base sign is made in front of the signer, and if the semantic feature [female] is to be added, the signing hand touches the back of the neck. For 'father' or 'mother' the sign begins with the thumb edge of the horizontal hand touching the upper edge of the brow. For the eldest sibling this sign is made lower; Smith, in a lecture at Gallaudet University (28 January 1987), said and showed in the film that the lowering may be as small as one-half inch. Signs for other siblings (with or without the feminine morpheme) are made lower, of course, some below the signer's face level. This might be support for a theory that signs are simple depictions of stature, except that these signs do not work that way. Instead, the relative position of the sign denotes the birth order of the brother or sister; a tall younger brother is denoted by a lower sign; eldest sister, who may be shorter than any of her brothers, is signed with the highest sibling sign. The system uses signs that are visibly graded along one dimension, but they are morphemes linked to an arbitrary system of ordering; they are not 'mainly aimed at depiction' of height.

The whole chapter, 'A "Phonology" of Sign Languages?' (pp. 39–51) is built on similar misrepresentations. Of the work of Poizner (1981 [*sic*], Poizner *et al.*, 1982), van Uden says, 'the proof cannot be found', (p. 50), that deaf signers and hearing tests subjects process signs differently. To support this denial he uses an example of his own: 'a manual movement running from top to bottom was interpreted by some deaf as an element of FALLING or LIGHTNING, and by some hearing as a vertical line' (p. 50). This has as much pertinence to Poizner's careful research as the assertion that the sound /uw/ is interpreted by some French speakers as 'where' and by others as 'or' but by English speakers as an interjection (Oooh!).

Of morphology? Van Uden says at the end of chapter 5: 'The morphology of the [*sic*] sign language, if this is not artificially influenced, seems extremely poor, particularly in expressing relationship' (p. 60). The seven-page chapter entitled 'Morphology' thus concluded purports to refute all serious treatments of sign morphology, especially the whole last section of Klima and Bellugi's book (1979), which devotes half of its 400 pages to the subject. Van Uden focuses, however, on the central facet of morphology; that is, morphology as it is presented in school grammars. Here too he misunderstands if he does not misrepresent; for example, 'Stokoe (1978) rightly says: "Sign languages do not have the inflectional call-systems of Indo-European and related languages"' (p. 60), intending this statement to support his claim that sign languages are not inflected. What I stated, of course, supports no such conclusion. Noun classes and verb classes in I–E languages are marked both as verbs or nouns and also into sub-classes by differences in the forms affixed to their stems. Even relatively uninflected I–E languages such as English retain elements to show number in nouns and tense in verbs. Sign languages do not have identical or even analogous systems for noun number or verb tense tense, but instead they inflect (i.e. change the base form of the sign, internally and not by affixation) for other kinds of meaning change; for example, adverbial (Klima and Bellugi 1979, pp. 243–71). Sign languages inflect some verbs to incorporate the number ('1' up to '5' or 'many'), but verb number is marked very differently in I–E languages (which add singular, plural, and sometimes dual marking morphemes to a verb stem). Sign languages have inflectional systems but not those of I–E languages: the former alter the performance of the basic sign (using facial change, head or body movement, or hand–arm actions) to inflect; the latter may change an internal vowel, but more regularly add a morphophonemic unit (e.g. -ing, -ed, -s). A further difference is that these rules for inflecting an English verb are obligatory, not optional as sign language rules may seem to be (But see below).

Of syntax?   van Uden claims: 'We cannot accept Bellugi's . . . thesis (Bellugi *et al.*, 1981): "We have found that the American Sign Language is one of the inflective languages of the world, like Navajo and Latin . . ."' (p. 72). This is found at the end of the one and one-half page chapter 6, 'A Resemblance to Latin?'. It ignores, of course, the many well-conducted studies of sign language syntax (see, e.g., Baker and Cokely, 1980. . . . Again my early work is traduced: 'Stokoe (1972, 1978), Schlesinger and Namir (1978) and Crystal and Craig (1978) consequently deny the existence of parts of speech in the Natural sign language used by the deaf, as they are found in spoken languages' (p. 72). The last clause of this incongrously grouped citation hedges against a charge of misrepresentation. Speaking for myself, I stand by the literal statement. Without appeal to the difference between the production of sound and the production of visible bodily actions, 'parts of speech' are differently expressed and differently recognized in signed languages and spoken languages. Furthermore, the term 'parts of speech' begs several of the most important questions linguists can address. Those psycholinguists without sign language competence, however, who set out to discredit sign languages and to find cognitive deficits and linguistic incompetence in deaf persons, will no doubt continue to use antiquated terms and methods to show that sign languages cannot accomplish what familiar (but not all) spoken languages use add-ons to accomplish. To a historian of science, many of the psycholinguistic experiments cited approvingly by van Uden must recall the notorious IQ tests required of immigrants to the United States 60 or so years ago.

Of semiology?   The claim is: 'The informative power of the Natural sign language of the deaf is extremely weak, both with children and adults' (p. 89). Again, to present a detailed examination of van Uden's argument for this conclusion would be beating a dead ass; one experiment will suffice to establish death. Van Uden asks 'Are deaf people able to make clear the difference between subject, direct object and indirect object in their natural sign language . . . ?' To answer, he cites the experiment of I M Schlesinger (1971), showing deaf adults' cartoons and asking for a sign translation of, for example:

> 'the cat throwing the fish to the pig' . . . The result was so pitiful that
> Schlesinger concluded that the Natural sign language of the deaf has no means
> of expressing these important linguistic functions . . . Oleron (1978) repeated
> about the same test as Schlesinger (1970) . . . [Oleron] was able to confirm
> Schlesinger's results . . . and one has to conclude: the French Natural sign
> language has no means either to express clearly enough the difference in
> function of subject, direct object and indirect object.
> (van Uden, 1986, pp. 87ff)

It is no doubt unnecessary to point out that adult deaf people whose primary language is a natural sign language have been giving, sending, throwing and showing things to others all their lives and reporting their and others' similar actions, with no more confusion than occurs in such reporting in any language. It is the experiments and the experimenters and not adult deaf persons and their sign language that must be examined for flaws.

The evidence?   Although only brief examples have been brought forward here, they suffice to characterize the evidence van Uden uses to support his negative thesis. Fair treatment of the literature is to be expected in 'a critical evaluation'. In this book, however, quotations are taken out of context; the conclusions of sign language researchers are alleged to have been overthrown by psychologists who demonstrably do not know any sign language; and the final resort is to authority—the author's own: 'We cannot see any proof in this . . .' (p. 50). 'We cannot subscribe to the following theses . . .' (p. 51). 'I deny the theses . . . that deaf people . . .' (p. 93).

Are claims supported?   Not only is evidence lacking to support denials that signing can be language and that 'the manual deaf' are of normal intelligence, but the tone of the book, perhaps unintentionally, reveals that this negative pleading is expected to fall on deaf ears. Reference has already been made to van Uden's categorical nay-saying. There is also the implication throughout that the author knows 'the manual deaf' and the other kind, and knows what is good for them better than any 'centres which are concerned particularly with research into sign language . . . (p. 13). A few paragraphs later: 'We shall evaluate some researches . . . and come to the conclusion that sign languages of deaf people, at least in their pure forms (i.e., not mixed with verbal elements), cannot be compared with any spoken language . . .' (p. 14).

The language and connotation of 'verbal' here is particularly revealing. In the last parenthesis, van Uden refers, of course, to the peculiar circumstance of adult deaf persons with more or less formal education. They possess not only a sign language, but in the United States and in many countries of Europe (though not in Israel), they have also a long-standing tradition of fingerspelling the words of their nation's official language. They can switch codes and do so, mastering perhaps several (reading, writing, sign language, sign translation of speakers' words, fingerspelling, etc.), but the code used depends on the perceived ability of the person they are communicating with (See Cokely, 1983). American Sign Language also contains a so far undetermined number of signs that have come into it as borrowings from fingerspelled English after undergoing changes imposed by the phonological and morphological rules of ASL. These borrowed words cannot be distinguished by most signers from native (or as van Uden might term them 'Natural') signs (See Battison, 1976). What van Uden is saying in the passage quoted above, however, is that the signs of a natural sign language are simple depictions (iconic or indexic) of meaning (ch. 3), but that signing 'mixed with verbal elements' is not pure signing, because only spoken languages can be 'verbal'.

The whole semiotics, or 'linguistic cosmology' as it were, of van Uden and his ilk begins with a strict dichotomy: Verbal–Non-verbal. This extends throughout their scheme of things; therefore they have a category language, which is spoken, and may be written. Only English, Dutch, French, etc. can belong to this category—can be verbal. Against this they place non-verbal communication, and they include mime, gesture, animal communication, body language, and the signing of 'the manual deaf' in the latter category. This usage of the term 'verbal'—referring only to spoken or written language—signals at once that the user belongs to the school of thought in which the verbal/non-verbal test divides man from all other creatures.

The manner.   Van Uden's theoretical foundations show throughout the book, but he can be commended for being dogmatic and opinionated without being sarcastic. Not as much can be said for Oleron, who contributes the bilingual Preface and is listed sixteen times in van Uden's Index. A typical reference is this:

> Oleron (1972, 1981) and many others found that deaf children and adults were significantly behind in thought processes . . . Oleron looks for the cause particularly in backwardness in language; apart from the difficulties in relations (see below), concepts such as thinness, length etc. are not identified as such in the 'pure' signs.
> (van Uden, 1986, p. 37)

It is worth noting that the earliest work by Oleron listed in 'Literature' (pp. 95–114) dates from another era in the history of sign language research: *'Etudes sur le langage mimique des sourds-muets. I. Les procedes d'expression'*, in *Annee Psychologique*, 1952. At that time the French psychologist had proved to his own satisfaction that the sign language used by deaf persons cannot express abstractions. Introducing van Uden's book 35 years later, he writes:

[. . .]

> Dr. van Uden here presents a work of primary importance to all who want to get a better idea of Sign Languages of the Deaf.
>
> It is essentially a criticial study. Numerous publications, mainly American ones but widely disseminated elsewhere, have appeared in the last fifteen years,—some by authors who have based their renown in this simple reproduction, resulting in the development of incorrect ideas about this language. These ideas have met with undoubted success, thanks to their repetition and to diffusion by means close to propaganda, and also by their resorting to scientific-type methods in collecting and analysing the observations. Hence the importance of examining them critically, and of indicating why, and in what respects, they are not valid.

This kind of innuendo at the front hardly encourages serious consideration of the eighty-four pages that follow, even as it signals the desperation of those who would like to turn back the clock and calendar—how far? Oleron and van Uden, and other supporters of oralism, were finding 'the manual deaf' defective well before 1960, when the first studies of sign language began to appear. But one suspects that they would like to have had the world stopped in 1880. It was in that year that educators promoting oralism and meeting in Milan shouted, *'Viva la parola!'* and decreed that sign language, as a dreaded interference with their methods of teaching the deaf, would no longer be tolerated.

Notes

1   Van Uden, Rev. Dr A. (1986) *Sign Language used by Deaf People, and Psycholinguistics: A Critical Evaluation*, Lisse, Swets and Zeitlinger.

2   In the Human Studies Film Archives, Natural history Bld. RE-207, Smithsonian Institute, Washington, DC 20560.

References

Baker, C. and Cokely, D. (1980) *American Sign Language* (4-vol. series), Silver Spring, MD, T.J. Publishers.

Battison, R. and I.K. Jordan (1976) 'Cross-cultural Communication with Foreign Signers', *Fact and Fancy, Sign Language Studies, 10*, pp. 53–88.

Bellugi, U., Klima, E. and Siple, P. (1975) 'Remembering in Signs', *Cognition, 3,* pp. 93–125.

[Bellugi *et al.* (1981). This does not appear in van Uden's bibliography, but the quotation cited thus is from]:
Bellugi, U. (1980) 'Clues from the Similarities Between Signed and Spoken Languages, in Bellugi, U. and Studdert-Kennedy (eds) *Signed and Spoken Languages: Biological Constraints on Linguistic Form,* Weinheim, Verlag Chemie, pp. 115–40.

Cokely, D. (1983) 'When is a Pidgin not a Pidgin? An Alternate Analysis of the ASL English Contact Situation', *Sign Language Studies, 38,* 1–24.

Crystal, D. and Craig, E. (1978) 'Contrived Sign Language', in Schlesinger, I. and Namir (eds) *Sign Language of the Deaf: Psychological, Linguistic and Sociological Perspectives,* New York, Academic Press, pp. 14–68.

Klima, E. and Bellugi, U. (1979) *The Signs of Language,* Cambridge, MA, Harvard University Press.

[Poizner 1981 also does not appear in van Uden's bibliography, but the reference may be to]:
Poizner, H. (1982) 'Visual and Phonetic coding of movement: Evidence from ASL', *Science, 212,* pp. 691-3.

Schlesinger, I.M. (1971) 'The Grammar of Sign Language and the Problems of Language Universals', in Morton (ed.) *Biological and Social Factors in Psycholinguistics,* London, Logos Press, pp. 98–121.

Schlesinger, I.M. and Namir, I.L. (eds) (1978) *Sign Language of the Deaf: Psychological, Linguistic and Sociological Perspectives,* New York, Academic Press.

Stokoe, W. (1978) 'Problems in Sign Language Research', in above, pp. 365–78.

6.5 What Sign Language Research Can Teach Us About Language Acquisition

Virginia Volterra (1986)

Introduction

Twenty-five years ago when research on gestural communication used among the deaf began, the main goal was to show that SL (in particular ASL) used by the deaf community could be defined as a language. As a consequence the effort of the first developmental researchers was to show that acquiring a SL (ASL) could offer all the advantages of acquiring a language, and in some cases even more. For example, the first studies considering age of acquisition of the very early 'signs' have reported that first signs emerged significantly earlier than first words. But overall in research conducted on SL acquisition from 1965 to 1975 (considering the particular handshapes used by deaf children, the first semantic relations expressed, etc.) the main goal was to demonstrate similarities to acquisition of spoken languages. In the last 5 years, together with new investigations of SL morphology and syntax and with a growing interest in the study of other SL's, the perspective has completely changed. As Margaret Deuchar (1985) has written 'the time has now come, for the results of SL research to feed back into linguistic theory'. At the present time, research on SL acquisition and more generally on deaf children's linguistic development can throw new light on many of the basic questions regarding language acquisition, helping us to clarify our notions of the general factors influencing such an acquisition. Comparison of the acquisition of various SLs with the acquisition of various spoken languages may help to delineate those aspects of acquisition which are universal over languages in general and those aspects which may prove to be specific to modality. In the following pages I will consider four general areas to which SL research has already brought interesting clarifications and might bring even better understanding in the future.

1   The role of inconicity in acquisition of language.

2   The transition from the prelinguistic to the linguistic period.

3   The fundamental sequence of language development and its timing.

4   The relevance of linguistic input and age of exposure for subsequent linguistic development.

Considering these four topics I will try to show some peculiarities of

European research in respect of the research conducted in the United States [. . .]

Iconicity

Unlike spoken languages a certain degree of iconicity is present in sign languages. Some iconic characteristics remain in the language despite their significant historical modification and grammaticalization. It is possible to perceive a relationship between the sign and its referent. The visual form of many signs resembles in some way that of their referents. At the same time each SL could chose to conventionalize in an arbitrary way a particular different iconic relationship (see for example the different signs for TREE). In SLs a certain degree of iconicity co-exists with one of the fundamental features of a language: arbitrariness. The question that immediately arises is: Does this type of iconicity play a role in acquisition?

Brown (1980) has shown in a very elegant way that inconicity does play a role in the acquisition of individual signs by older hearing children and adults. But the question still remains open as to whether iconicity plays a role in the acquisition of a SL as a native language by infants. If infants acquiring a SL would exploit the particular iconicity of the language, this could be taken as evidence of a more facilitating effect of iconicity in the acquisition of languages in general. Extensive evidence has been reported from various sources showing that this is not the case. The early signs of infants acquiring ASL as a native language are not particularly iconic. According to Bonvillian *et al.* (1983), only one third of the early signed vocabulary could be considered iconic. The earliest signs of children learning SL refer to the same referents of earliest words of children learning a variety of spoken languages: MILK, DOG, MOMMY, DADDY. Furthermore, what iconicity might be available to the young child in a sign like MILK in ASL, even if it is considered iconic by an adult? As Penny Boyes Braem has pointed out [Braem (1986)] iconicity ('the perceived relationship between the sign and its referent') depends on the knowledge of linguistic code, cultural background, etc. and consequently on age.

According to Pizzuto (1980; 1985) and Petitto (1983; 1985) the use of the pointing gesture (apparently more 'iconic' than personal pronouns in spoken languages) does not facilitate the mastering of the SL pronominal systems (see the following). Other researchers have pointed out that in the two-word stage, the dative relation emerges relatively late (as in children acquiring spoken language) even if the expression of the dative in SLs could be considered highly iconic. In a similar way Supalla (1982) reports that children produce errors in the acquisition of complex verbs of motion, despite the fact that these complex forms are highly iconic when viewed holistically. All this evidence taken together shows that iconicity does not have a facilitating effect on acquisition of SL as a native language by infants. As a consequence, many interpretations or explanations concerning acquisition of spoken languages must now be reconsidered.

Children seem to pay particular attention to the actions or functions of objects which are products of these children's activities carried out by themselves or in their interaction with adults. They use actions as a kind of recognitory label for the object. For example, the action to bring the telephone to the ear becomes a gesture that stands for or represents the telephone. It does not mean that the child exploits the iconicity of this gesture with respect to the phone. Simply, he uses the action more frequently associated to the object in the same way he could use the word 'hello' to label the phone, the word more frequently associated to that object.

The very first gestures or onomatopoeic words are adopted by children acquiring spoken languages not because of their iconicity but instead because they are the more 'simple' label associated with certain object or events. 'Simple' here means easier to reproduce according to the motor or vocal development of the children. This last point brings us to introduce the second topic: the transition from the prelinguistic to the linguistic period.

The transition from prelinguistic to linguistic period

It has been reported by many researchers (Schlesinger and Meadow, 1972; McIntire, 1977; Prinz and Prinz, 1979; Bonvillian *et al.*, 1985) that children acquiring SL produce their first signs (around 5–7 months) much earlier than hearing children produce words. This apparent sign advantage looks very 'strange' given the fact that none of the subsequent milestones are earlier in SL acquisition than in speech (as we will see in the following pages). In fact, if we look more carefully at the data reported by various researchers, we can suggest some alternative interpretations. First, it has been claimed that hearing children use gestures as a kind of prelinguistic communication before acquiring language and using words (Bates *et al.*, 1979). If we compare the production of the so-called first 'signs' of children acquiring SL with the production of what we call first 'gestures' in children acquiring spoken language, the difference in timing tends to disappear (for a detailed comparison see Caselli, 1983). Secondly, what researchers have called 'signs' has only a vague resemblance to the signs used by adults and are produced by infants only as imitative routines or in high ritualized contexts. In fact, if the same criteria are applied to define the first 'signs' and the first 'words' respectively, they tend to appear around the same time after passing through a similar decontextualization process (Volterra and Caselli 1985a).

In the past, we have had the tendency to consider gestures in hearing children as communicative but not linguistic, or as symbolic but not communicative. In contrast, gestures in deaf children were considered from the very beginning to be linguistic symbols. This is, we think, the source of the confusion about 'precocious signs'. In sign language acquisition, as in spoken language acquisition, we must distinguish a prelinguistic period from a true linguistic period. The fact that both could be expressed in the same modality must not obscure the distinction. A careful analysis of this transition in deaf children acquiring SL has brought us to a better understanding of the same phenomenon in the acquisition of spoken languages and of the role of gestural modality. Deaf children can use gestures in a very contextualized way, not yet as true symbols; and on the other side, hearing children can use gestures also as symbolic labels in the same way they use words. The gestural modality is exploited by infants acquiring spoken languages because it is used in the environment and the infant is not yet capable of distinguishing linguistic input from other types of input (communicative but not linguistic).

Our belief is that the 'sign advantage' observed in children exposed to a sign language does not reflect a true advantage in linguistic development but only an advantage of gestural modality in communicative prelinguistic development, the same phenomenon observed in children exposed to a spoken language. There is a slight preference for the gestural modality in the communicative prelinguistic period. One possible explanation is that the articulation with the hand which is temporally slower than the one with the tongue could offer greater perspicuity to the infant learner of gestures than the one who learns through words. However, in the following linguistic period there is equipotentiality between gestural and vocal modalities, the final choice depending on the modality in which linguistic input is offered to the child (Volterra and Caselli, 1985b).

In short, the transition from the prelinguistic to the linguistic period is constrained by deeper cognitive and linguistic factors and not by factors related to modality.

The sequence of language development and its timing

The data on SL acquisition have been collected for the most part in the United States. It has been particularly difficult to collect such data in European countries (for few exceptions see Ahlgren, 1981; Caselli *et al.*, 1984) mainly for two reasons:

— We did not have enough detailed knowledge of the structure of the SL used by the deaf parents.
— Deaf parents have often been persuaded to withhold SL from their children. Influenced by a strong oralistic tradition, they are often afraid that the use of SL could prevent their children from learning to speak.

Because of this situation, we will refer here primarily to data on acquisition of ASL (see in particular Newport and Meier, 1986).

The fundamental stages of SL language acquisition are the same and also the timing of milestones corresponds fairly well to their counterparts in spoken language acquisition. It has been reported that, as in the acquisition of spoken languages, infants acquiring SL 'babble' prior to the time of producing the first recognizable signs. They produce sequences of gestures which phonologically resemble signing (Prinz and Prinz, 1979; Maestas y Moores, 1980). Further research is needed in order to discover if this sign babbling is phonologically restricted to those forms which are possible in SLs generally or in the particular SL the children are exposed to.

As in spoken languages, language use begins with a one word stage. For several months, children produce gestures and later signs in isolation one at a time. Formationally the early lexical signs are uninflected citation forms. Furthermore, there are phonological errors characteristic of young children: in handshapes (unmarked simpler handshapes are substituting marked ones), in contact (they often use contact for signs in neutral space or replace one contact with an other), in movement (simultaneous movement often replaces alternating movement). Around the middle of the second year young children begin to produce two or more sign-utterances. The range of semantic relations expressed is as in spoken languages at the comparable time, and they emerge in about the same order: existence, action on objects, locative relations and, later, recipients, instruments, causes and manners of action. These first combinations have the same characteristics as telegraphic speech: no use of morphology; the signs are not marked by the adult inflectional devices. The few inflected forms used are unanalysed and unproductive. According to Hoffmeister and Wilbur (1980), young signing children tend to use word order prior to inflections and to maintain it for some time despite the fact that SLs seem to show considerable word order flexibility. With regard to negation in ASL, as in English acquisition the young child first acquires a single negative form which is used quite differently than in the adult language; only later is a range of more specific negatives acquired and used in their correct sentence internal positions (Newport and Meier, 1986). As for personal pronouns, which in SLs involve pointing to the addressee, studies by Pizzuto, and more extensively by Petitto, have shown a developmental schedule and types of errors which are similar to those of the acquisition of spoken language. Despite their apparent transparency in SLs, the formational aspects of these personal pronouns are the same as pointing gestures of hearing infants. According to Petitto (1983), non-linguistic pointing first occurs in deaf children at approximately 10 months of age as it is reported in hearing children. The child points at objects and persons, in the environment, but not to himself. Personal pronouns emerge at approximately 18 months with the first person pronoun (I or ME) produced first. Pointing at self begins at the same time as the first person pronoun is produced by hearing children. Proper names are often used instead of pronouns. Around 24 months a reversal error could occur, with *you* used to mean the child himself. By 27 months all the pronouns are used correctly.

According to Newport and Meier, acquisition of morphology begins at 2½/3 years and continues well beyond 5 years. A similar pattern of acquisition occurs across all the morphological subsystems: in the earliest stages, morphology is omitted entirely (uninflected citation forms or unalysed amalgams occur). In a subsequent period some of the morphemes are produced while others are omitted. There is a third period in which all of the morphemes are produced but sequentially rather than simultaneously. Finally, for subsystems where many morphemes are required, the production of fully correct forms occurs after age 5 (for example, errors on the morphemes of complex verbs of motion continue as late as at age 7 or

8). Once again it appears that the use of a different modality does not affect the course of acquisition of the linguistic system. The same cognitive and/or linguistic constraints seem to influence stages of acquisition.

Furthermore, the sequence of development in sign language acquisition makes us better understand some data on morphology acquisition in spoken languages. Slobin has reported that agglutinating morphology of Turkish where morphemes are syllabic, stressed and highly regular is acquired very early, for the most part prior to 2 years. Sign language agglutinating morphology, however, is acquired relatively late. What makes morphology of Turkish easier for children to acquire is that (as Newport and Meier underline) it is agglutinative but sequential. By contrast, the morphology of ASL is agglutinative but produced simultaneously. In fact errors made in the process of acquiring ASL morphology included sequentialization of morphemes which should be produced simultaneously.

The relevance of linguistic input and age of exposure for linguistic development

It has been stated that there is a critical period for the acquisition of language, and that the timing of linguistic input has a clear effect on the child's acquisition of language. But obviously research on language acquisition under conditions of no or limited input can be conducted very rarely. Deprivation manipulations of the linguistic environment cannot be performed deliberately. The case of Genie (Curtiss, 1977) is one of the few recent examples, but in this circumstance language was only one of many human factors missing. However, in the case of deaf children, hearing loss can create atypical language learning conditions, apart from other circumstances. Thus, deaf children could become 'exceptional situations' or 'experiments of nature'. The study of their linguistic development can be extremely relevant in order to understand better the relationship between early exposure and native fluency in a language.

Within the deaf community there is a number of individuals who are not effectively exposed to a conventional language until school age or even later. The majority of deaf children learn SL without input from the parents. They will first be exposed to SL at variable times, when they happen to meet other signers. In the past the first exposure tended to be at school age, from the other children, a small minority of whom had learned SL from their parents. Teachers did not sign, so the children might receive no adult signing input at school. Furthermore, these children also received spoken input quite late, when vocal training began in the school period. The question is: how do these SL users organize and process language in adulthood after having acquired it late from a limited input? The answer to this question can throw light on the significance of linguistic input and age of learning in language acquisition. In fact, Newport and Supalla have observed important differences between native and non-native ASL signers: non-native learners do not achieve the same levels of fluency in ASL. especially in the use of complex morphology. Those differences could be due either to age of exposure to the language or to the reduced input or both.

More recently the situation has changed in many respects. The shift in favour of introducing SL at an early age is due to many different reasons:

1   The acceptance of SL as a genuine language with the structural complexity and expressive potential of spoken languages.

2   The observation that some deaf individuals achieve little usable language after years of oral education and lipreading.

3   The other social, psychological and cognitive problems that can occur as a consequence of the lack of communicative interaction between the child and his parents and peers.

At the present time in many European countries there is a tendency to expose deaf children from the very first diagnosis of deafness to both spoken and signed input. This exposure can be realized in many different ways which are difficult to define and classify. Here, in order to clarify the situation, we will make an important distinction between *bilingual* and *bimodal* exposure. I will call *bilingual* the situation in which the deaf child is exposed to the two inputs in separate settings or from separate sources. I will call *bimodal* the situation in which the deaf child is exposed in the same setting and from the same source to both inputs. In the first case (the bilingual situation) the child is really exposed to two languages—one spoken language and one sign language. In the second case (the bimodal situation) the child is in fact exposed to only one language (signed or spoken) to which the other mode tends to be used as a support. In fact when a person signs and speaks at the same time he uses one of the two languages or a kind of pidgin language. Even in those oralist cases when the choice to offer both inputs to the child is not made, and deaf children receive intensive and formal training in spoken language, bimodal input prevails. In real life, that is in everyday communication, parents and teachers do in fact use unconscious gesturing with deaf children. In studies of 'home sign' by Goldin-Meadow *et al* (1979; 1982; 1984), the parents have chosen the oral approach; but it is clear from the data that mothers adopt informal supplementary gestures with their children.

In all those situations the question becomes: how much and by which strategies can deaf children make use of the limited gestural input or the limited oral input to which they are exposed from the early years? Just how little language input is sufficient to activate the child's linguistic creativity? Various studies (Ahlgren, 1981; Goldin-Meadow and Mylander, 1984; Volterra *et al.*, 1983; Pereira, 1985; Mohay, 1982) have recently shown (despite their different interpretations of data) that deaf children can go well beyond the information given to them in gestural modality, which indicates their inductive power. Unfortunately, we have at present very little or no information about the early progress of deaf children in oral languages. For example, researchers report no testing of the children's comprehension of spoken language. But the shift away from exclusively oral education and in favour of introducing SL at an early age makes it even more interesting to study the process by which they acquire oral language especially when they do this prior to formal schooling. One of Goldin-Meadow and Mylander's critical premises is that because their subjects are deaf they can make no use of the oral input to which they are exposed; this is not true, as the other studies above mentioned have reported. It becomes extremely relevant at this point to know more precisely how much of the mother's integrated speech and gesture system is taken in by their deaf children. What is the child's contribution to language learning? How much is innate and how much depends on a model? How much is original with the children? How much is derived from the spoken language and transferred to the gestural mode or, vice versa, borrowed from gestural input and transferred to spoken production?

Human children are active and creative participants in the language acquisition process and they go well beyond the data to construct successive theories of their language. Deaf children give us a unique opportunity to study this capacity.

References

Ahlgren, I. (1981) 'Parental Input and Sign Language Aquisition in Deaf Children', paper presented at the *Second International Symposium on Sign Language Research*, Bristol.

Bates, E., Benigni, L., Bretherton, I., Camaioni, L. and Volterra, V. (1979) *The Emergence of Symbols: Cognition and Communication in Infancy,* New York, Academic Press.

Bonvillian, J.D., Orlansky, M.D. and Novack, L.L. (1983) 'Early Sign Language Acquisition and its Relation to Cognitive and Motor Development', in Kyle, J. and Woll, B. (eds) *Language in Sign: An International Perspective on Sign Language,* London, Croom Helm.

Bonvillian, J.D. Orlansky, M.D., Novack, L.L., Folven, R.J. and Holley-Wilcox, P. (1985) 'Language Cognition and Cherological Development. The First Steps in Sign Language Aquisition', in Stokoe, W. and Volterra, V. (eds) SLR '83. *Proceedings of the III International Symposium on Sign Language Research,* Silver Spring, MD Linstok Press, and Rome, Instituto di Psicologia CNR.

Braem, P. Boyes (1986) 'Two Aspects of Psycholinguistic Research: Iconicity/Temporal Structure', in Tervoort, B.T. (ed.) *Signs of Life, Proceedings of the Second European Congress on Sign Language Research,* The Institute of General Linguistics of the University of Amsterdam, publication number 50.

Brown, R. (1980) 'Why are Sign Languages Easier to Learn than Spoken Languages?', keynote address presented at the *National Symposium on Sign Language Research and Teaching,* Chicago. Published in Stokoe, W.C. (ed.) *Proceedings of the First National Symposium of Sign Language Research and Teaching,* Washington, DC, National Association of the Deaf.

Caselli, M.C. (1983) 'Communications to Language: Deaf and Hearing Children's Development Compared', *Sign Language Studies, 39.*

Caselli, M.C., Ossella, T. and Volterra, V. (1984) 'Sign and Vocal Language Aquisition by two Italian Deaf Children of Deaf Parents', in Loncke, F., Boyes-Braem, P. and Lebrun, Y. (eds) *Recent Research on European Sign Languages,* Lisse, Swetz and Zettlinger.

Curtiss, S. (1977) *Genie: A Psycholinguistic Study of a Modern-Day 'Wild Child',* New York, Academic Press.

Deuchar, M. (1985) 'Implications of Sign Language Research for Linguistic Theory', in Stokoe, W. and Volterra, V. (eds) SLR 83, *Proceedings of the III International Symposium of Sign Language Research,* Silver Spring, MD, Linstok Press and Rome, Instituto di Psicologia CNR.

Goldin-Meadow, S. (1979) 'Structure in a Manual Communication Sytem Without a Conventional Language Model', in Whittaker, H. and Whittaker, H.A. (eds) *Studies in Neurolinguistics,* New York, Academic Press.

Goldin-Meadow, S. (1982) 'The Resilience of Recursion', in Wanner, E. and Gleitman, L.R. (eds) *Language Acquisition: The State of the Art,* New York, Academic Press.

Goldin-Meadow, S. and Mylander, C. (1984) 'Gestural Communication in Deaf Children: The Effects and Non-Effects of Parental Input on Early Language Development', *Child Development Monographs, 49.*

Hoffmeister, R.J. and Wilbur, R. (1980) 'Developmental: The Acquisition of Sign Language', in Lane, H. and Grosjean, F. (eds) *Recent Perspectives on American Sign Language,* Hillsdale, NJ, Lawrence, Erlbaum Associates.

Maestas y Moores, J. (1980) 'Early Linguistic Environment: Interactions of Deaf Parents with their Infants', *Sign Language Studies, 26.*

McIntire, M. (1977) 'The Acquisition of ASL Hand Configurations', *Sign Language Studies, 16.*

Mohay, H. (1982) 'A Preliminary Description of the Communication System Evolved by Two Deaf Children in the Absence of a Sign Language Model', *Sign Language Studies, 34.*

Newport, E. and Meier, R. (1986) 'Acquisition of American Sign Language' in Slobin, D. (ed.) *The Cross Linguistic Study of Language Acquisition,* Hillsdale NJ, Lawrence Erlbaum Associates.

Pereira, M.C. (1985) 'An Interactional Approach in the Study of Gestural Communications in Hearing-Impaired Children', in Stokoe, W. and Volterra, V. (eds) SLR '83, *Proceedings of the III International Symposium on Sign Language Research,* Silver Spring, MD, Linstok Press and Rome, Instituto di Psicologia CNR.

Petitto, L.A. (1983) *From Gesture to Symbol: The Relationship Between*

Form and Meaning in the Aquisition of Personal Pronouns in American Sign Language, unpublished Doctoral Dissertation, Harvard University.

Petitto, L.A. (1985) 'From Gesture to Symbol: the Relationship of Form to Meaning in ASL Personal Pronoun Acquisition', in Stokoe, W. and Volterra, V. (eds) SLR '83, *Proceedings of the III International Symposium of Sign Language Research,* Silver Spring, MD Linstok Press, and Rome, Instituto di Psicologia CNR.

Pizzuto, E. (1980) *Indexes of Various Types in ASL Acquisition,* working paper, The Salk Institute, La Jolla, California.

Pizzuto, E, (1985) 'Sign Language Iconic-Indexical Features and Language Learning Processes', in Stokoe, W. and Volterra, V. (eds) SLR'83, *Proceedings of the III International Symposium of Sign Language Research,* Silver Spring, MD, Linstok Press, and Rome, instituto di Psicologia CNR.

Prinz, P. and Prinz, E. (1979) 'Simultaneous Acquisition of ASL and Spoken English in a Hearing Child of a Deaf Mother and Hearing Father', *Sign Language Studies, 25.*

Schlesinger, H.S. and Meadow, K.P. (1972) *Sound and Sign: Childhood Deafness and Mental Health,* Berkeley, CA, University of California Press.

Supalla, T. (1982) *Structure and Acquisition of verbs of Motion and Location in American Sign Language,* unpublished Doctoral Dissertation, University of California, San Diego.

Volterra, V. and Caselli, M.C. (1985a) 'From Gestures and Vocalisations to Signs and Words', in Stokoe, W. and Volterra, V. (eds) SLR '83 *Proceedings of the III International Symposium of Sign Language Research,* Silver Spring,, MD Linstok Press and Rome, Instituto di Psicologia CNR.

Volterra, V. and Caselli, M.C. (1985b) *First Stage of Language Acquisition Through Two Modalities in Deaf and Hearing Children,* paper presented at the SRCD Meeting, Toronto.

Volterra, C., Massoni, P. and Beranesi, S. (1983) 'Quando Communicazione Diventa Lingugaggio?' in Attilli and Ricci-Bitti (eds) *I Gesti e i Segni,* Rome, Bulzoni.

6.6 A Stimulus to Learning, A Measure of Ability

T. Stewart Simpson* (1990)

Prior to 1982 a national system of training and examinations in sign language did not exist. Sign language classes offered in Centres for the Deaf were few, aimless and usually of short duration. It is an indictment of past provision that there are still specialist social workers who cannot communicate with their clients, and 'interpreters' who cannot interpret. This was not always so.

Until the early 1970s, the Deaf Welfare Examining Board (DWEB) had, for some 50 years, supervised in-service training and examined candidates in sign language interpreting as part of the Board's Certificate and Diploma examinations for missioner/welfare officers to the deaf. This earlier provision required the trainee missioner/welfare officers to spend much of their time in the company of, and interpreting for, deaf people, with a consequential emphasis on good communication/interpreting skills (Lysons, 1977). The missioner/welfare officer's function was wide ranging and in common with prevailing attitudes—which would now be regarded as paternalistic. As such, the major emphasis was on the welfare rather than on developing the potential of deaf people. Even so, this limited provision remained virtually without parallel in any other country throughout the entire life of the DWEB.

Demise of the DWEB was brought about by implementation of the Younghusband Report[1] and the Seebohm Report[2] which, by the early 1970s initiated a rapid transition to generic full-time training and qualifications, with many of the specialist missions and their workers being brought into the generic social service departments. Though attempts were made to ensure continuance of specialist training, henceforth the required professional qualification for all social workers was the Certificate of Qualification in Social Work (CQSW). Subsequent provision of post-qualifying courses for Social Workers with Deaf people—at North London Polytechnic and Moray House College of Education—had difficulty in recruiting students.

In effect, the introduction of full-time generic social work training was not only instrumental in closing down specialist training for social work with deaf people, it diminished the value of specialist work with deaf people and destroyed one, albeit restricted, national system of training and examinations in sign language.

*Council for the Advancement of Communication with Deaf People.

Elsewhere, particularly in the USA research into sign language, the influence of Gallaudet[3]—and its proximity to and close links with the Capitol—as well as the aspirations of deaf people, provided a catalyst for change which culminated in the 1973 Rehabilitation Act.[4] This far-reaching piece of legislation provided for the equal rights and opportunities of disabled people. One of its effects was to ensure the payment of interpreters, as well as to boost substantially the training of sign language interpreters and provide for the formation of a Register of Interpreters.

Aware of developments in North America, and actively conscious of declining specialist provision in the UK, there was widespread concern amongst individuals and organizations concerned with and for prelingually profoundly deaf people. It was argued that the number of competent sign language interpreters was declining at a time when deaf people were seeking greater educational, economic and social opportunities. Against this background, in 1976 the British Deaf Association (BDA) applied to the Department of Health and Social Security (DHSS) for funding to develop communication skills. The application was for a grant which would:

1   Encourage interested people in the community and particularly those concerned with health and social services, to acquire some skill in communicating with the deaf.

2   Set up training centres to enable those already possessing communication skills to qualify as interpreters, and to this end to set up a Registry of Interpreters.[5]

Grant aid for a 3-year project-known as the BDA/DHSS Communication Skills Project—was awarded in April 1977. The post of Consultant Director was taken up by Willard J. Madsen, an Associate Professor and former Director of Sign Language Programmes at Gallaudet College, Washington, who remained with the Project until early 1978. He brought to the Project a wealth of material and experience on the training and assessment of interpreters in America.

At an exploratory meeting of prominent deaf people and leading sign language interpreters held in September 1977, it was agreed to establish the Standing Conference of Interpreter Trainers (SCIT).[6] From this initial meeting the SCIT focused on interpreter training/assessment and membership of the Registry of Interpreters to almost a total exclusion of the Project's other major aim. With benefit of hindsight, the SCIT was seduced by the promise of an interpreting service and failed to recognize that American achievements stemmed from active lobbying and legislation.[7]

In attempting to ensure minimum standards of competence, the SCIT agreed that entry to the Registry of Interpreters would be only by those who had satisfactorily completed the assessment. This was not acceptable to some DWEB Certificate and Diploma holders who already held an 'interpreting qualification' and who argued they had been interpreting satisfactorily for many years. Also they, and some members of the SCIT, expressed disquiet about the examination format which gave entry to the Register. This anxiety was exacerbated by lack of formal representation of interested organizations, for, although the SCIT comprised eminent individuals, it did not include official representation of national organizations. As a consequence, the National Council for Social Workers with the Deaf—whose members provided most interpreting services in formal settings—withdrew their support from the Project until such time as there had been satisfactory consultation (Simpson, 1980).

In May 1979 a new director was appointed and, at meetings of the Standing Conference of Interpreter Trainers, gained agreement on the need for an independent review of assessment procedures together with the involvement of all interested organizations. An independent review by a team of academics helped restore confidence in the Project and, at subsequent meetings, led to formation in December 1980 of the Council for the Advancement of Communication with Deaf People (Simpson, 1981).

The inaugural meeting agreed a Constitution allowing two representatives from each of the member organizations, at least one of whom should be deaf. This involvement of deaf people as equal partners was a major platform of the Communication Skills Project. Whilst commonplace in the 1990s, it was innovative in the 1970s when hearing people controlled, or were dominant on, the executive committees of virtually all national organizations. There were twelve founding member organizations of the Council. By 1981 the Registry of Interpreters had been established by giving interpreter status to holders of the DWEB's Certificate and Diploma. Their membership of the Register was for a period of 5 years by which time DWEB holders were expected to take CACDP's examination if they wished to remain as members of the Register. Recognizing that there were a number of experienced and competent interpreters—mainly Social Workers with Deaf people—who did not hold DWEB qualifications in 1981 CACDP introduced training courses for 'interpreters of known ability' and initially sought out their involvement to ensure the Register's success (Simpson, 1981).

In Scotland, the Scottish Association for the Deaf (SAD)—and later the Scottish Association of Interpreters for the Deaf (SAID)—frustrated by the Communication Skills Project's early attempts to establish a Register, had developed a three stage scheme of training and examinations in Sign Communication Skills,[8] and played a major part in forming CACDP. It was agreed that this scheme be adopted for use by CACDP in England, Wales and Northern Ireland.

Until the Project ended in December 1981, CACDP was based in the BDA's headquarters in Carlisle. On becoming independent, CACDP's staff (then a director and part-time secretary) ran the organization from a number of temporary addresses, returning to the BDA in 1983 before moving to its present address in the University of Durham in January 1985. The move had long been advocated for a number of reasons: first, CACDP was committed to the improvement of all communication skills, not just sign language. By April 1984, eighteen organizations were members of

CACDP, not all of whom preferred sign language as a means of communication. Some of the new members were interested in developing communication with deaf-blind people, or in the provision of lip-speakers. As such, given the historical differences between the member organizations and the range of communications needs, it was important that CACDP be impartial, and be seen to be impartial, in the development of communication skills—a policy difficult to sustain when based in an organization promoting a single means of communication. Second, until recently, sign language and other means of deaf communication has had relatively low status. Basing CACDP in an educational establishment compensated for this and recognition of its qualifications was more easily achieved. There was an added advantage in having training facilities—including residential accommodation—close to the organization's administration. The choice of Durham was relatively easy for, apart from the Open University, it was the only university providing a full-time service for hearing-impaired students, as well as having research interests in deaf studies.

Whilst the DHSS provided annual starter finance from 1982, it was not until 1984 that CACDP received a 3-year grant of £40,000 a year. With greater support from the Government, and member organizations' support, CACDP was able to employ a full-time development officer and, as its work continued to grow, additional office staff.[9]

The DHSS grant was awarded on the understanding that CACDP would look to member organizations and other sources for continued funding. Most member organizations did not raise sufficient funds to support their own objectives, let alone those of CACDP. Of the few which did, it was unfortunate that the largest donor in the year ending 31 March 1987, suddenly changed its policy of awarding grants and ceased providing financial support for CACDP. This withdrawal of support did not go unnoticed when DHSS consideration was given to CACDP's application for continued and enhanced funding as from April 1987:[10] the application, subject to considerable delay and subsequently described as 'totally unrealistic', was followed by an offer of £40,000 for one year only. Under these circumstances CACDP could not continue. Examinations were cancelled, staff were warned of impending closure, and there followed a campaign to save CACDP, with strong support from the 'Panel of Four'. In essence, the DHSS argued that member organizations should fund CACDP, whilst they in turn argued that funding should come from central Government.[11] Both sides wished to see CACDP continue but neither was prepared to fund it.

Prompted by coverage on the BBC Television News of the imminent demise of CACDP, a private benefactor donated £100,000 'for CACDP's good work to continue'. Continue it did, until the financial year commencing April 1988, when the DHSS awarded CACDP a grant of £60,000 a year for 3 years, and there was increased recognition of its work.[12]

Funding remains an overriding problem for CACDP. Most examination boards are financed from fees and CACDP's examination fees are comparable with those of other examining boards, but it is unable to derive sufficient income from its examinations. There are two main reasons: high costs and relatively small numbers. Unlike most examinations—which are written—there is a basic requirement for examiners and candidates to meet face-to-face. In addition, the need to use both deaf and hearing examiners, and to recruit nationally (thus involving travel and accommodation costs) adds to the expenditure. Leaving aside the higher costs of its examinations, the relatively small number of candidates (under 3,500) compares with City and Guilds 700,000 and RSA's 600,000 per year.[13]

There is also the added cost of deafness. Since its inception CACDP has involved both deaf and hearing people at every level of activity: as representatives on the Council, as Committee members, as tutors and as examiners. Those who are prelingually, profoundly deaf come from a grouping which has a normal range or intelligence but the majority of whose members left school at the age of 16, with an average reading age of 9 years. The implication of this is best illustrated by comparison with another examining board. For example, the normal requirement of a GCSE 'O' level examiner in, say, French, is that he or she should have an appropriate language degree plus a teaching qualification, followed by 3 years' full-time teaching of the subject area and 10 years' of full-time further/higher education and teaching practice.

The majority (some two-thirds) of CACDP's examiners are deaf, and the overwhelming majority of them left school at the age of 16. Though CACDP selects the most able, they have had little opportunity for further/higher education, and, at this stage of development, none to teach sign language full-time. Preparation of an examiner for French 'O' level is paid for largely by the State, from the age of 16 and over a period of 10 years. By comparison, CACDP has to train its examiners—in days rather than years—from whatever resources are available.

Training, selection and registration of examiners is critical to the fair and efficient conduct of examinations. It is even more so in examinations which are face-to-face, and in which candidates and examiners, moving within a relatively small social framework, may have met previously and even know each other. It is a major weakness in CACDP's development that there has never been sufficient funding to provide adequate training for examiners. In other spheres of education such training is rarely of length for it relies on extensively educated, trained and experienced teachers, a provision not yet available to CACDP. In 1989, with funding from monies provided by the DHSS and the UK Carnegie Trust, CACDP began the long and continuing process of training, selecting and registration of its examiners.[14] There is no doubt that the introduction of a progressive system of training and examinations has stimulated the learning of sign communication, and the trend is one of continuing growth.

It has been suggested that CACDP is solely concerned with signing, and, amongst those who advocate signing, that its interest is in British Sign Language. Whilst recent developments in lip-speaking and in communication with deaf-blind people would appear to deny that charge, it is true that examinations in Sign Communication Skills have increasingly moved towards British Sign Language. This reflects not only a public awareness of the language, it is also related to the demands of deaf people and the organizations who represent them. Recently, some teachers and parents of deaf children have expressed disquiet about such a trend and argued the need for children to develop language skills through the use of Sign Supported English. It is a function of CACDP that it will respond to such needs if they are clearly identifiable, national in character and sustainable.

Of particular importance has been the advocacy of training in colleges of further and higher education. Prior to CACDP, the few sign language classes available took place in Centres for the Deaf—hidden from and unrelated to general provision in tertiary education. Now most sign language classes take place in colleges of further and higher education— thus claiming parity with other subject areas and gaining recognition for the language, the skill and the people who teach it. In addition, CACDP has played a major role in initiating training agency-sponsored full-time communication skills training within such colleges, to provide support services for deaf trainees on its youth and adult training programmes. By 1990, seven colleges were providing up to a year of full-time training for some eighty students.

Overall there has been a continual and rapid growth in the number of candidates taking CACDP examinations in Sign Communication Skills as Table 1 illustrates.

Table 1   Candidates taking sign communication skills assessment 1983–1990

Year ending 31st March	No. of candidates taking sign communication skills			Total no. of candidates
	Stage I	Stage II	Stage III	
1983	188	—	9	197
1984	614	27	25	666
1985	1174	63	22	1259
1986	1506	116	15	1637
1987	1902	218	53	2173
1988	3104	118	46	3268
1989	2404	317	47	2768
1990	2416	488	88	2992

Even the down-turn in candidates entering for the Stage I examinations from 1989 is explained by the introduction of a new and more demanding curriculum and examination format requiring a considerably longer period of learning than previously. At Stage II and Stage III levels the fluctuations reflect not only a shortage of tutors and classes at Intermediate and Advanced levels, but also funding difficulties for students wishing to undergo training, and for CACDP which, at times, has had to restrict or cancel entries. Availability of suitably qualified and confident tutors will remain an impediment to development for some time to come, but the Universities of Bristol and Durham are making considerable progress in the training of tutors and of interpreters.

More recently (from 1985) CACDP has developed training and examinations in communicating with deaf-blind people and, in conjunction with the British Association of the Hard of Hearing (BAHOH), lip-speaking. In both these skill areas the numbers of candidates have grown, and though not comparable with sign communication skills, their provision has undoubtedly stimulated interest and learning.

With the increased awareness of deafness and the needs of deaf people came a recognition of CACDP's qualifications. In particular, local authorities and voluntary organizations employing social workers, teachers and, increasingly, sign language interpreters, recognized the need for a measure of attainment in their employees. Similarly, deaf and hearing consumers of interpreters wished to employ interpreters of a known standard. The Open University Professional Diploma in Social Work with Deaf People emphasizes a need for specialist workers to have a minimum level of skills,[15] a view reinforced by the DHSS Inspectorate's report *Say it Again* (1988).

The Register of Interpreters

Development of a register of qualified sign language interpreters was of paramount importance to the BDA/DHSS Communication Skills Project as it is to CACDP. Competent interpreters provide access to social, educational and economic opportunities—as well as the means of safeguarding the interest of individuals in such fundamentals as health care and justice in the legal system.

Despite rapid growth in the numbers successfully completing sign communication examinations, the Register of Sign Language Interpreters has not yet shown a marked increase in numbers, though the numbers of those passing CACDP's Stage III (Advanced) Certificate in Sign Communication Skills (now the prerequisite for interpreter training) has shown a marked increase (Table 2). Whilst not all who hold this qualification will wish to train as interpreters, there are many who do, given the resources and the opportunity. In part, the figures reflect a decision in 1986 to require specialist training beyond Stage III. It was 1988 before such training and examinations were introduced and—as with so much of CACDP's development—training was limited by costs. With DWEB membership of the Register ending in December 1986, and delays in implementing interpreter training and examinations, the number of interpreters has fallen at a time when demand has risen rapidly. Only recently has the number of qualified interpreters begun to increase, and only recently have more interpreter training opportunities occurred, most notably at the Universities of Bristol and Durham.

Despite the many impediments to progress, CACDP has an impressive record of growth, achievement and recognition. In so doing it has brought together national organizations for a common purpose: the improvement of communication skills.

It has helped relieve the isolation of deafness through the provision of a system by which hearing people can learn to communicate with those who

Table 2   Stage III holders and registered interpreters 1983–1990

Year 31st March	DWEB qualifications	CACDP* qualifications	Total register	Numbers holding Stage III certificate
1983	112	9	121	9
1884	112	18	130	29
1985	90	37	127	44
1986	83	51	134	54
1987	—	62	62	97
1988	—	62	62	137
1989	—	69	69	172
1990	—	70	70	240

*Includes Stage III Holders—Stage III is a prerequisite to taking the interpreting examination.

are deaf, hard of hearing, or deaf-blind—be they friends, neighbours, relatives or work-mates. CACDP has also helped enable specialist social workers and teachers of deaf children to make full use of their professional skills. In addition, It has established a register of qualified interpreters which will provide deaf people with the rights and opportunities available to those who are hearing. Finally, CACDP has provided opportunities for deaf, hard of hearing and deaf-blind people to teach and to examine in communication skills-situations, which give both income and status and which, without CACDP, may not have come so readily.

Notes

1 The Younghusband Working Party was appointed in 1955 to enquire into the proper field of work, recruitment and training of social workers, and in particular, whether there is a place for a general purpose social worker. Its report in 1959 led to setting up The Council for Training in Social Work (now the Central Council for the Education and Training of Social Workers) and the development of full-time generic training in social work.

2 The Seebohm Committee was appointed in 1966 to consider the organization and responsibilities of the local authority social services, and what changes were desirable to secure an effective family service. Its report *Local Authority and Allied Personal Social Services* was published in 1968 and recommended that all major local authorities should have a social services department administering all the various welfare services.

3 Gallaudet College, now Gallaudet University, Washington, DC, founded as a school for deaf (and blind) children in 1857. It became a college for deaf students and was given powers by Congress to award degrees in 1865.

4   Section 504 of the Rehabilitation Act of 1973 provides that: 'no otherwise qualified handicapped individual in the United States . . . shall, solely by reason of his handicap, be excluded from participation in, be denied benefits of, or be subjected to discrimination under any program or activity receiving federal financial assistance'.

5   Application to the Department of Health and Social Security, 1976.

6   Report of the British Deaf Association Conference on Interpreter Training 16–18 September, 1977.

7   See 'Deaf Persons and the Political Process', *Gaullaudet Today,* Fall, 1979.

8   The Training and Certification of Interpreters for the Deaf in Scotland. Report of the Scottish Association for the Deaf, 1979.

9   Annual Report of the Council for the Advancement of Communication with Deaf People for year ending 31 March 1985.

10   Report of the Council for the Advancement of Communication with Deaf People for the two years ending 31 March 1988.

11   Ibid.

12   Annual Report of the Council for the Advancement of Communication with Deaf People for the year ending 31 March 1989.

13   The practical (and possibly prohibitive) effect of a *£10* increase in fees for each candidate theoretically could yield an extra £35,000. With City and Guilds 700,000 entries a *10 pence* increase in fees would yield an extra £70,000.

14   Report on Project to train deaf people to become CACDP examiners in sign communication skills, CACDP, 1989.

15   Stage II is required for the Open University's Professional Diploma in Social Work with Deaf People.

References

Department of Health and Social Services (1988) *Say it Again*, a report on contemporary social work practice with people who are deaf or hard of hearing.

Lysons, K. (1977) 'The Development of Training for Work with Adult Deaf Persons', *British Deaf News*, April and August.

Simpson, T.S. (1980) 'The Development of Communication Skills', *Supplement to British Deaf News*, June.

Simpson, T.S. (1981) 'Council for the Advancement of Communication Skills with Deaf People', *Supplement to British Deaf News,* July.

6.7 British Sign Language Tutor Training Course (Formerly British Sign Language Training Agency, BSLTA, Project[1])

A. Clark Denmark* (1990)

The present interest in the teaching of British Sign Language (BSL) may be traced back to the late 1970s when the British Deaf Association (BDA) established a Communication Skills Project in 1979. One aim of the project was to produce a teaching manual for tutors of BSL. Consultative meetings and workshops were held before and after its publication in 1981. The interest in BSL generated by these meetings, together with that created by sign language research projects at Moray House College of Education (Edinburgh) and the University of Bristol, and the transmission by the BBC of a television series ('See Hear') presented in sign, resulted in a demand for more information on teaching methods and materials appropriate to the teaching of BSL. This was reflected in a significant increase in the number of enquiries received by the BDA from (Deaf) members seeking information on how they might become sign language tutors.

In 1982, the Association carried out a national survey of sign language classes.[2] The survey revealed that only seven of the fifty-seven classes on which information had been received claimed to be teaching BSL; the other fifty were engaged in teaching sign systems based on English (such as Sign Supported English). It also revealed that the tutors engaged in teaching these classes were predominantly hearing tutors. The few Deaf people involved were, for the most part, bilingual Deaf persons with speech. The Association concluded that there was an urgent need to establish introductory BSL classes across the country, where those seeking to learn the language could be certain that it was BSL. Equally important was the need to provide Deaf people with the opportunity to become tutors of BSL. The establishment of a BSL tutor training course for Deaf tutors was seen as a way of addressing both needs. The announcement by the

---

*This paper was prepared in collaboration with David Brien.

BBC that it was to produce a language series aimed at introducing BSL to non-signing hearing people, further confirmed the necessity and urgency of establishing such a training course. The Association was unsuccessful in its initial attempts to create a full-time post to provide such training. The British Sign Language Training Agency (BSLTA) was established to take the project forward. Rather than base the project within the Association, it was decided that it would be more appropriate to locate it within an institution of higher education. This would, it was anticipated, enhance the status of BSL by placing it alongside other languages being studied and taught at university level. It would enable links to be established with other colleges and universities engaged in sign language research as well as language departments engaged in second language teaching and tutor training. The BDA was, at this time, engaged in sponsoring work in the Department of Sociology and Social Policy at the University of Durham. The Department agreed to accept responsibility for the project and it commenced in January 1985.

Aim of the project
The aim of the project was to establish a training course which would enable Deaf users of BSL to become tutors of their own language (at foundation level). The following objectives were identified:

1   To develop a curriculum for a foundation level BSL tutor training course for Deaf tutors.

2   To establish a tutor training course based on the above curriculum: the course to be taught in BSL by the Deaf staff member(s) of the project team.

3   To devise an appropriate examination and assessment procedure for the BSL tutor training course (given that BSL does not have a conventional written form).

4   To develop a syllabus for an introductory BSL course to be taught to non-signing hearing people (as well as deaf and hearing-impaired people wishing to learn the language) by tutors trained on the BSL tutor training course (1–3 above).

5   To develop a direct experience method for the teaching of the introductory BSL course (an approach based on using the target language, BSL, as the language of instruction).

6   To prepare and produce course study materials (including the introductory BSL syllabus) in BSL on video and in written English.

Tutor training course
It was decided at the outset that the course would be conducted in BSL and taught by the Deaf member(s) of the project team. It was recognized that most Deaf adults, fluent in BSL, would not wish to undertake a course based on written English materials. Video provided the means by which

course study materials could be presented in BSL (rather than written English) enabling students to engage in private study.

The course was organized as a part-time, distance learning and residential course. Each course lasts 25 weeks, during which time trainees attend three residential, one-week (7 days) blocks in Durham. In between the residential blocks, trainees are required to engage in home study based on the video study materials. These provide summaries of lectures, etc., presented in BSL by the Deaf course tutors during the residential weeks of the course. The introductory course syllabus is also made available in BSL on video. One student described the videos as '. . . like having someone from the training course in the living room to guide me along . . .'—a view expressed by many of those who have attended the course. The videotapes enable the students to study in their first or preferred language (BSL)—an experience never available previously. The videotapes compensate in part for the limited time available during the residential weeks of the course, and for the lack of local tutorial support which is the major disadvantage of a national distance learning course of this type. Consideration was given to organizing the course on a regional basis, but lack of resources has made this impossible to date.

In addition to home study and attendance on the residential weeks of the course, trainees are required to carry out a 10-week teaching practice placement in their home area. This usually takes the form of ten classes each lasting two hours, in which the trainees use the introductory BSL syllabus to teach a group of hearing non-signers. The placement is normally carried out between the second and third residential blocks of a course.

Course examination

The course examination is in two parts: an assessment of the students' teaching practice placement, and a formal examination at the end of the third block of the course. Students must pass both parts of the examination to be eligible for the award of the University's Certificate in British Sign Language: Tutor Course (Foundation Level).

Teaching practice placement Each trainee receives two visits from a member of the project staff during his or her teaching practice placement. The first is a guidance visit during which the member of staff observes the trainee teaching his or her class. After the class, the member of staff will offer advice and discuss with the trainee any matters he or she wishes to raise. It is felt important that each trainee has the opportunity to discuss his or her placements directly with a member of staff before assessment—particularly as many trainees do not have access to a video camera and therefore are unable to contact staff by video letter (in BSL). After the guidance visit, each trainee receives a report summarizing the staff tutor's observations and recommendations. The second visit is the assessment visit. Each trainee is granted one opportunity to retake their teaching practice placement should they fail.

Final examination   The formal final examination is conducted in BSL—a written examination in English would obviously be inappropriate. The examination questions are presented in BSL on video. The trainee views the examination on a TV monitor, controlling it through the use of a hand-held remote control. When the trainee is ready to answer a question, he or she informs the invigilator who records the signed answer by video camera. Each trainee is granted one opportunity to resit the examination should they fail.

Innovative use of video

It was clear from the beginning that the use of videotapes would play a crucial role in encouraging suitably qualified members of the Deaf community to train as tutors of their own language. A large section of the Deaf community, through no fault of their own, do not feel comfortable in situations where they are required to work in English (a consequence of their school education). For this reason, priority was given to ensuring that study materials would be available in BSL and that the final course examination would be conducted in sign language. This was only made possible through the use of video.

A syllabus for teaching BSL

A syllabus was developed for an introductory BSL course to be taught by those who had been trained on the tutor training course. This was based on an American Sign Language (ASL) syllabus developed by Vista College, California, USA. At the start of the project, consideration had been given to various teaching syllabi that were available at that time. None were found to be appropriate and work had commenced on developing a syllabus based on Dorothy Miles' Manual for BSL Tutors.[3] However, on a visit to the USA in 1986, A, Clark Denmark, one of the authors of this paper, learned of the Vista College series 'Signing Naturally', and the Rochester Institute of Technology's 'Basic Sign Communication' course. Both were based on a similar approach to that which we had intended to use for our introductory BSL syllabus. The Vista syllabus incorporated the latest sign language research findings and had been developed by a team of contributors working over a number of years. As it had been tried and tested, and appeared ideally to meet our requirements, we accepted Vista's offer to make use of their syllabus. The Vista syllabus was translated from ASL, into BSL, and changes were made to reflect cultural differences. We found its approach very positive: it enabled us to introduce BSL as a second language to non-signers; it enabled us to use a direct experience method of teaching; it created greater understanding of language use in context; we found it developed positive attitudes in both Deaf tutors and their students, enabling tutors to overcome the patronising attitudes that so often characterize hearing people's attitudes towards Deaf people.

The syllabus was prepared and produced in BSL on videotapes (forming an integral part of the trainee's BSL study). A written guide to the syllabus accompanies the demonstration tapes, which feature the Deaf course tutors teaching the syllabus (using the direct experience method) to a group of hearing beginners. A series of written English handouts are provided as part of the package (giving background information about BSL, the Deaf community in Britain, Deaf culture, etc.) which the tutors distribute to their students as course study materials.

Funding of the course

In the first eighteen months, difficulties in obtaining funding made it impossible to plan courses on other than an *ad hoc* basis. We were unable to confirm courses until ten persons with funding had enrolled. It was clear that it would be impossible to establish the course properly without block funding. The BDA agreed to subsidize the early courses but did not have the financial resources to do so indefinitely. The process of applying to local authorities involved the individual preparation of each application. The project simply did not have the staff to continue to pursue funding in this way. In a number of cases, local authorities made reference to the fact that they had not received applications previously for funding from Deaf adults and/or had difficulty in accepting that their regulations permitted them to fund the attendance of Deaf adults on a course of this type. Compared to other certificate courses (of similar duration, etc.) the cost per student (unsubsidized) was expensive. This was due to the necessity to produce course materials on video, and the fact that the project staff were not funded through the University Grants Committee (UGC) and therefore staff costs had also to be found. An application for funding was made by the BDA and the University of Durham, in October 1986, to the (then) Manpower Services Commission. This application, and subsequent applications in 1988 and 1989, were successful and enabled the project to make enormous advances: without these grants progress would have been slow and difficult.

Contribution of the course to the Deaf community

The tutor training course has given the Deaf community in Britain a great boost in confidence. It has given the Community a sense of Pride—Pride with a capital 'P'—a pride in their own language, which in the past has often mistakingly been a matter of shame: shame in their 'difference' (use of BSL) and their 'weakness' (lack of competence in English). It has strengthened their sense of their own positive Deaf identity. If we consider the experiences of the Deaf people who have been through the training course, and compare their pre-training and post-training circumstances (both socially and in terms of employment), the change is readily apparent. In many cases the change has been incredible, with many, in the view of the chief course tutor (Denmark), demonstrating for the first time their true potential (having previously been denied the opportunity to do so). The project has, we believe, enhanced the employment and training opportunities of the Deaf people who have attended the course (both directly and indirectly). The training and qualification provided by the course has encouraged them to apply for jobs which previously they would not have considered. A number of advertisements have specifically invited applications from Deaf people who have attended the BSL tutor training course. About 5 per cent have become self-employed sign language tutors. The great majority of them have discovered a new found confidence in themselves. Their attitude towards hearing people has changed, now that they are aware of the obvious respect in which they are held as tutors. The fact that Deaf people are now engaged in teaching BSL to hearing people will, we feel, make a major contribution to enhancing (in general) the employment opportunities of Deaf people in this country. It provides Deaf people with the opportunity to address what has been described as their greatest obstacle in obtaining employment (in particular employment commensurate with their abilities), namely the attitude of hearing people. Hearing people who attend BSL classes taught by trained Deaf tutors will, we believe, form a very different perception of Deaf people from that which as prevailed in the past. Such change is, we believe, a necessary prerequisite to Deaf people gaining equality of opportunity in obtaining access to training and employment. We are only in a position to refer to the short term successes (given the course has only been running for a relatively short period of time)—one can only wonder what long-term benefits this new found confidence will bring.

It's not all roses! And Pandora's box
The major expansion of the project in the last few years has been made possible through funding from the Department of Employment. The BDA has continued to contribute to the cost of the course but does not have the financial resources by itself to fund a course of this size. Recent changes in government policy have led to Department of Employment funding being available only to unemployed Deaf persons attending the course. The future funding of the course is a matter of grave concern to us. This uncertainty means that staff can be employed only on short-term contracts. In turn, this limits the number of courses, and the waiting list of Deaf people who wish to attend the course grows longer.

A criticism that has been made of the BSL introductory syllabus is that it inhibits, or it does not encourage, trainees to be inventive in developing their own teaching materials and approaches to teaching. It has also led a number of trainees to think that this is the only possible way to teach! We need to find the time to address these issues to ensure that trainees do not become rigid in their approach to teaching. The course provides a base—it is not in itself the 'end'. It is but one of many possible approaches to the teaching of BSL.

The new found confidence of some trainees has, however, resulted in some unforeseen negative consequences. Some are forever arguing, or being provoked into debating (with other deaf people who do not share their views) the pros and cons of BSL, and the teaching of BSL by the direct experience method. At times, when they are unable to support their arguments, they reply that 'Durham University says/signs so'—instead of swallowing their pride and replying, 'I don't have the answer to that at present but I will come back to you'. A lecture entitled 'Learn to Walk before You Run' has been included in the training course in an attempt to address this issue.

The reaction of the long-oppressed majority who make up the Deaf community (those who have been described as 'oral failures') has had serious repercussions for relationships within and without the community. A bitter battle is going on within the Deaf community with regard to the issue of language preference: BSL, or English (and the use of both languages by Deaf/deaf people). The minority, that is those who have been traditionally considered 'successful' by hearing society and who were also viewed as 'superior' by members of the Deaf community, are now 'having to look over their shoulders', as Deaf people (defined in terms of their use of BSL) come to the fore. Not that this tension is necessarily unhealthy but it has, to some extent, had a damaging affect on the campaign to advance the use of sign language in both the Deaf and the wider community. We do not view the languages as alternatives: in Britain both BSL and English should be 'languages of the Deaf community'.

Conclusion

The project has, we believe, achieved a lot—but not without considerable difficulty. It has placed excessive demands on staff in relation to the number of hours worked. The course itself is not perfect—there is room for improvement in a number of areas. But if we were asked to start again we would have done much the same thing (though would insist on more staff to ease the workload). We hope you will agree that the opportunities the course has provided for Deaf people (and in turn for non-signing hearing and deaf people) has made the project well worth undertaking.

Notes

1   The name was changed in 1987 when the course was granted certificate status by the University of Durham.

2   The survey was carried out for the BDA in 1982 by Ms L. Lawson.

3   Miles, D. (1981) *British Sign Language: A Teachers Manual,* British Deaf Association.

Section 7
Social Welfare: Enabling or Disabling?

Discussions within social policy reflect the recurrent themes of deafness viewed as disability, or deaf people seen as a cultural minority group. Social work with deaf people had its beginnings in early Church of England voluntary societies. The combined aims of evangelism, mutual aid and philanthropy reflected a perception of deaf people as disabled and in need of care. It is argued in some of the papers which follow that the shadow of this Victorian paternalism persists, and current debate focuses on whether social work aims at providing assistance to inadequate members of society or facilitating independence and empowering a minority group.

Related to the view of deaf people as a cultural minority is the issue of the role of interpreters in social welfare provision. Traditionally, social workers with deaf people have combined the roles of providers of social services and of interpreters; more recently it has been suggested that these are incompatible.

Finkelstein argues that negative associations are not a necessary correlate of disability. He advocates a bringing together of all disabled groups to effect a radical change in perspectives on disability in society. He believes that if deaf people disassociate themselves from the label of disability they are, albeit implicitly, reinforcing the negative ideas of disabled people held by other members of society rather than helping to promote a positive approach. Finkelstein's rejection of the view of deaf people as a cultural linguistic minority group may be contrasted with Kyle's model.

The national voluntary organizations of The National Deaf Children's Society (NDCS), the British Deaf Association (BDA) and the Royal National Institute for the Deaf (RNID) have played an important part in defining deafness in the UK, particularly in attempting to influence public images of deaf people and in representing the views of deaf people in negotiations with other official bodies. The BDA has traditionally not only represented but also developed and safeguarded a cultural model of deafness. It is the voluntary organization with which Deaf people themselves identify.

The RNID is the largest organization in the field of deafness and sees as its constituency all people with a hearing loss. This concern with a wide range of deaf people, including hard-of-hearing and deafened people, has led to a bias towards audiological models of deafness which focus on hearing loss, and has resulted in an emphasis on the assimilation of deaf people into a hearing world—although this emphasis may currently be shifting.

The NDCS represents deaf children and their families, and is essentially a parents' organization. Parents of deaf children are often in a particularly vulnerable position. The deficit view of deafness, which focuses on how deaf people differ from the hearing norm and emphasizes normalization through amelioration of the perceived deficit of hearing loss, places on parents a double burden: that of having a disabled child and pressure to make their deaf child as much like a hearing child as possible. The cultural view of deafness, on the other hand, which emphasizes the common values and language of Deaf people, inevitably places hearing parents in an anomalous position. In ethnic minority groups, acculturation generally occurs through primary socialization, whereas deaf people often acquire their socialization into the Deaf community outside the home. What then is the role of hearing parents of deaf children within the cultural minority group model of deaf people?

Debate within social welfare may be characterized by the competing ideologies of deaf people viewed either as disabled or as a cultural minority group. This polarization of views has perhaps inhibited exploration of common middle ground. It may be that technological advances, normally associated with a disability model, may come to be seen as facilitating access for a minority group in a pluralist society. It remains to be seen, however, whether the two competing ideologies in fact represent incommensurable paradigms.

7.1 The Development of Local Voluntary Societies for Adult Deaf Persons in England

Kenneth Lysons (1979)

It is not possible to state with certainty when or where the first mission for the adult deaf in the United Kingdom was founded beyond stating that the work seems to have originated in Scotland. Kathleen Heasman[1] mentions that the first deaf mission was started in Glasgow when, in 1822, John Anderson held religious services for the deaf in his own house 'in a way they could understand'. The present writer, however, has evidence[2] that mission work commenced in Edinburgh in 1818 when a Miss Elizabeth Burnside noted that a number of deaf and dumb men congregated each evening at the corner of Lawnmarket and Bank Street because they had 'no meeting'. Miss Burnside therefore obtained a room for which she paid the rent, acted as door-keeper and also preached at the meeting 'in a conversational way'. Later she consulted Mr Kinniburgh, the Principal of the Edinburgh Deaf Insitution, who agreed to organize the meeting under the name of the 'Edinburgh Deaf and Dumb Meeting'.

In the above incident there are two elements which are characteristic of the founding of most early societies for the adult deaf. Firstly, the congregating of groups of deaf persons drawn together by the desire to meet with others in like condition. Secondly, the intervention of an individual or individuals motivated by a mixture of compassion, evangelistic zeal and charitable concern who endeavoured to obtain and maintain premises where the deaf could assemble for social and religious purposes. Subsequently, there was the inevitable fund raising, election of a management committee and organization of activities which, as they became more complex, required the appointment of a 'missioner' on whom responsibility for the 'mission' devolved.

For well over a century these 'mission' or welfare societies constituted virtually the only provision for deaf persons in post-school life. With the development of local authority welfare services for the deaf there is the danger that the impressive contribution of voluntaryism in this field may be forgotten.

[. . .]

**The motives prompting the establishment of
local voluntary societies for the deaf**
Three motives inspired the founding of societies for the adult deaf, namely
Evangelism, Mutual Aid and Philanthropy.

The first two of these motives is implied by the use of the terms
'mission' and 'benevolent association' in the titles of the earliest organizations for deaf persons in post-school life.

Philanthropy did not play the same part in the development of agencies
catering for the spiritual and material needs of adult deaf persons as it did
in the case of persons suffering from handicaps such as blindness or even in
the founding of some schools for deaf children.

In addition to the factors such as their sparsity as a population group
and community attitudes to the disability, several supplementary reasons
may be adduced for the comparative neglect of the deaf by philanthropic
sources. The deaf and dumb could only appeal effectively to the charitably
minded through interpreters. The baser incentives to the dispensation of
charity towards the adult deaf were largely absent.

[. . .]

Unless the donor of charity was prepared to master the manual
language as used by deaf and dumb people, he would be unable to make
contact with the deaf and dumb and obtain the warm glow of 'doing good'
which he received from the gratitude of the poor, lame and blind. With the
deaf schools prestige might be derived as a member of a 'voting charity'
where, in return for financial assistance the subscriber was given the right
to nominate pupils for the school. The missions conferred no such
privileges. The Deaf missions were also, in general, obscure organizations
and membership of their committees did not afford an opportunity of
associating with the rich and powerful. Philanthropy in the case of missions
to the adult deaf seems to have been extended almost exclusively by
persons who were themselves deaf, related to someone deaf, or brought by
chance or business into contact with the deaf. Thus at Southampton Sir
Arthur Fairbairn, himself deaf, and others raised funds for the erection of
a church for the deaf. The foundation of the Wolverhampton Mission was
due to Miss Jane Mesemeres 'who, inspired with a love for the deaf and
dumb and having had much experience in educating a deaf and dumb boy,
started the work. . . early in 1886 at the advanced age of 60 and at her
own expense'.[3]

When, in 1907 The Rochdale Society for the Deaf separated from
Bolton to become an independent mission, an Institute was provided by Sir
J.E. Jones whose interest in the deaf was due to the fact that his son, Ellis
Llwyn Jones, had been born deaf.[4]

The demise of local voluntary effort for the adult deaf
In the above ways a network of missions was established in various parts of
the country.

[. . .]

Not until 1960, however, did the Minister of Health direct 'the Council of every County and County Borough to . . . exercise these powers under Section 29 (of the National Assistance Act 1948) in relation to persons ordinarily resident in their area who are deaf or dumb or are substantially and permanently handicapped by illness, injury or congenital deformity'.[5]

A local authority was able to provide for the deaf either directly: i.e. by establishing a service under the authority's auspices or indirectly: i.e. by entering into an agency agreement with one or more voluntary societies. Some local authorities preferred to retain direct responsibility for certain aspects of deaf welfare while entrusting other duties to the voluntary societies thus establishing a divided as distinct from a unified service for the deaf.

At first the County and County Borough Councils were glad to use the expertise of the missions and in 1962 at least 101 out of the 128 Authorities in England and Wales had full agency agreements. Of the remainder 11 and 6 respectively had a partial agency or directly operated services while information from 10 other Authorities was incomplete.[6]

The future of voluntary work for the deaf was already under threat as a result of the recommendations of the Report published in 1959 by the Working Party on Social Workers in the Local Authority Health and Welfare Services under the chairmanship of Dame Eileen Younghusband which had been appointed by the Ministry of Health and Secretary of State for Scotland in June 1955.

The Report made a number of general recommendations regarding the role of local authorities in the provision of welfare services for the deaf.

[. . .]

The working party expected that, following its Report, there would be a rapid increase in the number of County and County Borough Councils in which the welfare of the deaf was provided for by a divided service in which individual case-work would be undertaken by the local authority whilst such groupwork activities as recreation and spiritual ministration would be either wholly entrusted to or shared with the voluntary organizations for the deaf.

This prognostication has been fulfilled and today (1978) only about twenty of the local authorities in England and Wales now entrust all aspects of deaf welfare to a voluntary society. Whether the deaf are better served by a voluntary or a directly provided service is a matter for further research.

Notes

1   Heasman, K. (1962) *Evangelical in Action*, Geoffrey Bles. Chapter XI, p. 203.

2   Lockhart, Alexander, late Session Clerk to the Deaf Church in Albany Street, Edinburgh in a letter dated 5 August 1938, to Selwyn Oxley, Esq.

3   Walsall—Church Mission to the Deaf.
Extracts from a Pamphlet issued at the Annual Meeting and official opening of the new Extension to the Headquarters of the Mission, 5 December 1959.

4   Rochdale Deaf and Dumb Society, Annual Report 1907.

5   Younghusband Report table 28, p. 226 and para 802, pp. 226–7, Ministry of Health Circular 15/60, 18 July 1960.

6   Survey undertaken by the writer, 1962.

7.2 Deaf People, Ethnic Minorities and Social Policy

George Taylor (1986)

Welfare services for deaf people have evolved separately and significantly differently from those for other sections of society. In examining the reasons for this, I shall outline the establishment and growth of the 'missions' and the central role they have played as a model for working with deaf people. Supported by a specialized form of professional training and a specialized professional association, the 'missioner' model determined the way that the voluntary societies and, eventually, the local authorities provided welfare services to deaf people. Because of the isolated situation of deaf people in British society, they have been virtually ignored by policymakers, thus allowing welfare services to be developed in a way that is out of step with mainstream social services provision.

It is often stated that the nature of deafness has determined the way that services are provided. I will argue that this is not the case, and to demonstrate this I will refer to the way that welfare services, through social policy, have been established for ethnic minorities. Whilst there are many differences between immigrant communities and the deaf community they both share the disadvantage of being a linguistic minority group in Britain. For this reason I shall be concentrating upon immigrant groups that bring with them a different culture and language, and on profoundly deaf people, users of British Sign Language. There has been much controversy about the status of British Sign Language as a recognized language, but it is now being accepted that it has its own structure and form and therefore does qualify as a language.

> British Sign Language (BSL) is one of several natural human languages which are produced in a visual/gestural medium. The language user, the signer, makes gestures, including movements of the hands, arms, eyes, face, head and body, which are watched and decoded by the other participants in the communication. If we do not know the significant types of patterning within the gesturing activity of the signer, we cannot decode, and hence understand, the linguistic information imparted by the signer.
> (Brennan *et al.*, 1980)

Whereas language has been seen as a problem, and it does complicate the provision of services, it can also provide a partial solution. If deaf people were to be aligned with other linguistic minorities, welfare services for deaf people could be improved through current and recommended social policies. I shall be considering the implications of this approach and also the implications of altering those elements of welfare provision that are historically determined, rather than a response to either a needs assessment or social policy.

Missions

Long before the phrase 'Welfare State' was first used, voluntary organizations were involved in social welfare. The earliest schools, hospitals and poor relief came from private charities. Indeed, the existing health and education services, and to a large extent the child care and social welfare services, all emerged from a pioneering voluntary effort, at first unaided by government, then assisted by government funds, finally leading to a direct statutory service. As far as deaf people were concerned, the earliest 'welfare' intervention was by church based organizations. It is not possible to identify positively where or when this took place, but it is likely that it happened in Scotland in the early part of the nineteenth century. Throughout the nineteenth century, 'missions' for deaf people were established by a variety of religious bodies, for two main reasons:

1   Deaf people had no place of their own where they could mix socially with other deaf people, and

2   Enthusiastic members of the local church wished to carry their religious message to groups of deaf people.

In order to achieve this, it was necessary to find premises, establish administration and organizations, and appoint somebody to be responsible for it all. These people, known as 'missioners' were always men, never women, either directly employed by an organized religious body or otherwise active in parish affairs. Just as organized religion travelled on the back of colonization to instruct the ignorant masses of the Dark Continent, so deaf people were viewed as 'fair game' for domestic missionary work.

As these early missions gathered pace they identified targets for intervention by voluntary societies. Broadly speaking, the three main aims were:

1   Employment

2   Education, and

3   Religious instruction

However, the main element of early voluntary work was almost certainly the religious element. Asylum-type schools for deaf children started appearing in the early part of the nineteenth century and mission-centred voluntary organizations were not involved in any significant way. In fact, the major education input was also part of the employment element. Deaf people were received into refuges where they learned and were required to work at a trade or a handicraft. These workshops were intended to be supported by voluntary subscription and the sale of their produce. They mostly failed to achieve any sort of financial stability, however, and fell into disuse. One of these organizations, the 'Institution of the Employment, Relief and Religious Instruction of the Adult Deaf and Dumb' (originally founded in 1841 as 'The Refuge for the Destitute Deaf and Dumb') was forced, for financial reasons, to cease its activities in this field. The same year, 1854, the Institution re-emerged as 'The Association in Aid of the Deaf and Dumb'. The constitution of the Association contained no reference to employment or education, but concerned itself exclusively with spiritual and moral affairs.

[. . .]

Strategies
In this section I will outline some of the strategies used to provide welfare services to ethnic minorities, and recommendations for improving service delivery, and apply them to the deaf community to see if they offer a viable alternative to present methods.

Policy review procedure
One of the conclusions of the Association of Directors of Social Services and the Commission for Racial Equality report 1978 was that, overall, services for ethnic minorities had been provided in a patchy, piecemeal fashion. They recommended that, whilst the spread of population of ethnic minorities was not evenly distributed and services should be determined locally, that more co-operation was needed between local authorities. And, that a government funded review procedure should be implemented to examine the policies of local authorities and the DHSS. The scattered deaf community also, suffers from uncoordinated services and would benefit from the sort of policy-making and review procedures recommended for ethnic minorities. Nobody knows how many people are involved in providing welfare services to deaf people in this country, neither is there a coherent philosophy discernible amongst service providers in a small geographical area.

Positive discrimination
In recent years many local authorities have introduced a policy of matching, that is, employing staff of the same ethnic origin as a group they are working with. There are problems with this approach, however, that, if not overcome, can be quite destructive. It is first necessary to identify the group the worker will be working with in terms of culture, language and social status. It is not enough to appoint a person with a black face to work with black groups. It is all too easy for Social Services Departments to appoint someone whom they think is respectable and agrees with their general overall policies. Whereas, in fact, this is a nonsensical approach, given that they are appointing somebody to work with a group that the Social Services Department does not understand, and with whom their policies have largely failed. For instance, it is not a good idea to appoint a Nigerian worker for a community drawn mostly from Jamaica, or a Punjabi Sikh to work with a Hindu group.

Likewise, when appointing deaf workers to work with the deaf community. To be born profoundly deaf puts you in a significantly different position from someone who lost their hearing at a later age. How many local authority social services departments could contemplate interviewing a profoundly deaf person? Where local authorities appoint a hearing-impaired person to work with deaf people they usually appoint someone who is hard of hearing or partially hearing. This is rank tokenism. If the object of the exercise is client matching, it is simply not acceptable to appoint a worker with a partial hearing loss who may have been educated in an ordinary comprehensive school, and expect that person to identify with profoundly deaf people who were (or are), more than likely, educated at a residential school for the deaf and whose life experiences will be significantly different.

[. . .]

Conclusions

The foundations of welfare provision for deaf people were laid in the early nineteenth century. The 'mission' became the centre of social, employment and educational activity for deaf people, and in deaf people grew a strong dependency on the mission. Since that time the religious and employment aspects have largely disappeared, in fact, many social workers with deaf people do not operate from a mission or a centre for the deaf, but from a local authority social services office. What has been retained, however, is the central importance of the mission/social worker and the dependency of the deaf community upon that person. This has been reinforced by the nature of the training available to welfare workers with deaf people, and the professional association to which they belong. The lack of any significant change of direction has been made possible by the lack of any meaningful legislation, and the reluctance of local authorities to involve themselves, in any informed and informative way, in the operation of voluntary societies working with deaf people.

Whilst ethnic minorities have only recently been seen as a 'problem' in this country, legislation has appeared relatively quickly compared with that for disabled groups. A large influx of commonwealth immigrants during the 1950s and 1960s raised a moral panic. West Indians and Asians were accused of having 'dirty habits', threatening English women and taking jobs. The consequential legislation was aimed at reducing the numbers of immigrants and integrating those that were here, thus reducing the element of 'threat' implied by their presence. The ineffectiveness of the legislation is witnessed by the riots of 1981 in the depressed areas of Britain populated by black majorities. Nevertheless, whilst social policies have not ensured racial equality there have been improvements in this respect experienced by ethnic minorities. The main problem as far as deaf people are concerned, is that they feature hardly at all in British society, and being hidden has meant that very little attention has been paid to their needs by policy makers.

There are, however, many similarities between the experience of deaf people and some ethnic minorities in this country. Primarily, a language and culture that differs from that of the majority of the population, and also, just as the British social system encourages institutionalized racism, it also encourages institutionalized prejudice towards disabled people.

That deaf people would benefit by being considered in the same legislation as ethnic minorities has been demonstrated by my arguments. Examples of how they could benefit from current legislation and planned/ recommended future social policies can be outlined as follows:

● **The Local Government Act 1966, Sec. 11.** Identifies funds for the provision of staff to work with ethnic minorities. At a time when local authorities are reducing their overall staff numbers, this legislation could ensure provision for deaf people.

● **Policy review procedures.** More co-operation between local authorities in the way that they provide services to deaf people would enable social services departments to provide a more appropriate service. For instance, social services department A could employ a social worker to cover both their responsibilities plus those of social services department B. Meanwhile, social services department B could employ a community worker to cover the same area. At present they would both, more like, employ somebody called a 'social worker with the deaf', whose job description would be vague and whose activities would be even vaguer.

● **Positive discrimination.** In local authorities, deaf people should be preferred to hearing people for employment involving contact with the deaf community and issues related to services for deaf people. Special education schemes should be initiated for deaf applicants without the relevant educational qualifications.

● **Access to information.** Local authorities should address themselves seriously to the question of access to information for deaf people in public places. Clear, visual symbols in bus stations council offices and the like, will alleviate some of the anxiety. Properly trained receptionists will also help. Because of the low level of English of some deaf people, and the difficulty of access generally, local authorities should take positive steps to bring public information to the deaf community.

● **Interpreters.** Local authorities should employ, on a full-time basis, sufficient interpreters to satisfy the needs of the deaf community in that area. The local authority should also co-operate with CACDP[1] in recruiting, training, examining and regulating a list of interpreters.

● **Deaf advisory groups.** Local authorities should make provision for such a Deaf Advisory Group to be included in planning exercises where deaf people may be affected.

There are two major problems to overcome before any of these recommendations can be implemented with any hope of improving services for deaf people:

1 As has been witnessed with legislation for ethnic minorities and disabled people, discretionary social policy without clearly identified funds and specific instructions for implementation will either not be implemented, or will be axed as soon as local authorities come under financial pressure.

2 The very nature of existing welfare services to deaf people will present problems.

> The problem facing policy-makers is to effect 'real world change' in intended directions. The degree to which they succeed in doing so is a measure of policy impact. Yet policy is rarely applied directly to the external world. Characteristically it is mediated through other institutions or actors. Thus the impact of policies is affected as much by the mediation of other key actors—the 'implementers'—as by the intrinsic merits or feasibility of the policy itself.
> (K. Young in Adler and Asquith, 1981, p. 34–5)

The history, the training and the professional identity associated with providing welfare services to deaf people has a stranglehold upon the way in which services are provided, and the tasks involved in that provision. Services must not be dictated by voluntary societies or quasi-official bodies managed by charismatic hearing people. Local authorities have been grossly irresponsible in allowing this state of affairs to develop. Workers involved in providing services to deaf people must identify primarily with the organization that employs them, and that organization, in my opinion, should be the local authority.

The term 'social worker with the deaf', is a misnomer. It does not signify that the person has any skills or qualifications as a social worker, neither does it signify that the person has any skills or qualifications to work with deaf people. Of course, there are social workers with the deaf who have skills and qualifications in both areas and this merely serves to further confuse the issue. Whilst this confusion exists any improvements in welfare services to deaf people will be ad hoc, unco-ordinated and vulnerable to the whim of the provider.

Implementation of these proposals has its consequences, were local authorities to accept 'real responsibility for provision of welfare services to deaf people' then the workers would become much more a part of the organization. Also, promotion through social work grades would be more closely linked to that of Generic Teams. The situation where workers with minimum qualifications and experience are appointed to highly paid senior positions would not occur.

Policy review procedures would ensure a greater co-operation between local authorities and also a greater understanding of the problem. Coupled with the implementation of Deaf Advisory Groups, this would mean a more specific focus of activity for workers. Caseloads would be more closely controlled and areas of operation more closely defined. No longer would the social worker with the deaf be a free agent, seeking out and banishing evil like some latter-day Robin Hood. No longer would the social workers with the deaf be a 'friend' of the deaf. She or he would simply be an employee of the local authority whose job was to provide appropriate services to deaf people. No longer would the difference between personal and professional involvement be blurred. Work with deaf people would be clearly defined.

The employment of full-time interpreters by local authorities would create the single most radical departure from current practice. The combined roles of the social worker/interpreter have for too long been an unholy alliance, and there is a fierce resistance to altering the status quo. Many social workers were originally attracted to the job because of the interpreting element, and operate almost exclusively in that role. This may mean that some social workers would switch to being full-time interpreters if they reached the required standard, others would simply drop interpreting from their work load. Of course there is the option of community work, with either local authorities or voluntary societies, where some element of interpreting/facilitating would still be a feature.

The final significant change would be the recruitment of deaf people into key positions. There are a handful of deaf social workers with the deaf in this country but they are far out numbered by hearing social workers. A policy of positive discrimination would reverse this situation and therefore jobs for hearing people involved in welfare provision for deaf people would be greatly reduced.

[. . .]

This is not to say that I see no place for voluntary societies in the provision of welfare services to deaf people. Voluntary societies have proved their worth as pressure groups both at a local and a national level, and their pioneering and advocacy roles have led to improvements. However, I am concerned about voluntary societies growing too large, and appearing to be more interested in their own maintenance rather than the concerns of the group they claim to be representing. I believe the state should be the main provider of services, implemented through effective and relevant social policies.

Note
1   CACDP—Council for the Advancement of Communication with Deaf People.

References
Adler, M. and Asquith, S. (1981) *Discretion and Welfare*, London, Heinemann.

Brennan, M., Colville, M.D. and Lawson, L. (1980) *Words in Hand,* Edinburgh B.S.L. Project.

Cheetham, J., James, W., Loney, M., Mayor, B. and Prescott, W. (1981) *Social and Community Work in a Multi-Racial Society,* London, Harper and Row.

Grimshaw, A. (1979) 'Social Problems and Social Policies', in *Social Problems, 26,* no. 5.

Higgins, P. (1980) *Outsiders in a Hearing World,* London, Sage Publications.

Lysons, K. (1984) *Hearing Impairment,* Cambridge, Woodhead-Faulkner.

Morrison, L. (1976) *As They See It,* Community Relations Commission.

National Council of Social Workers with the Deaf (1970–1984) *Minutes of South East Branch Meetings.*

National Council of Social Workers with the Deaf (1980) *Submission to Barclay Report.*

Rodda, M. (1970) *The Hearing-Impaired School-leaver,* London, University of London Press.

Schackman, J. (1984) *The Right to be Understood,* Cambridge, National Extension College.

Stephenson, O. (1981) *Specialisation in Social Service Teams,* London, Allen and Unwin.

Stein, L.K., Mindel, E.D. and Jabaley, T. (1981) *Deafness and Mental Health,* London, Grune and Stratton.

7.3 The State, Social Work and Deafness

David Parratt and Brenda Tipping (1986)

[. . .]

The history of services to hearing-impaired people

There are two major works on the history of the provision of services to deaf people. Kenneth Lysons (1977/79) gave us a history of the voluntary sector's contribution to the services. In compiling this, he used records and minutes of several local and national organizations. Stephens (1982) gives a history of state provision for deaf people based on legislation, parliamentary records and supported by personal accounts of the process of legislation. Both works are of major importance, but what they gave us is the hearing policymaker's side of the story. Sheila Rowbotham (1973) has described women as being hidden from history. Lysons and Stephens have both hidden deaf people from history. We need a book based on oral history with deaf people being interviewed in sign language through the use of video before we can understand the history of missions and social work from their point of view. Taylor (1986) relied on the work of Lysons and in so doing regarding deaf people simply as the passive recipients of welfare services and made such statements as 'Just as organized religion travelled on the back of colonization to instruct the ignorant masses of the dark continent, so deaf people were viewed as "fair game" for domestic missionary work'. We would contend that no missioner had absolute power or influence.

Deaf clubs have always had deaf leaders who have fought back against anything they considered to be inappropriate. Deaf people have always striven to resist oppression and to use services to their own advantage. Any history which ignores the role of deaf people is similar to a history of colonial Africa which ignores black resistance.

We perceive an underlying implication in Taylor's work, though this may not have been his intention, that deaf work is degraded by having its origins in religion. This suggestion is both unrealistic and unfair. Virtually all the caring services in this country were initially established by religious orders—the oldest hospital in the county, St Batholomews in the City of London, is still proud of being founded by the monk Rahere. Services for the mentally ill and the probation service also have religious roots. Even today, many of the organizations caring for ethnic minority groups are run by religious leaders within these cultures. The church is and was a wealthy and benevolent institution and we see no reason why deaf people should not have had access to the resources of the church. It can also be an important force for social change as is evident in South Africa today. We must remember too that although in many cases the church officially began welfare services, they were simply responding to the demands of deaf people. Nor was missionary zeal the only force at work. The Victorian obsession with overcoming pauperism was also an important element. Lysons recognized this when he pointed out that one of the main aims of missions when they were set up was either to help deaf people to find open employment or to find sheltered employment for them. In our own experience of working in voluntary societies, the pressure to find work for deaf people was very strong both from the deaf themelves and from management. We both need convincing that the impact of religion on the day to day work of both missioners and deaf people was very great. While many missioners were of high religious motivation, very little of their time was taken up in religious instruction or in administering the sacraments. It is important not to confuse Christian motivation with active evangelism. We have used the term 'missionary model' as did Lysons and Taylor, but we are not really sure what this actually means. Does it suggest the location of welfare services in church-based centres, or does it mean a particular type of relationship with deaf people? The term missionary model could be applied to people today who see themselves as saving deaf people from the evils of either manualism, or oralism, as the case may be!

[. . .]

The role of social workers with the deaf

With the exception of Sainsbury (1986) there have been few works that look at services for deaf people from the view point of deaf people themselves. Without such research, it is almost impossible to define what the task of social worker with deaf people is. Taylor does not define this task but by implication indicates that he sees social work in terms of that which is done with deaf people by local government social services departments. Even if we accept this as a definition of social worker, each individual agency, authority and even social worker, sees their particular priorities uniquely. A social worker with the Social Services Department does very different things from a social worker in, for example, a family welfare association. Further, the definition of the social work task is not the exclusive remit of social workers. It must involve a dialogue between deaf consumers and the employing organizations. The present looseness of the definition results in deaf people receiving a service which fluctuates from area to area. The problem is one of power and relationship to the state. The social worker decides his own definition and then argues with his superior that this is what deaf people need. Deaf people usually have very little to say in the job description of the social worker with the deaf and this is often defended in terms of professional autonomy. In fact it is largely due to a lack of accountability to the consumers. Hearing people complain to councillors and MPs. Deaf people traditionally have not done so.

[. . .]

The ethnic minority model

Taylor (1976) and linguists both in this country and in the USA have pointed out that deaf people are a linguistic minority group. Similarities are drawn between deaf people and the Chinese or other similiar minorities. It is true that BSL is a language in its own right and that use of that language defines membership of the deaf community. However, we see many difficulties in accepting this ethnic minority model. First, deaf people could not learn English even as a second language as easily as other minority group members simply because they are not physically equipped to do so. Second and third generation immigrants almost invariably learn English immediately they start school. For second and third generation deaf people, the task of learning and comprehending English is no less difficult that it was for their parents, despite the advances made in education. In saying this, we do accept that though black people may learn English more easily than people with a hearing loss, they may be the subject of greater discrimination. As we have said already, when we consider services for hearing-impaired people we must consider the needs of all categories. Deafened and hard of hearing people are native English speakers and as such cannot be included in the ethnic minority model. Taylor suggests that unlike the concentration of black people geographically, deaf people are scattered. This may or may not be true, but in class terms deaf people are concentrated in Registrar General Classes IV and V. In geographical terms, deaf people may be less randomly distributed than we think if we consider the influence of recessive genes aetiology of deafness. Groce argues that there is evidence there was a disproportionate number of deaf people in the Weald of Kent. We would accept that there is no strong evidence for the scattered argument or the concentration hypothesis, although surely it is only logical to assume that deaf people will have moved into areas where they could find employment.

The analogy with the Chinese community breaks down for other reasons. Chinese people in Britain are not as culturally homogenous as implied. The 'Chinese' came from Malaya, Singapore, Korea, Indonesia, Hong Kong and the Republic of China. There is no one spoken Chinese language. Another important difference is that Chinese people often work for one another. They are an economic community; deaf people are not. The idea of obtaining Section 11 money for deaf people is very attractive but unlikely to have been acceptable to those administering such funds, even when they were available, since it was clearly intended for immigrants from the New Commonwealth. To argue for obtaining such funds would also suggest that deaf people do not see themselves as part of English life and culture. We would say that although the deaf community is rich in language and culture, deaf people also have a part to play in their national culture and in English society. Kyle has shown that deaf people see English skills for deaf people as having high status. We accept that this may well be due to the historical oppression of deaf people, but before that can be stated categorically, much more research is necessary.

Ethnic minorities model and policy

Taylor writes 'The scattered deaf community also suffers from uncoordinated services and would benefit from the sort of policy-making and review
procedures recommended for ethnic minorities. Nobody knows how many
people are involved in providing welfare services to deaf people in this
country, neither is there a coherent philosophy discernible amongst service
providers in a small geographical area'. We are not sure if this is as
negative as it sounds. Surely services have to be established and organized
to meet local needs. Surely, on a local basis, we have the best chance of
providing services that deaf people want. If you live in areas with an ageing
deaf population, afternoon clubs would be more popular than rock-
climbing groups. What is a bigger problem is the variation in philosophy
among social workers with the deaf. The danger is that social workers with
the deaf may refuse to provide services that deaf people want; for example,
interpreting or holding 'surgeries' at the local deaf club. Services should be
based consistently on the needs and aspirations of deaf people. We would
stress, however, that we believe that central government should ensure
that local authorities' expenditure on services to deaf people should meet
set targets.

The idea that deaf people should be accepted for training even if they
do not have the required educational qualifications is patronizing as well as
impractical. In order to cope with training courses with their hearing peers,
deaf people need to have reached higher than the minimum entrance
requirements if they are to have sufficient background knowledge to fill the
gaps. The alternative would be to develop a course specially for deaf
students, but to make such a course viable it would be necessary to find
relatively large numbers which would create a danger of channelling deaf
people inappropriately along one route. Being deaf does not necessarily
make a person suitable for a career in a caring profession, and graduates of
such a course would be open to the criticism of being less well qualified.

Interpreters and the consumer

In Britain we lack central and local government commitment on a large
scale to interpreting provision. However, many social workers with the
deaf see this as one of their key roles. Training of interpreters is available
through the CACDP.[1] Surely we should publicize this form of certification,
which does provide protection against the type of abuse listed by Taylor.
The choice of interpreters is a difficult issue, as surely the hearing
consumer has rights as much as the deaf person. These issues need careful
exploration. The availability of interpreters is even more vital for deaf
people than it is for ethnic minority groups in that there are very few deaf
lawyers, accountants and doctors. Asian people in inner city areas usually
have access to Asian professionals. Deaf people do not have this facility.

The way forward

Sociology and social work literature is full of accounts showing the
difficulties clients have in relationships with both the central and local

state. Taylor argues that services for the deaf should not be an appendage to a Social Services Department but an integrated part of the department. Social workers with deaf people would have their own roles clearly defined and be no longer a friend of the deaf. This situation, we feel, would result in services to deaf people being bureaucratized without allowing for flexibility and joint working. Surely we should be aiming at a service that is controlled by the deaf community and the deafened and hard of hearing. What about job opportunities for these last two groups?

Taylor strongly supports a social work model which he fails to define, nor does he examine the appropriateness of that model for providing services to deaf people. The social work model is clearly one based on pathology and social problems approach. We need to look again at what the needs of deaf people are—not what we as social workers think they are—through research and dialogue with deaf people. May we suggest that deaf people may not need social workers but interpreters and advocates. These services are clearly nearer deaf control than is social work, where we are 'trained to assess needs'.

We would see a service based on the following principles:

1 Services that fulfil a need defined by both deaf people and service providers.

2 Geographically accessible to deaf people, e.g. through local deaf clubs.

3 Services for deaf people and the deafened and hard of hearing that are democratically managed and accountable to local hearing impaired groups.

4 Service providers are trained in the skills that the clients need. Training in social work may not be a good basis for providing welfare services.

5 It is important to consider the dangers to deaf people of professionalization. The problem is that duty to the profession can interfere with duty to the consumer.

Acknowledgements

May we gratefully acknowledge the help of Diana Atkins and Kathy Hall in the preparation of this paper.

Note

1 CACDP—Council for the Advancement of Communication with Deaf People.

References

Groce, N.E. (1985) *Everyone Here Spoke Sign Language: Hereditary Deafness on Martha's Vineyard*, Harvard University Press.

Kyle, J., Woll, B., Llwellyn Jones, P. and Pullen, G. (1983) *British Sign Language in the British Deaf Community*, University of Bristol.

Lysons, K. (1979) *The Development of Local Societies for Adult Deaf Persons in England*, BDA.

Rowbotham, S. (1973) *Hidden from History*, London, Pluto Press.

Sainsbury, S. (1986) *Deaf Worlds*, Hutchinson. 'Interpreters Forward Please', *Community Care*, 1 May 1986.

Stephens, S.D. (1982) 'The Role of the State in Hearing Health Care', *British Journal of Audiology 16*, pp. 255–63.

Taylor, G. (1986) 'Deaf People, Ethnic Minorities and Social Policy', *Journal of NCSWD 2*, no. 2. [See this volume, article 7.2.]

Tipping, B. (1986) 'The Ever-Changing Need', *Journal of NCSWD, 2*, no. 1.

7.4 Sign Language Interpreting: An Emerging Profession

Liz Scott-Gibson* (1990)

Introduction

In 1989, the United Nations General Assembly, as part of its World Programme of Action concerning Disabled Persons for the decade 1983–1992, issued a set of 'Guidelines' to promote effective measures to enable 'full participation and equality for persons with disabilities';[1] the 'Guidelines' recognize that 'disabled persons are agents of their own destiny rather than objects of care', and refer to the need for educational provision to be made available through interpreters who are 'proficient in the indigenous sign language', as well as more general access to information by means of sign language interpretation.

Whilst there are those members of the British Deaf community today who continue to feel uncomfortable bearing the label of 'disabled person', it is true that the Community welcomes the recognition that their specific linguistic needs may be met by the provision of sign language interpreters, by such prestigious bodies as the United Nations General Assembly, and, nearer to home, as contained in the resolution unanimously accepted by the European Parliament in Strasbourg in 1988, calling for the official recognition of sign languages. However, whilst it may be accurate to say that sign language interpreting is indeed an emerging field, it is, in addition, one which is not only under-resourced, but one which has struggled with its identity.

In order to examine this more closely, it is necessary to look at the development of this fledgling profession.

Historical development

Sign language interpreters have been present in the Deaf community for generations. Traditionally they were perhaps religious workers or teachers who had acquired some knowledge of sign vocabulary by association with Deaf people, but more frequently it appeared that they were people who had grown up in a family with at least one Deaf member, who had reasonable fluency in both sign language and English, and who had thereby assumed the role of the 'go-between' in a variety of settings between the

*Director of Sign Language Services, British Deaf Association, Carlisle.

Deaf and hearing communities. Such people had been brought up to share the values of the Deaf community, were perceived by them as less likely to threaten or try to change it, and were, accordingly, highly valued.

Such individuals were, for many Deaf people, the only channel to wider hearing society, and this often resulted in their acquiring positions of power and influence, either informally, or more formally, as the 'missioner' for the many clubs and societies for the Deaf which were founded in the late nineteenth and early twentieth centuries. These missioners not only offered sign language interpretation when needed, but acted as the brokers between one community and another, providing advice and support as necessary to enable Deaf people to, for example, find employment, seek medical treatment, hold religious services, and enjoy leisure activities. However, by the mid-twentieth century, Britain was beginning to become aware of the existence of a range of minority groups—including that of the Deaf community—in its midst: there was a growing belief that such groups should be enabled to become part of mainstream society, and not continue in what was a perceived ghettoization of service delivery. This liberal philosophy regarded the missioner, with his monopoly of power (albeit at times unsought) over the Deaf community with horror.[2] Local authorities began to take over the welfare services offered by the missions and societies, and workers were increasingly encouraged to seek professional social work training, and to clarify their own roles and responsibilities.

Whilst this professionalization was welcomed by many Deaf people, there was some sadness at what was thought to be a decline in sign language skills, as many social workers, being removed from the hub of Deaf community and cultural life, found difficulty in developing and maintaining a minimum competence in sign fluency. There were others who, whilst recognizing that there were members of the Deaf community who were less advantaged and in need of the specialist help that a trained social worker could give, began to articulate a resentment at being labelled a social work client when all that was necessary for them to function independently in most situations was access to appropriate interpreting assistance.

In an attempt to respond to this, the British Deaf Association established a major project (funded by the DHSS) in 1977 to examine the whole area of sign language learning, interpreter training and assessment. It became clear that, for many Deaf people, to have to rely on a friend, neighbour or relative to 'help out' with interpreting support when required, was an anathema; it implied that Deaf people were incapable of taking care of their own affairs, and because this type of interpreting assistance was provided on a voluntary basis, Deaf consumers felt unable to complain if dissatisfied with the service provided. In addition, there was no guarantee that such an individual was performing the task adequately, far less that the 'interpreter' was aware of the rights of the client to expect impartiality and confidentiality. Deaf people wanted to have access to a pool of people who would be competent, aware of their professional responsibilities, and thereby paid professional rates. From this initiative evolved the two Registers of Interpreters in existence today (that for the Council for Advancement of Communication with Deaf People, established in 1980, and that for Scotland, presently maintained by the Scottish Association of Sign Language Interpreters, which was founded in 1981). The work being done to expand the numbers of interpreters available to function in a wide range of settings—medical, educational, legal, religious, political, employment related, on television and in the theatre, and at meetings and conferences—coincided with the work being done by research teams at the University of Bristol and Moray House College in Edinburgh in the late 1970s, into the structure of British Sign Language (BSL). This established that the sign language used by deaf people was not, as it had been labelled, 'inferior' and 'ungrammatical', but rather should be viewed as a fully fledged language, with its own grammatical rules and structure. It therefore was necessary to ensure that sign language interpreters were fully fluent in both this (and not merely some manually coded form of English) and English. Efforts were accordingly made (with both greater and lesser success) to implement these research findings into sign language courses, and Deaf native users of BSL were trained to teach the language.[3] The number of sign language courses increased, helped in part by the funding of a number of full-time 'Communicators' courses around the country by the Training Agency, who were beginning to recognize that there was a desperate need for communication support for Deaf people in employment training, but such courses in themselves were insufficient to provide the level of skills required by interpreters.

Current situation
To function as an interpreter it is necessary to not only have good BSL skills, and, as stated by Koser[4], '. . . the ability to intuit meanings, the capacity to adapt immediately to the subject, speaker, public and conference situations, the ability to concentrate, a good short and long term memory, a pleasant voice, above average endurance, and very good nerves . . .', but excellent English language skills. Interpretation is not merely comprehension of a message, but is the process by which one is able to express those thoughts understood in one language in a second language, in the same way that a native speaker would express him- or herself, in style, and in intent. It is an understandably complex process, and one which requires additional high level training (presently being offered by the Universities of Bristol and Durham). In addition to being bilingual, interpreters must also strive to become bicultural, for accurate transmission of information may take place only if based on a deep knowledge of both languages, both cultures, and the cultural differences involved, and it is this awareness that current training seeks to provide.

Over and above this, however, is the requirement stated by Deaf people (based on observation and anecdotal evidence in this country, and the results of a survey conducted in the USA in 1988[5]) as having prime consideration—something labelled 'attitude'. In an attempt to ensure that consumers of an interpreting service receive a professional service delivered by interpreters with the right 'attitude', a Code of Conduct and Practise was established for registered sign language interpreters to adhere to, which embodied principles of impartiality (to assist interpreters—said to apply to particularly to children of Deaf parents—overcome the impulse to be helpful, and possibly controlling), responsibility and confidentiality. The former was also especially intended to enable a clear distinction to be drawn between the perceived advice giving, counselling, advocacy role of the social workers with Deaf people, and that of the interpreter as a mechanism to enable information exchange between two languages and cultures to take place.

Whilst some clarity is now developing about the respective roles and responsibilities of social workers and interpreters, there continue to be problems. In the apparent absence of sufficient numbers of independent interpreters, Social Workers with Deaf People are still obliged to carry out the function of interpreter, accompanying Mr/Mrs Smith for a job interview, and Mr/Mrs Smith to the doctor. Not only does this lead to confusion in the minds of the consumer of such a service, but it would also appear to result in a certain amount of resentment and frustration from trained social work personnel who are unable adequately to utilize their skills and knowledge with this particular client group, as an inordinate amount of their time has had to be expended on non-social work tasks, such as interpreting for people who should not be termed 'clients', and who, by so doing, are performing a task for which they may have received no training whatsoever. (Indeed, it is in fact possible to become a specialist social worker without ever having been assessed in one's ability to communicate with one's client, far less interpret for them.)

The situation is far from satisfactory, and it is not helped by the insistence of some employing authorities that interpreting is an integral part of the social work task. It is inappropriate to expect that all sources of information should be channelled through a Social Worker with Deaf People in this way, and it is to be welcomed that there are now some more enlightened authorities which are beginning to differentiate these functions and establish separate interpreting services to promote equality of access and opportunity for the Deaf community. Nevertheless, such developments are by no means widespread, and, apart from particular and individual negotiated provision made by the Training Agency, some employers, organizations and individuals, Deaf people have neither access to, nor the means to pay for, an interpreting service.

Future trends

It is encouraging, nevertheless, to see that the Deaf community is becoming more sophisticated in its approach to interpreting services: there is a move away from the insistence on the 'interpreter as machine' image— the 'non-person'—which assumes that any two people involved in a dialogue are equal, to a recognition that sign language users are employing a minority language in an interaction with people who are using the language of a dominant, power holding majority. It is therefore essential that an interpreter recognizes this and the cultural differences involved in order to ensure that successful dialogue takes place. The extreme swing away from the former benevolent/paternal interpreting of the traditional 'missioner' or other 'helper' to a rigid interpretation of the Code of Practise on issues of neutrality and responsibility, is being tempered by a more mature move towards a humanistic model, involving greater cultural awareness and respect.[6]

The Deaf community is also developing to become much more politically active and to be aware of the need to lobby to have its demands met. Thanks to on-going consumer education programmes, Deaf people are increasingly knowledgeable about the standards of service delivery which they can expect from social workers, interpreters and other professions, and are prepared to articulate any dissatisfaction. The Deaf community, therefore, has a major responsibility to press for more and better trained social workers, and an increase in the number of, and the means to pay for, professional sign language interpreters.

Regrettably, this growing awareness on the part of the Deaf community is not always matched by parallel enthusiasm in other spheres. Although the recent *Say it Again* report,[7] published by the Social Services Inspectorate, recommends that local authorities should consider the provision and funding of interpreter services, it makes no clear statement about the nature of such services, and there is no government funding available to pay for interpreter training. Furthermore, as long as Social Workers with Deaf People continue to perform interpreting tasks outside the remit of their professional role, they continue to paper over the cracks in the system and deny Deaf people the opportunity for greater and improved access to a wider hearing society.

It is true that there is still a very small number of registered sign language interpreters throughout the UK (some seventy in England, Wales and Northern Ireland, and twenty-one in Scotland); even fewer are functioning exclusively as interpreters. However, there is within this emerging profession a wish to work to improve the type and standard of service they can offer. Professional associations of sign language interpreters have been established (in 1981 in Scotland and in 1988 in England, Wales and Northern Ireland) which it is hoped can provide support and access to information and on-going training for interpreters, as well as working to promote knowledge about the profession. Links are being forged with sign language interpreters in other countries (for example, through the European Forum of Sign Language Interpreters) in order to learn from different experiences. Whilst it is undoubtedly the case that sign language interpreting in this country is indeed an emerging profession, it would appear to be one which is ready to respond to the challenges which will be presented to it in the coming years. For the consumers of such a service, this can only be welcome news.

Notes

1   The Tallin Guidelines for Action on Human Resources Development in the Field of Disability, UN, 1969.

2   See, for example, 'Hearing Impaired or BSL Users? Social Policies in the Deaf Community', by P. Ladd in *Disability, Handicap and Society*, vol. 3 no. 2, 1988.

3   The British Deaf Association sponsored the Deaf Studies Research Unit at the University of Durham, which has to date trained 143 people to teach BSL at foundation level and is currently offering the opportunity for Deaf people to take an Advanced Diploma/MA in BSL teaching.

4   Quoted by Liz Scott-Gibson, British Deaf Triennial Congress, Rothesay, 1986.

5   From *Sign Language Quarterly*, Sign Language Associates, Inc., Silver Spring, MD, USA, 1989. Quoted by Betty Colonomos in Bi-Cultural Seminar held at University of Durham, October 1989.

6   *Rebuilding Bridges to the Deaf Community*, by M.J. Bienvenu in *TBC News*, no. 4, June 1988.

7   Social Services Inspectorate, *Say it Again,* Department of Health and Social Security.

7.5 Social Work and Interpreting

David Moorhead (1990)[1]

The connection between social work and interpreting is a key one in the relationship between deaf and hearing people in the UK. Historically, these two roles, however they have been defined, have been combined in a single service provider. This amalgamation has been the subject of considerable discussion and argument.

I do not intend to go over these issues again, as they have been outlined clearly in the previous paper. Rather, I wish to present a different analysis of this connection. This can be framed by two questions:

1 How do social work and interpreting address the issues of equality, independence, self-determination, respect and choice for deaf people?
2 Does combining the two roles in a single deliverer detrimentally affect deaf people's experience of these human rights?

Considering these two themes will mean looking at a number of issues: the nature of the relationship between hearing and deaf people; helping; the nature of welfare; the meaning of social work; social workers as public servants; the role of interpreters; and the perspectives of deaf people.

These issues need to be set against a changing context of social policy in the UK. This change has implications for the role of social workers, though a greater emphasis being placed on social control in legislation and a heightening awareness of citizen choice and empowerment. Those functions of social work that previously rested in the element of social care, such as interpreting/advocating for deaf people, now sit more uneasily in the new control framework—whether that control is from society or from citizens.

First, let me define some terms and make some preliminary statements:

Who are deaf people?
What do I mean by interpreting?
What do I mean by social work?
What is deafness?

I shall be using the term 'deaf people' in this paper to refer to both Deaf people, a linguistic and cultural minority, and to previously hearing people, whether deafened or hard of hearing.

I shall use the term 'interpreting' as a generic one, encompassing the activities of interpreting, translating and reflecting as outlined by Kyle (1989). This may not be very proper, but it does allow me to include in my analysis those groups of previously hearing people who may be more part of the majority culture than the minority Deaf culture. Activities such as text-transcribing, lip-speaking and note taking, although more accurately described by Kyle as reflecting rather than interpreting, will then be included.

My meaning of 'social work' is encompassed by British Association of Social Workers (BASW) principles of practice, outlined later. These principles provide a basis for seeing social work as an individual activity, in relation to personal power and control, and a group activity in relation to social power and control.

I wish to distinguish between meanings of 'deafness' on two levels: pathological and social.

Much of our understanding of deafness and the experience of deaf people is based on the perception of deafness as a sensory handicap. Definitions are based on developing, or not developing, speech and upon decibel loss (Myklebust, 1964), on hearing and not hearing sound, to what degree and at what age (Sainsbury, 1986), and on impairment of intellectual and emotional development (Ballantyne, 1977).

Causes are seen as physiological in nature, whether hereditary or as a result of illness, accident or age, while effects are seen largely as functional, and in terms of individual's or family's adjustment to the loss.

The purpose of rehabilitation and support is seen as mitigating the effects of hearing loss, and in attempting to narrow as far as possible the gap or difference between hearing and deafness. Hearing experience is taken as the norm, and deaf people's handicap is seen as their inability to communicate normally within a hearing world.

The perspective that gives rise to these definitions is that of people who have experienced hearing, not deafness. It is largely pathological, and so in many ways is a medical, male, middle class, white hearing perspective. This limits the base of knowledge and understanding on which the definitions are based. To a person who has never heard, the concept of hearing has a different meaning to that of a person who has always heard. So too, therefore, has the concept of deafness.

However, in a social analysis, as writers such as Oliver (1986), Finkelstein (1980, 1981) and Abberley (1987) have argued in relation to disability, the emphasis changes onto the key role of disabled people's perspectives in forming meanings of disability, and onto the difference between their experience and that of non-disabled people. In this perspective, deaf people's experience may provide them with the basis for forming their own group and individual identity. Their handicap is the control exercised over them by a dominant group that does not permit them full and equal use of their own language, nor allow them to value their different experience and understand their lives in terms of that experience.

This change in emphasis alters the relationship between deaf and hearing people. The norm is people's experience, rather than a specific physical state, and understandings have to encompass differences between experiences, rather than homogenize them. This places deafness on an equal footing with hearing, not as a second-rate experience.

This may be a difficult concept to grasp. Surely, one may ask, deafness is not a state that people would choose to have? But then, would one say that about being black? Or being a woman? Both of these groups also suffer oppression by a dominant group that bases its understandings on limited knowledge and experience. Whether a person has never heard, or has been previously hearing, any perspective that undervalues that person's experience will be oppressive, denying as it does that person's individuality, dignity and rights.

Where do social work and interpreting stand in this relationship?

The first four principles of practice in BASW's Code of Ethics (BASW, 1975) are as follows:

1 He (*sic*) will contribute to the formulation and implementation of policies of human welfare and he (*sic*) will not permit his (*sic*) knowledge, skills or experience to be used to further inhuman policies.

2 He (*sic*) will respect his (*sic*) clients as individuals and will seek to ensure that their dignity, individuality, rights and responsibility shall be safeguarded.

3 He (*sic*) will not act selectively towards clients out of prejudice on the grounds of their origin, status, sex, sexual orientation, age, belief or contribution to society.

4 He (*sic*) will help his (*sic*) clients increase the range of choices open to them and their powers to make decision.

Kyle (1989) from the University of Bristol, Deaf Research Unit which had looked in detail at sign language and interpreting, defines an interpreter as someone who 'presents the message of the first person in the language of the second person in a form which the first person would if he/she could use the language of the second person'. He identifies four elements that emerge from this definition:

1 The interpreter, 'stands between' the two parties, 'representing' neither.

2 The interpreter should be functionally bilingual.

3 The interpreter is concerned with meaning and how this is to be represented in each language.

4 The interpreter works in 'real time'; that is, there is a time constraint on the transfer of the message.

I do not wish to compare elements in these two descriptions, and identify specific causes for the role confusion that Kyle points out arises in combining interpreting with social work. But let me draw out one key issue. How can a worker 'standing between two parties, representing neither' also 'help clients increase the range of choices open to them and their powers to make decisions'?

What I do wish to do is address the issue of how far Deaf people and previously hearing people can maintain control over the circumstances that allow them to exercise their rights of equality, dignity, self-determination, independence and choice.

I will do this by looking at helping, at the control of language, at dependence and at the nature of welfare and social workers as public servants, within the dual frameworks of a pathological model and a social model of deafness.

So what is helping?

> I suspect that our real motives and attitudes, the ones that most affect what we actually do as social workers, are derived from experiences of helping and being helped.
> (Jordan, 1979, p.3)

Three issues seem to me to emerge from this observation. First, that there may be a difference between what we *actually* do as social workers, and what we are *meant* to do. Second, that helping is a two-way process, which thirdly, is a common experience for all of us.

Let us first consider further this issue of what we are meant to do. Social work practice is defined by a number of sources: by its professional standards, by legislation, by the policies of local authorities and voluntary agencies, by central government guidelines and by the ethos of public concern that underlies these sources. These definitions will not all be complementary, as they will be addressing different interests.

Public concern will not necessarily be wholly altruistic, motivated solely by concern for and care of less fortunate members of society. It may also be motivated by guilt, that the social and economic system creates poverty, disadvantage and oppression. Concern is exercised to assuage that guilt— but not necessarily to remove the poverty, disadvantage and oppression.

Social work, and social workers, are often caught in this dilemma between safeguarding their clients' individual and group interests, and being obliged to meet the expectations of their employers to exercise control over their clients' behaviour and over the allocation of scarce welfare resources to them. The dilemma places constraints on helping, by making it a one-way process, and increasing dependence. Helping becomes the means of implementing the definitions of the physical state of deafness that have emerged from a limited base of knowledge and experience in the welfare structure.

Helping deaf people under a model where problems and solutions are defined from this limited, non-deaf, experience, places the helper in a dominant position, and the helped in a passive role. The two helping roles, social work (helping the deaf person to adjust) and interpreting (helping the hearing world to communicate with him or her) are based on the same understanding: that deafness is a lack of hearing and communication is the means of narrowing the gap between deaf people and the hearing norm. In this model the two roles may logically be combined as they are both fulfilling the same function—control.

The deaf person, however, remains a passive receiver of a service that does not derive its validity from his or her experience; and his or her opportunity to exercise language use, or communication method[2] is restricted by the very helping structure set up to provide communication access—combining the two functions in a single provider, one of whose key functions is to administer limited public welfare.

How does this understanding of interpreting and social work fit in with those definitions and principles outlined earlier? A key element in the definition of interpreting is that of linguistic independence; that is to say, that the language is owned by the user, not the interpreter. Equally, in considering the principles of practice set down by BASW, the social worker's obligations towards his or her clients can only be met in an equitable relationship between the two parties, in order to safeguard their dignity, individuality, rights and responsibilities.

Within a social model, helping is recognized as a two-way process. Problems and solutions are defined by reference to deaf people's experience, and deaf people are able to exercise their full language and communication rights; difference is recognized. Social workers and interpreters are able to fulfil their obligations *separately*, as control and choice rest equally with the deaf person, and not solely with the helper and the helping machanisms. If the two roles are combined, both the interpreter and social worker become unable to fulfil their functions (because of the role confusion identified above), deaf people are denied full use of their language, and are therefore deprived of their rights of self-determination, independence, choice and equality.

Both social work and interpreting, under the definitions outlined here, can provide deaf people with the means to control the circumstances that allow them to exercise their rights of equality, dignity, self-determination, independence and choice. These circumstances are: the full and equal use of language and communication method, recognized as different from the majority non-deaf group's use; acknowledgement of the type of services and how they are provided; acknowledgement of deaf people's experience, and the validity of Deaf and previously hearing identities based on that experience.

The treatment of deaf people as dependent and passive, which emerges from a pathological model of deafness, lessens considerably their ability to exercise their rights. It denies deaf people the opportunity to explain their deafness in terms of their experience, and denies them use of their different language and communication method.

Interpreting as an independent function may give deaf people back the use of their language and communication method, and therefore the opportunity to explain their experience to themselves and to others. However, if social work and other human services continue to operate within the same limited, non-deaf knowledge boundaries that come out of the pathological model, the opportunities for exercising this use will be restricted.

Where social work has a dual purpose of care and control, as in the UK, any combination of interpreting with social work, whichever model of deafness it operates under, will deny deaf people the use of their own language in their own way, and will therefore be denying them control of the circumstances under which they may exercise their rights. We need to ask ourselves as social workers, whether this form of oppression is acceptable to a Code of Ethics whose first principle is that a social worker 'will not permit his (*sic*) knowledge, skills or experience to be used to further inhuman policies'.

Notes

1   This paper is presented from the perspective of a hearing person.

2   'Communication method' is used here to describe means of communicating by deaf people, such as lipreading, using a hearing aid, writing or signed English, that are to be treated equally with the different language of deaf people; that is, British Sign Language.

References

Abberley, P. (1987) 'The Concept of Oppression and the Development of a Social Theory of Disability', *Disability, Handicap and Society, 2*, 1.

Ballantyne, J.C. (1977) *Deafness*, London, Longman.

BASW (1975) *A Code of Ethics for Social Work*, Birmingham, BASW.

Finkelstein, V. (1980) *Attitudes and Disabled People*, New York, World Rehabilitation Fund.

Finkelstein, V. (1981) 'Disability and the Helper – Helped Relationship', in Brechin, A., Liddiard, P. and Swain, J. (eds) *Handicap in a Social World*, Beckenham, Hodder and Stoughton.

Jordan, B. (1979) *Helping in Social Work*, London, Routledge and Kegan Paul.

Kyle, J.G. (1989) 'Some aspects of British Sign Language – English Interpreting', *Deafness, 3*, 4.

Mykelbust, H.R. (1964) *The Psychology of Deafness*, New York, Grune and Stratton.

Oliver, M. (1986) 'Social Policy and Disability: Some Theoretical Issues', *Disability, Handicap and Society, 1*, 1.

Sainsbury, S. (1986) *Deaf Worlds*, London, Hutchinson.

7.6 'We' Are Not Disabled, 'You' Are

Vic Finkelstein (1990)

I have always accepted that there are critical differences between the assumptions that lead to race and gender discrimination. Similarly, there seem to be important differences in the source of discrimination against disabled people (including deaf people) and other forms of discrimination. If, for example, there was an operation that could turn black people into white (or women into men) and this was universally applied, then there could be no discrimination based upon skin colour (or gender). However, in the first place, such an operation would be universally rejected by the oppressed groups. Secondly, in the case of race, the oppressor nations would simply find other ways of identifying the racial groups against whom they wished to discriminate; or in the case of gender, if the operation was successful, the human species would die out. With regard to race and gender, therefore, performing surgery (or intervening in any other direct physical way) on individuals could never be a route to the removal of the discrimination faced by these groups. Not so in the sphere of disability. In the first place, every (!) disabled person would welcome such an operation (or other forms of personal intervention) which guaranteed successful elimination of the impairment (whether this was a spinal injury, visual impairment, hearing impairment, or birth defect, etc.). In the second place, direct personal interventions of this type, where the body defect is eliminated, also places that individual into a new social status which is not subject to the former oppression.

From this perspective, deaf people have more in common with other disability groups than they do with groups based upon race and gender. In this respect, the language oppression imposed on deaf people is more in line with, for example, the *'mobility oppression'* imposed on people with motor impairments, than with other language oppressed peoples. This is not to deny that all oppressed groups do share some common features, but I would suggest that a deeper discussion on discrimination against disabled people needs to be based upon a theory which clarifies the link between body impairment (and ways of intervening to eliminate this) and the discrimination (or oppression or disability) faced by the group.

The fact that most deaf people do not want to be regarded as disabled seems important, but the meaning of this is not necessarily obvious. I think most disabled people (people with a physical impairment) also do not like thinking of themselves as disabled! Part of this has to do with disability being interpreted as a synonym for physical impairment (with all its negative associations). On the one hand the term seems to be used in the above sense, but in other places it seems to have a different meaning and to be linked to the idea of social discrimination against people with body defects. The desire of deaf people to distance social discrimination (in the particular form they face as a linguistic minority) from body impairment (hearing defect) is, I think, exactly the same issue that other disability groups are facing.

At first it seems a mystery why, if most people who have obvious bodily impairments such as spinal injuries or hearing loss (and their very many able-bodied sympathisers) object so strongly to the label 'disabled', it has been so difficult to change negative attitudes towards the term. Yet disabled people have remained persistently reluctant to put energy into changing the meaning of the word 'disabled'. They have preferred to distance themselves from the label. At the same time campaigns to change public attitudes towards disability have also been remarkably unsuccessful.

This would suggest that there must be some very good reasons why disabled people reject the label. After all, disabled people are not stupid! If attitudes towards disability remain strongly negative—even amongst ourselves—despite all the efforts to change these attitudes, then perhaps we should change our assumptions and accept that negative attitudes are not due to ignorance or misunderstanding. On the contrary, perhaps negative attitudes are appropriate and reflect the real position of disabled people in society.

Given that there are good objective reasons for viewing disability in a negative way, and as long as these objective conditions survive, we can expect negative attitudes to survive, regardless of what disabled people like to think about themselves. One set of (objective) facts immediately stands out when looking at disability in its negative form. As far as I can see, from government statistics, independent research projects and personal experiences, on nearly every parameter which might be regarded as indicating participation in mainstream life, disabled people come out extremely badly: on attainment results in education, on numbers of disabled people in employment, on income levels, on suitability of housing and on access to public transport, public buildings, public information (newspapers, radio television) and public leisure activities. Being disabled, then, has clear negative implications.

If we look at history I believe we can trace the development of objective conditions which gradually drove all physically and mentally impaired people (i.e. 'cripples') out of active participation in their communities and into their current negative status.

Contemporary literature over the centuries shows that, although people with physical and mental impairment have continuously occupied an inferior status in society, they have, nevertheless, as cripples also lived in periods when they were integral members of society (as is still the case in very many Third World societies). The cripple begging in the street, or the deaf person working in some menial job, were still members of their communities. The disappearance of cripples from the streets and places of ordinary employment was a slow process which involved increasing public acceptance of physical and mental 'normality' as a criterion for participation in society.

That the progressive acceptance of signing as a means of communication for deaf people was suddenly halted and then rejected may be historically true. But how are we to explain this change in attitude towards what is acceptable as a means of communication? In other words, 'what objective conditions *disable* people who use signing as their means of communition despite their wishes?'

I believe that the meaning of disability is determined by the way our society is organized. In this respect it is not only the oppression of British Sign Language that is socially determined but also the dominant interpretation of deafness. If the meaning of deafness is socially determined as a form of disability then this will utlimately assert itself regardless of what deaf people want. The only way to change the meaning of deafness would be to change the social determinants of the meaning. From this point of view, changing the meaning of deafness (or the meaning of disability) it is essential to understand the social nature of deafness (i.e. the social context in which the meaning is created). Logically this suggests understanding the nature of our society (the general) before understanding its impact on hearing impaired people (the particular),

One argument is that the predominant factor contributing to the disablement of different groups of people is located in the way in which wealth is created and the possibilities for people to participate in this process. For example, at a time when small scale manufacture was carried out in the individual home, or when transport was individualized with the horse and cart, or when products were exchanged in small stalls in the market place, then there might have been some scope for these activities to be carried out by people of different shapes and sizes. Being deaf and working a hand loom at home could be a viable means of livelihood.

However, the invention of the steam engine introduced the possibility of working with large machinery which could produce more efficiently than, say, the operative working on a home-based hand loom. But the new machinery of the industrial revolution had to be designed not for a specific individual but for an *'average'* person who might be hired off the streets (i.e. the *'hands'*). People who deviated from this *'norm'* were in increasing danger of being unemployed as more and more machinery was introduced into the productive processes. In addition, as the machinery was not something to become familiar with in one's one home, the potential worker had to be able to follow instructions accessible to the *'normal'* worker (i.e. oral instructions) on the factory floor.

Under these conditions of production it seems clear that the increasing dominance of large scale manufacture created objective conditions which progressively raised the importance of *'normality'* and all forms of normal behaviour. Being normal became the dominant criterion for employment and so there was an imperative to suppress non-normal behaviour, including signing. If this means certain groups of people progressively lose their prospects for earning a living then they have no alternative except to beg and rely on charity.

Undoubtedly this led to the appearance of large numbers of beggars on the streets and made a policy for their removal a necessity. Once the process of removing these unemployed from the physical and social environment was well under way, particularly into the alms houses and later the large institutions, then I think there must have been pressure to provide food and shelter *only* to those who were regarded as unable to work because they were not normal. The other unemployed must surely have had pressure maintained on them to find jobs.

From this perspective the unemployed had to be separated into two categories: the infirm and the indolent (thieves, vagabonds and the so-called lazy, etc.). This need for classification provided the setting for diagnostic experts to intervene in separating the infirm from others. The experts in identifying the infirm were, of course, doctors. I believe this marked the beginning of a process of classifying disabled people and interpreting disability in medical terms.

Once disabled people were collectively defined as unemployable it was logical for the defining experts, the doctors, to concentrate their attention on ways of making these people *'normal'*, or as normal as possible. After all, the machinery of large-scale manufacture was designed to be worked by *'normal'* people. If disabled people could be returned to normality (rehabilitated) then they might obtain work and cease being dependent upon charity and state handouts. This meant the development of different types of professional intervention and the provision of specialist aids for different disability groups. To facilitate this, disabled people had to be classified into the mentally ill, lame, mental handicapped, blind and deaf, etc. By the middle of the twentieth century all disabled people were being routinely classified and registered by many different agencies according to medically defined categories.

Being labelled disabled became an objective fact of life for all disabled individuals. Once treatments (e.g. physiotherapy), special services (e.g. provision of hearing aids) and specific benefits (e.g. mobility allowance) proliferated, the need to sharpen boundaries between different categories of *'disability'* became increasingly important, and, in the 1970s and 1980s, we saw a rapid increase in scales and measures for defining and classifying disability groups. Disabled people were identified both in general and in specific sub-groups. Disabled people, of course, played very little part in this process (although some organizations campaigning for financial benefits, such as the *Disablement Income Group*, needed to provide their own categories of people who would be eligible for the benefits for which they were campaigning).

Regardless of personal wishes, therefore, being labelled disabled in the contemporary world is a fact of life for all disabled people. As long as there is no possibility of gaining access to services or social and welfare benefits without surrendering to the label disabled (or one of the sub-categories), there will be no possibility of convincing the general public that an individual or group is not disabled. The use of certain equipment such as wheelchairs, and aids not used by *'normal'* people, only confirms the user as a disabled person. I believe signing is viewed by non-disabled people in this way, as a special aid to communication.

Another factor in not seeing oneself as disabled is that, subjectively, the living experience of most disabled people is that the closer one is to being normal the better one's social status and employment prospects. If forced to acknowledge an impairment, then the incentive is at least to distance one's own personal condition from that of another thought to be lower down the scale of normality. Thus people with the impairment thought to be below can be labelled 'disabled'. This then frees the individual, or group, to consider themselves as only a variation in the pattern of normality.

For example, people with a spinal injury can think of themselves as reasonably normal (only restricted by the failure of society to accept their form of mobility—wheelchairs—that is, they are mobility oppressed), while those with learning difficulties can be regarded by wheelchair users as *'really'* disabled. Similarly, people with a hearing impairment can think of themselves as reasonably normal (only restricted by the failure of society to accept their form of communication—British Sign Language—that is, they are language oppressed), while those with a spinal injury can be regarded by BSL users as *'really'* disabled!

Assumed levels of employability separate disabled people into different levels of dependency and this, in turn, leads to different types of services and provisions. At the bottom, those regarded as hopelessly unemployable are offered places in residential homes where they can have total care. Whereas those who can work may have access to special equipment and adaptations funded by the state.

This objective ranking of disabled people into different degrees of employability, with consequent access to different provisions, provides the context for disabled people to fear constantly that they may be identified with those whom they see as worse off than themselves (i.e. less employable and more dependent). By distancing themselves from groups that they perceive as more disabled than themselves, they can hope to maintain their claim to economic independence (i.e. employment) and an acceptable status within the community.

Subjective and objective factors in the lives of disabled people, then, constantly encourage them to distance themselves from each other, denying that they are disabled while readily defining others with this label. In this behaviour, disabled people are, of course, acting exactly like able-bodied people who, for their part, see the need to distance themselves from those who are disabled.

It seems that when people with a hearing impairment identify themselves as language oppressed but not disabled, while at the same time they see people with a mobility impairment as disabled (but not as mobility oppressed), they are attributing medical labels to others in exactly the same way that they reject such labels for themselves!

I believe that despite the wishes of people with physical or mental impairments to distance themselves from the label 'disabled', there are two contemporary service approaches which persist in contributing towards the general public image of disabled people as a unified social group. These approaches are based upon the medical model and the administrative model. It is, perhaps, these service approaches which contribute most to the construction of a common identity amongst disabled people.

I have already mentioned the role of medical diagnosis in providing the historical lawful separation of disabled people from their unemployed peers. This role provided the medical profession with a powerful base for the determination of the status of disabled people in society. Once disabled people were separated out of society and considered the legitimate concern of doctors, the stage was set for the growth of new professions (in particular physiotherapy, occupational therapy and speech therapy) to service the developing disability-related medical specialisms (ortho-paedics, ophthalmology, audiology, psychiatry, etc.).

The growth of these specialist professions and their highly public visibility as gate-keepers to medical, social and welfare services provides a powerful reinforcement to the view that disability is a medical problem. This coupled with the fact that being '*normal*' is still a major consideration in obtaining employment and promotion, and thereby gaining an independent livelihood, means that the role of medicine in the lives of disabled people remains extremely significant.

Publicity and public acclaim given to rehabilitation efforts aimed at making disabled people behave or look more normal (like dramatic surgical operations to make children with cerebral palsy walk, or electronic implants to make people with auditory impairments hear) confirm the public's attachment to the medical interpretation of disabled people's needs. The medical approach towards disabled people has been much discussed and criticized, but it still dominates current legislation and provides the main criteria for defining categories of people who shall have access to services and benefits.

The over-riding feature of the medical approach, again despite any wishes of the recipients, is that it brings all disability groups together under a single medical interpretation: the medical model of disability.

Criticism of the medical model has led to some changes and there are increasing signs that disability-related services are beginning to move away from medical control in the health service, to the social and welfare umbrella in community-based services. The problem is, however, that this shift in control has not resulted in disabled people necessarily exercising more control over their lives. On the contrary, service providers in the community generally have a wider perspective than their medial colleagues in identifying areas of disabled people's lives for their professional assessments and interventions.

This wider perspective, unfortunately, often leaves very little that disabled people can do without feeling that an expert is waiting in the background to intervene. The community-based disability worker is there to provide expert assessments and advice on nearly everything, from the shape and architecture of the home, and the whole range of equipment that all people need for modern living, to advice and counselling for intimate personal and sexual problems.

In this respect these experts are usually trained to see the lives of disabled people in terms of problems to be solved, and their role as providing solutions, or guidance towards the solution. The existence of this vast army of workers daily reinforces the impression that disabled living is an exercise in problem solving.

Nationally, then, the existence of large and expensive social and welfare services provides ample evidence that a characteristic of all disabled groups is that they face a series of problems which they cannot solve on their own, and which the state has had to administer through the provision of specialized services.

In my view, understanding the growth of local authority administrators and workers in *'disability units'* orchestrating community services, provides the key to identifying this new *'administrative model'* of disability as the *'medical model'* declines in power and influence. And it is the administrative model of disability that objectively draws different groups of disabled people together in the assessment forms for problem solving and service provision. From this point of view, disabled people can be identified as a distinct social group (with several disability sub-groups—see for example the World Health Organization's *Classification of Impairment, Disability and Handicap*).

Curiously, one feature of the medical and administrative models of disability, perhaps above all others, that does indeed seem to unite all groups of disabled people, is the hostility felt by disabled people towards these interpretations of disability!

The modern disability movements which are bringing together different groups of disabled people and developing a common identity, not only represent a united front against medical and administrative dominance over a fragmented social group, but a historical leap forward in redefining disability in more positive terms. It seems to me that it is this new situation that is creating prospects for the removal of social and physical barriers that disable different groups of people with physical and mental impairments.

The significant factor is that, by coming together in the new political organizations of disabled people, the new arts organizations and the new organizations providing services (e.g. Centres for Integrated Living), disabled people can identify themselves not only as disabled people but, at the same time, provide mutual support for the removal of language oppression, mobility oppression, information oppression and other forms of oppression that particularly impact on them.

7.7 Deaf People and Minority Groups in the UK

Jim Kyle (1986)

[. . .]

Deaf people

What hope is there for deaf [people]? According to the general societal and educational mood, one can see very little reason why society should accept deaf people as another minority group. Given the present position of these minorities, it's questionable whether deaf people would wish to be another minority group in their position of subservience to English. Nevertheless, it is as a minority group that we have begun to conceive of the deaf community. Our research[1] indicates the same bonds of language and social gathering, the same attitudes towards community identity as in any other group.

Not all deaf people associate with one another all the time and the deaf club itself is not the only feature of the community. Profoundly deaf young people are more likely to be members of their local deaf club than partially hearing (79% as compared to 37%). Attendance also is variable as one would expect in any community, some are more centrally involved than others. Fifty-three per cent of profoundly deaf people attend once a week or more, while only 25 per cent of partially hearing young people do. If we look in detail at those who never attend (Table 1) we see the clear effect of hearing loss.

Table 1 Lack of attendance and hearing loss (*N* = 205) %

	dB				
	−65	66–85	86–95	96–105	106+
People who rarely or never attend	74	49	31	20	13

Not surprisingly, it is profoundly deaf people who would be more upset and affected by the closure of the deaf club and who also value their social life more highly than hearing people (Table 2).

Table 2 Evaluation of deaf and hearing social life (*N* = 205) %

Deaf social life is:	−85dB	86dB +
Better or much better	16	63
The same	51	29
Worse or much worse	33	8

Deaf people show all the characteristics of minority group membership. Central to it is attitude and commitment and use of the community language. However, there are important differences between deaf people and other communities:

1 Deaf people do not live together in a geographic area (though they do choose to marry one another).

2 They do not use a 'spoken' language (which gives them a lower status almost by definition in comparison to English).

3 Their language is not usually passed on from generation to generation but rather transmitted by peers or associates.

4 Normally deaf people are not proficient in this first language before they reach school as other minority group members would tend to be (however, the Linguistics Minorities Project shows this situation to be not uncommon in some linguistic minority groups).

5 They do not acquire high status positions in society and so have no easy way to legitimize the language use (in fact this may not be a difference but a key determining feature of the minority language status).

Having said that these differences exist, the factors are explanatory rather than disallowing in terms of the coherence of the community. If we can accept for the present the integrity of such a community, and our linguistic research has established validity of its language, we can begin to piece together an explanatory framework for the position of deaf people in the UK today.

Deaf bilingualism in the UK

According to the main definition of bilingualism adopted by the Linguistic Minorities Project, deaf people can be considered functioning bilinguals in English and BSL even though we have come to question their level of facility in English and may in some cases question their skills in BSL. The options for deaf people in education and society are therefore rather similar to those of South-Asian or West Indian minority groups.

We know, in addition, the general laws of power in history: when two groups come together then it is the weaker which learns the language of the stronger. According to Skutnabb-Kangas (1984), bilingualism becomes a halfway house between the monolingualism of the weaker group and the acceptance of the monolingualism of the stronger group. In effect, this type of assimilationist policy may lead to an ultimately well-ordered society . . . but a monocultural one. When this policy of integration does not seem to work, or works only slowly, then racial tension begins to arise as it has now done again in the UK, and as it has been recognized officially in the Swann report's conception. Monolingualism is nothing unusual. It's happening all over Europe at the present time. With 3,000 languages in the world and only about 200 states, some languages are treated as poor minority language. Skutnabb-Kangas (1984) has provided a way of conceptualizing the educational approaches when bilingual situations arise in different countries and it is a useful way of considering deaf people in the UK.

Type 1 is what takes place in most educational environments—education of the majority in their native language. It is usually termed mainstream education.

Type 2 is described as a submersion programme; the sort of situation which Bullock (1975) said should not occur in the UK.

> No child should be expected to cast off the language and culture of the home as he crosses the school threshold . . .

In this type of education, the classes are mixed but the minority children do not have equal rights and do not usually even have the satisfaction of having their native language taught to the majority in the school. This is one of the features the Swann report wishes to remedy. It will be interesting to see how many programmes of BSL for hearing children emerge. In practice, even if we reach the stage of making education aware of deaf children's position as ESL (English as a second language) learners, there are still factors which ascribe low status to the first language: if media programmes for minority languages are restricted to unsocial hours or:

> If teachers of English as a second language do not use or refer to the pupils' mother tongues as an aid to learning, then this may signal a low evaluation of the minority languages.
> (LMP, 1983, p. 10)

[. . .]

In addition, the type 2 practice has tremendous social overtones for the minority group member.

> One of the more implicit goals in this type of programme is also that those minority children who succeed in the programmes at the same time are socialized into accepting those values which are connected with that part of the majority society which controls the schools. In that way, those minority children who succeed are pacified: they are alienated from their own group and they do not feel solidarity with those minority children who do not suceed . . . It is the 'we-made-it-and-they-can-do-it-too-if-they-work-hard-enough' syndrome. Those minority children on the other hand who do not succeed are pacified by shame: they are made to feel that it is their own fault that they don't succeed—the 'blame-the-victim' technique.
> (Skutnabb-Kangas, 1984, p. 128)

This type of approach is used throughout the world, even in supposedly bilingual environments like Canada where non-French, non-English speakers are not catered for.

Type 3 education is less likely to occur in the UK, being one usually reserved for workers in transit, though it could be used to describe some of the sign language education to which oralism was the reaction, 100 years ago.

Type 4 is the equivalent of mother tongue maintenance rejected by the Swann report but increasingly taken over by minority groups themselves. There are as yet no classes for deaf children or children of deaf parents to teach them their language.

Type 5 is an approach popularized in Canada where it is the majority who attend an immersion school in order to develop their second-minority language. It is directly excluded by the Swann report—in fact it is hardly even considered on the basis that the multilingual situation in the UK is far more complex than the bilingual situation in places like Canada. In practice, it seems to be one of the most effective ways of creating bilingualism.

Type 6 is perhaps the nearest the Swann report comes to using minority languages. What is most interesting is that it is exactly the position of most countries in relation to sign language. Use of sign is a vehicle towards competence in the spoken and written language. In effect it is a transitional tool towards an assimilationist goal. It is easy to accept since it seems kind to the minority deaf people. In practice, it may be a trap for direct integration.

> It is said, often even officially that the children need not be taught bilingually anymore . . . when they have learned enough of the majority language to be able to follow instruction through the medium of the majority language. The criteria for when they can be transferred to majority-medium instruction are often based on loose evaluations of when the child can manage orally in simple face-to-face interaction, discussing concrete everyday things, situations where contextual clues help the child to understand . . . Often children at this stage still do not have any chance of succeeding as well as majority children in cognitively and linguistically more demanding decontextualized tasks . . . The result often is that they fail miserably at school regardless of superficial oral fluency.
> (Skutnabb-Kangas, 1984, p. 131)

Type 7 programmes demand meaningful examination of the type of support required to teach each language. When the language is at risk then it will require greater attention within school. But it is vital in this approach that *both* groups become bilingual and not revert to the situation of the majority learning a few vocabulary items of the minority languages.

It is not too difficult to place minority languages in the UK at present. It is also easy to see that BSL has been subject to type 2 treatment for a long time and perhaps unwittingly we have now accepted type 6 as the meaningful goal for teachers and for deaf people. In doing so, and even if there were a successful conversion to it throughout the UK, we would not be successful. Deaf people are not yet well enough understood for us to specify their needs adequately to achieve competence in English. To use a signed version of English as a means of 'bilingualism' cannot be linguistically acceptable and ultimately will lead to success and failure in the way that type 2 approaches have done.

Linguistic minorities have always been under pressure in the UK and, according to what will be treated as a very influential review (the Swann Report), there is no likelihood that this will change markedly in the forseeable future. Deaf people do not have the ethnic roots of these other minority groups to fall back on and so have been even more at risk. Mainstreaming policy is being implemented because they are treated as handicapped as well as because they are a minority. One can see that society must be alerted to the major problem for deaf people since they are ultimately unlike the other minorities in an assimilationist situation—it has been shown that they do not learn English simply by exposure. Because of this and the corresponding reduction in access to sign language which occurs in a mainstream monolingual situation, deaf people face a real risk of becoming semi-lingual not only in English but also in sign language.

This sort of situation of semi-lingualism would confine deaf people's language and communication to specific domains such as school, or deaf club and never really allow adequate productive language. Deaf people have reported this sort of problem, describing other deaf as 'going low'; in effect being unable to communicate adequately even with other deaf people. Deafness as a handicap would then be very severe indeed.

The deaf community will be required in the near future in the UK to develop a coherent policy for bilingualism if any change is to occur. There is no evidence of a major shift in UK policy in the treatment of minorities even though there will be greater recognition of pluralism. Deaf people do form a community in most senses of the concept but it is their development of a 'community image' for the hearing world which is most likely to convince the hearing world of this status. The process has begun in the UK through sign language research, interest in deaf education and exposure in the media but there is still a very long way to go.

Deaf people can form a coherent and identifiable linguistic and social minority in the UK. However, given the current problems of understanding and using the multilingualism of other larger minorities, this realization is something of a mixed blessing. When policy-makers in the UK begin to understand the true nature of multiculturalism, then we may see effective involvement of deaf people and BSL in education.

[Note

1   The findings reported here are based on the author's study of 205 young deaf people from all over England and Wales.]

References

Bullock, A. (1975) *A Language for Life*, London, Department of Education and Science, HMSO.

Linguistics Minority Project (LMP) (1983) *Linguistic Minorities in England*, University of London Institute of Education, Tinga Tanga.

Skutnabb-Kangas, T. (1984) *Bi-lingualism or Not*, Avon, Clevedon.

Swann, L. (1985) *Education for All*, London, Department of Education and Science, HMSO.

7.8 The British Deaf Association: The Voice of the Deaf Community

British Deaf Association (1990)

> We have served notice that the Deaf Community in Britain is no longer prepared to be a silent minority.
> *Murray Holmes, BDA Vice Chairman, 1983*

The British Deaf Association (BDA) is distinguished from other organizations by its historical links with Britain's indigenous Deaf community and the democratic way in which it is organized to represent the community's interests.

History

The BDA was founded in 1890, at a time of intense controversy about the use of sign language and fingerspelling in the education of deaf children, and about the exclusion of Deaf people from national decisions that affected their lives. The immediate cause of its birth was the failure of an 1889 Royal Commission on the education of deaf children to consult Deaf people. This led the magazine *Deaf Mute* to urge Deaf people to unite in defence of their own interests. A National Conference of Adult Deaf and Dumb Missions and Associations was duly held in London in 1890, which called for the formation of a national society to 'elevate the education and social status of the Deaf and Dumb in the United Kingdom'. The 1890 conference was also a belated response to the notorious international congress held in Milan 10 years earlier, when hearing teachers of deaf children passed a resolution banning the use of sign languages in schools throughout the world. The newly formed British Deaf and Dumb Association (BDDA) thus entered a fiercely hostile world, one dominated by hearing people acting on behalf of the Deaf but not representing their true interests or sharing their aspirations.

With the appointment of its first salaried General Secretary in 1972, the BDA became more professional and, as well as providing a number of services to the community, began to promote its beliefs more publicly, especially its commitment to Total Communication in the education of deaf children.

Aims and principles

The broad aims of the BDA are to advance and protect the interests of

Deaf people, to develop pride, identity and leadership qualities, awareness of their rights and responsibilities; thereby strengthening their own community and enabling them to take their place as full members of the wider national community.

The BDA is a grass-roots organization of Deaf people, with over 18,000 members, almost all of whom are deaf and use sign language. It is they who elect the BDA's governing body, the Executive Council, with its twenty Deaf Councillors who are seen as leaders of their community. BDA members are organized through a network of 178 local branches and eight regional councils. National policy is determined at an annual delegates conference. A week-long Congress held every 3 years usually features prominent Deaf people from home and abroad addressing major issues of current concern to the Deaf community.

The BDA has a strong commitment to being an equal opportunities employer and an increasing number of Deaf people are being employed. In 1989, 30 per cent of all staff were Deaf.

Sign language services

One important milestone in the BDA's work towards achieving recognition of sign language was the establishment of a Communication Skills Project (funded by the DHSS) in 1977; this not only examined the need for the training, assessment and registration of sign language interpreters, but also looked at ways to encourage the acquisition of basic sign communication skills amongst the general public. From this BDA initiative grew the organization known today as the Council for the Advancement of Communication with Deaf People (CACDP) which was formally constituted in 1980.

A further development was the British Sign Language Training Agency (BSLTA), established by the BDA at the University of Durham in 1985 with the aim of enabling Deaf people to become trained tutors of BSL. This foundation level BSL tutor training course is unique; all teaching is carried out by Deaf staff using BSL, with course study materials presented in BSL on video. By the end of 1989, some 143 Deaf tutors had completed the course, and were able to offer sign language teaching to hearing people all over the country.

The BDA recognized, however, the growing demand for sign language tutors at advanced levels, as well as the need for more trained sign language interpreters. In an attempt to meet this demand it entered into partnership with the Deaf Studies Research Unit at Durham University to develop an Advanced Diploma/MA qualification in Sign Language Studies. The course can be seen as a response to the BDA's concern not only to improve provision of sign language tutors and interpreters, but to give social workers, teachers and others working with Deaf people, an opportunity to develop sign language skills.

The BDA won the agreement of the main political parties to pay for sign language interpreters at their annual conferences, and has ensured the growing availability of interpreters at other public and leisure events, as well as providing expert advice and awareness training to central and local government authorities about sign language services. It was the driving force behind the establishment of the professional Association of British Sign Language Tutors in 1989, and continues to provide workshops for its members about interpreting and other issues.

Further afield, the BDA, with other National Associations of the Deaf within the European Community, made representations which resulted in the European Parliament voting unanimously in June 1988 for the official recognition of all indigenous sign languages in the European Community. It provided major support to the European Forum of Sign Language Interpreters in October 1988 to enable a European Charter for Sign Language Interpreters to be drawn up, and has worked energetically to contribute its knowledge and expertise to the Scientific Commissions of Sign Language and interpreting to the World Federation of the Deaf.

Advocacy
The BDA has four advocacy roles:

- To take up directly, individual cases of discrimination and justice;
- To act on the whole Deaf community to influence the content of government policy and legislation;
- To develop Deaf people's own advocacy skills so that they can represent themselves and other Deaf people;
- To make the hearing public better informed about deafness and to encourage positive attitudes towards Deaf people.

Personal advocacy
The BDA handles about 200 cases a year, most of which involve discrimination, injustice of problems of access to information or services. Although many are resolved successfully, results are frequently achieved only after protracted negotiations and efforts to educate and persuade the individuals, companies or institutions concerned to change their policies, practices or attitudes towards deaf people. The barriers to equality of treatment, opportunity and choice for deaf people are formidable. The inadequacies or inflexibility of legislation and policies prevent more positive or speedier outcomes to the problems referred by Deaf people to the BDA. Legal sanctions alone would not provide a comprehensive remedy but they would strengthen the BDA's hand in dealing with injustice. However, three attempts in the early 1980s to legislate against discrimination on the grounds of disability all failed.

Community advocacy
Promoting the needs of deaf people on particular issues, or in a particular locality is a recurring feature of the BDA's advocacy support to the Deaf community. One example is the several campaigns mounted to prevent the closure of deaf schools, regarded by the Deaf community as crucial to the

survival of the Community, its language and culture. Another example concerns the reaction to the Government's public awareness campaign on AIDS. The publicity and subsequent public debate in the media created confusion amongst some deaf people and failed to get its message across to others. The BDA acted quickly in forming a consortium of sixteen organizations in the deaf field and the Terence Higgins Trust to secure government funding and to devise and implement a programme of education on AIDS in the Deaf community.

Advocacy on policy and legislation

The needs of any minority group may easily be overlooked by legislators and policy-makers, so a major concern of the BDA is to monitor government policy and legislation and examine their implications for the Deaf community. In recent years the BDA's representations have succeeded in ensuring that some provision was made for deaf people in the 1983 Mental Health Act, the 1984 Police and Criminal Evidence Act Codes of Practice, the 1986 Disabled Person's (Services, Consultation and Representation) Act and the Youth Training Scheme. In essence, these provide access to appropriate communication services to enable deaf people to exercise their rights and responsibilities enshrined in the particular legislation or policy. Pressure for implementation of the 1986 Disabled Person's Act and in support of a Private Member's Bill to outlaw discrimination (1983) saw mass lobbies of Parliament by people with disabilities. On both occasions over 500 BDA members attended the lobby and were the largest group present.

Children and young people

Education

The BDA's education policy and programme for Deaf children and young people is aimed at raising standards and extending choice. Amongst the specific objectives are: enabling their access to sign language, Deaf adult role models, the Deaf community and its culture; developing their self-confidence and campaigning to end the restrictions which prevent many Deaf people from training as teachers of Deaf children.

Whilst some local education authorities (LEAs) now accept that Deaf children can benefit from special schools that use a Total Communication approach, many still place them in mainstream schools or special units that rarely use sign language, or have inadequate support services for Deaf pupils. A number of parents of Deaf children have turned to the BDA for help in such situations, which have been successfully resolved through determined intervention and have led to the child being allowed to go to a school of its choice. The BDA has also intervened on behalf of Deaf young people whose LEAs have sought to restrict their choice of further education. On national policy, constant attention is needed to ensure its appropriate application to the needs of Deaf pupils and students, and to campaign for equality of treatment, access and choice.

Direct services include courses to help Deaf pupils prepare for leaving school; outdoor adventure courses, activity weeks for younger children and sign language courses for parents.

Finding new families for Deaf children in care

Following a Delegates Conference motion, a BDA working party was established, in partnership with British Adoption And Fostering (BAAF), to look into the needs of Deaf children in care, with particular reference to the role of Deaf people as foster/adoptive parents, and other support the Deaf community might provide for these children and those who care for them.

Following nationwide consultation with professional workers and the Deaf community, two major themes emerged. The first was that the needs of Deaf children in care could often be met by Deaf people because of their experience, their sign language skills and their roots in the Deaf community.

The second major finding was that neither Deaf people nor fostering/ adoption agencies were fully aware of the special contribution that Deaf parents could make to the lives of Deaf children in care. Accordingly, it was decided to publish a book for fostering/adoption workers, setting out the needs of Deaf children and the potential of the Deaf community as a resource; and to produce a sign language video for the Deaf community, explaining the needs of Deaf children in care and how they could help to meet them. The book for professionals, *The Deaf Child in Care,* was published by BAAF in 1990, and the sign language video was expected to follow later in that year.

Young people

A resolution by the 1986 BDA Congress called for greater efforts to address the needs of young, deaf people and their participation in the Deaf community. This was a response to growing concern about the future of the Deaf community. Traditionally, knowledge of the access to the adult Deaf community was acquired from attendance at 'Deaf Schools'. However, implementation of the 1981 Education Act has resulted in the closure of some of these schools and in an increasing proportion of children being placed in units attached to, or in the mainstream classes of, ordinary local schools. Such children leave school with little, if any, knowledge of the Deaf community, its language and culture—'marginalized' young people with no 'Deaf' identity.

A study commissioned by the BDA (*Opportunities for Leadership Training*, BDA 1986) prompted action through a programme, making a clear commitment to young people and to the development of future Deaf leaders. The first step—a pilot project begun in 1987, to train a group of Deaf part-time youth workers—was followed by the development of a national course for Deaf Trainers and Youth Workers, launched in 1989. The same year saw the establishment of a BDA Youth Services department, headed by a qualified Deaf Youth and Community Worker, a 5-year project based in the West Midlands, and two further initiatives aimed at empowering Deaf young people, enhancing their involvement in the BDA and setting an agenda of their needs.

Information services

The BDA's information Service has three distinct groups to address—the Deaf community, professionals in the field, and hearing people. For most people, meaningful access to information is influenced by how it is delivered and presented. For Deaf people, who are members of a linguistic and cultural minority group, presentation is a very important consideration because their access is through BSL via television and video.

The BDA has been producing information on video in BSL for at least 10 years. It has a commitment to develop this area of work over the next 5 years. However, unless significant changes occur, access to information via television and video for Deaf people will continue to be severely and unnecessarily restricted.

To address this situation, the BDA supports the work of the Deaf Broadcasting Council and runs another television project—the London Deaf Video Project. This innovatory project, which produces videos and promotes 'video awareness', has, since 1985, been the cutting edge of video services for Deaf people. It was, for example, the first unit to produce a video about the AIDS HIV virus to inform the Deaf community.

The BDA is committed to enabling more Deaf people to gain access to public information. It believes that the Government should be responsible for information it generates—on benefits, health, legislation, etc.—to be translated into BSL on video. The Government already produces printed versions of information leaflets in ethnic minority languages.

The main print-based information vehicle of the BDA (and the Deaf community) is the monthly *British Deaf News (BDN)* which has a Deaf readership of 18,000. This magazine has, in various guises, been published without a break for at least a century and in recent years it has invested in a programme to ensure that the content and control of the magazine is in the hands of Deaf people. However, on its own, *BDN* is difficult for some Deaf people to read and does not enable access to wider 'non-deaf' information. It should be one part of a wider range of accessible sources of information to give Deaf people a choice.

For many years, the BDA has recognized the gap in information provision for professionals in the field of deafness. In 1988, it became joint publisher of *Deafness*—previously the journal of the National Council of Social Workers with Deaf People. Since 1988, the BDA and the Council have been developing this into a 'journal of the sociology of deafness'.

For the largest group, the general public, the BDA communicates largely in print. The main channels of communication to them are the Annual Report and Newsletters mailed during the year.

There is also a growing demand from the general public for information, particularly about sign language. To respond to this, the BDA runs the *Into Sign* information service that provides the facts, figures and details of local courses with Deaf sign language tutors.

The underlying message that the BDA has to put across in all of its information to this group consists of:

- the needs and continuing concerns of the Deaf community;
- the aspirations and rights of the Deaf community;
- the ability of Deaf people to contribute to and participate in society on equal terms;
- the fact that Deaf people are often ignored and under-used as active citizens;
- that Deaf people are best placed to inform the direction of their own future.

7.9 The Development of The Royal National Institute for the Deaf

The Royal National Institute for the Deaf (1990)

The Royal National Institute for the Deaf (RNID) was founded in 1911 as the National Bureau for Promoting the General Welfare of the Deaf—a title which now has a distinctly period flavour but is still an accurate description of the Institute's work. At the time there were about 140 local organizations in the U.K. concerned with education and welfare of the deaf, each pursuing its aims with very little reference to the others. In the previous 10 years there had been a growing realization that this fragmentation was a serious obstacle to progress and what was needed was a central organization to co-ordinate and encourage activity. The funds which enabled this concept to be put into practice were provided by Leo Bonn, a merchant banker who was himself deaf.

There is no formal definition of 'the deaf' in the account of the Bureau's inaugural meeting in its first annual report, but it is clear that the term was regarded as embracing anyone with a hearing loss, irrespective of whether they were born deaf or become deaf. This has always been the case. Although the RNID has on various occasions been accused of doing more for the born deaf than the hard of hearing, and vice versa, neither accusation is borne out by an objective survey of its activities over time.

The history of its first 50 years, as described in the annual report for 1961, followed a pattern of development typical of many voluntary organizations in the early to mid-twentieth century. Initially, the Bureau was heavily dependent on the efforts of concerned individuals with professional, social and political influence. It suffered a near demise during the First World War when personal concern was diverted elsewhere, but was reconstituted in 1924 as the National Institute for the Deaf, with a small administrative staff to provide operational continuity.

The Second World War was also a vulnerable period for the Institute, but again it survived and in 1948 acquired formal legal status when it was incorporated under the Companies Acts of 1929 and 1947, its Committee members becoming the equivalent of a board of dirctors and redefined as a Council of Management. The Council is elected from the Institute's voluntary members who are equivalent to shareholders. It functions via a number of committees elected from its membership plus co-opted non-members in the role of advisers where appropriate. From the viewpoint of the Institute's staff, the situation closely resembles local government, with paid officers responsible for implementing the Council's policy decisions and reporting to committees composed of voluntary members.

The RNID's current legal definition therefore is 'a company limited by guarantee and not having a share capital'. As regards its charitable status, when the General Register was set up following the Charities Act of 1960 there was no provision for backdating charities already in existence, so it is a technical point whether the status of the RNID as a charity goes back to the date of its governing instrument, in this case the Memorandum and Articles of Association of 1948 when it was incorporated as a company, or to the date it was officially notified of its charitable status in 1963.

During the 1960s and 1970s the number of paid staff grew rapidly as the RNID (which had acquired its 'Royal' prefix in 1961) consolidated existing services and developed new ones. Its organizational style during this period of its history is reflected in the tone and content of the review of its activities in the 1971 Annual Report, which is extracted here:

> Social Services and Training, under the simpler title 'Welfare' has been in existence as long as the Institute itself for this word, condescending as it might now seem, was a warm and helpful one and indeed still defines the raison d'etre of any voluntary society—welfare, in the old sense of all those it seeks to help. Every activity of every department of the RNID is directed towards this end. But from the strict committee-work angle the objects are keeping a watch on matters affecting the adult deaf, particularly in respect of jobs and training, making the most of State services and other helpful schemes, and encouraging new recruits into Social Work with the Deaf. A matter of considerable importance to the Social Services and Training Committee and in which they co-operate closely with the Children's Committee is after-school development, further education, careers, vocational training and, most difficult of all perhaps, what to do about the misfits. With our school for maladjusted deaf children and our training centre for maladjusted deaf youths, the question of what to do about those deaf youngsters who will never be able to stand on their own feet becomes much more immediate. Sheltered workshops might well be the answer.
>
> There should be plenty of productive work for them if only making the helpful devices for other deaf people that our own Technical Department invents.
>
> Publicity needs no explanation except in addition to press advertising it embraces all the printed matter put out in booklet form, including annual Reports, our magazine *Hearing*, films and TV appeals and relations generally with the BBC, Press and Public.
>
> Library and Information has increased in scope and importance enormously. The RNID Library is now generally admitted to be the greatest in the world on hearing, sound, speech and language, but it began humbly enough with books made homeless when a body called the Oral Foundation closed its premises in Fitzroy Square and became integreated with the Institute. Later in 1957 a huge increase came with a bequest from Mr Selwyn Oxley one of the pioneer deaf workers who had during his lifetime acquired a vast collection. After valuable work by first Honorary (notably Mr H.G.M. Strutt) then full-time librarians, (notably Dr Gorman) order was made out of chaos, and visitors, students and borrowers soon came to regard this as the fountain head for all deaf knowledge. So much information has to be passed out nowadays,

that a full-time Information Officer was appointed to leave the Librarian free to manage her own speciality. This has enabled a more positive approach to be made to information—instead of merely waiting for requests, digests and summaries from international papers are made and sent out where they are needed or are likely to make an impact in Government, medical, teaching and such circles.

The Homes committee is responsible for the well-being of residents in all the RNID Homes, ensuring that the fabric of the buildings, internal fittings and furnishings are well maintained . . . It too, as a Committee, goes far back to when our first Home, Poolemead near Bath, started by a local clergyman's daughter in 1868, was taken over in 1934. The financial responsibility also for all of these is great; most of the houses are old but solidly built and modifications like central hearing, fire alarm systems, modernising of sleeping and living quarters as well as routine painting and decorating call for constant attention.

As in so many other aspects of modern life, the emphasis today is on professionalism. Warm hearts and good intentions alone are no longer sufficient and we are following the new directions laid down by Government Reports, including secondment for some of our existing senior staff to the courses on Care in Residential Homes at Ipswich Civic College, School of Social Services.

One property that is not the concern of the Homes Committee is, perhaps, the most important one of all—Larchmoor School for Maladjusted Deaf Children. This was brought into existence through the Children's Committee, formed in 1960 under the Chairmanship of Dr Margaret Scott Stevenson and vigorously developed by Mr Micahel Reed. It had already been realized that no facilities existed for helping the deaf child who through some second handicap was not able to make progress even at a school for the deaf . . .

The first children were taken in in 1966. Now, five years later we are able to see with pardonable pride, young deaf children once regarded as 'uneducable', rehabilitated and on their way to success in more normal schools—often indeed the very schools which a few years earlier had been unable to cope with them.

Finally the Medical and Technical Committee—more technical than medical perhaps although there is a high proportion of doctors upon it—for it is responsible for the large and busy Technical Departments in London, and Glasgow where, over the years, many practical devices to help deaf and hard-of-hearing people have been invented or improved upon, and often put into production. This actual making of things has had a valuable side benefit in providing opportunities for young deaf men to learn the basic of electronics assembly, the visual alarm clock, battery tested, flashing light warnings, vibrators, etc. all being made or tested and repaired by trainees under the supervision of qualified staff. Chassis wiring contracts are also accepted when available and the patience and concentration of out trainees soon turns them into fast reliable workmen.

The most popular service provided by the Technical Department is the hearing aid advisory service under which any hearing aid user who suspects his aid might be faulty can bring it in for a check over. After it has been examined and put through response tests he is given a written report indicating what, if anything, is wrong and how it can be put right . . .

Medical research is something the Institute has not attempted yet. The cost has been far beyond us for one thing, but we co-operate with hospital research departments in any way we can, evolve instruments and advise on sound proofing and noise measurements. Research into hearing aids is a simpler matter and we are becoming more and more involved in this, especially in regard to Medresco improvements.

A very important development has been our audiometer calibration and repair scheme, under which almost every hospital hearing clinic as well as individual users, send this essential instrument for checking once a year . . . At the present moment we are conducting an official survey into the use, maintenance and condition of audiometers in hospitals all over the country.

The nearest we have come to real medical assistance is in supporting the Department of Psychiatry for the Deaf at Whittingham Hospital, Preston, where Dr John Denmark, the only psychiatrist in the United Kingdom able to communicate manually with pre-lingually deaf people tries to help (and indeed can often completely re-assess) deaf patients who have been considered to be in need of mental care. The Institute has also set up an out-patient clinic in London for deaf people needing psychiatric help.

This historical snapshot incorporates much of the thinking and many of the features of voluntary sector provision in the early 1970s. The picture that emerges is fairly representative. There are some areas, however, in which the RNID can claim to be unique—for example, the Scientific and Technical Department with its emphasis on research and development; similarly, the unusually high priority given to the Library, which has no equivalent either in or outside the voluntary sector in the scope of its collection and the range of services it offers.

By the early 1980s the wind of change was blowing through the voluntary sector and, in common with other major disability organizations, the RNID began to re-examine its organizational role and structure. The changes which were contemplated were given impetus by the appointment of a new Chief Executive in 1986 and an influx of senior managers with business-oriented management training. The Institute's new image was unveiled by the Chief Executive in the following extracts from a policy statement published in *Soundbarrier* in March 1987:

How best can we achieve our objective of ensuring that deaf people have, as of right, a quality of life equal to that of the hearing community? As a voluntary organisation, free to choose our priorities and style, it goes without saying that we must encourage deaf people to become involved at all levels with our work.

In comparison with the national network of health, education, social and employment services, the resources of the Institute are minute. We must, therefore, seek to influence the policies and practices of those people, be they in the public or private sector, who have the resources and the authority to change and improve the quality of life of deaf people.

Such a strategy, compared with just providing services ourselves, has impli-cations for the style and shape of the organisation. The Council of the RNID in October 1986 agreed two basic criteria for determining our future work:

● Work which develops direct services and opportunities for hearing impaired people.

● Work which is aimed at the hearing community and thereby directly or indirectly develops or improves services and opportunities for hearing impaired people.

In order to implement the first of these criteria, a substantial part of the Institute's work will be concerned with innovation and research. The RNID will need to develop services appropriate to specific groups in such areas as health, education, employment, social work, communication and 'rights'. In order to implement the second criterion, the RNID will need to devise strategies for identifying areas of concern and advocating ways of overcoming the problems . . .

Since arriving at the institute as Chief Executive ten months ago, I have been asked to consider the following issues which the Institute is now actively pursuing:

The shortage of interpreters

Employment for deaf people

Communication with hearing people

Deaf people in prisons and secure hospitals

Training for social workers working with deaf people

The development of deaf-hearing telephone communication

The problems faced by elderly hard of hearing people

Services for deaf-blind people

The total list is much longer and we cannot deal with all of these matters alone. We will seek to work with others so as to maximise effort. The challenge is there, and I believe the approach I have outlined will ensure that the RNID has a clear and powerful role which can be appreciated and understood by everyone involved with it.

The areas where change has been most noticeable are campaigning and regionally based activity. Public relations had long been acknowledged to be the Institute's weak point, and the necessary staff expansion in this area has been amply rewarded by the success of its recent Fair Hearing Campaign aimed at improving National Health Service provision of hearing aids, by reducing hospital waiting lists through the introduction of 'community dispensing' via general practitioners (GPs). Although some of the Campaign's proposals have been labelled impractical by professionals in the field, the Government will be taking them on board for consideration in its forthcoming review of the hearing aid service.

Given that the Institute was set up specifically to be a central organization, it is not surprising that it has never had a strong regional presence, and was becoming increasingly conscious of its lack of grass-roots contacts. This is now changing, with the establishment of five regional offices—not to act as mini-RNIDs in the provinces, but to concentrate on developing local provision through training. The Griffiths report on community care will have a profound influence on the development of community services, with local authorities in future contacting many of their services to voluntary organizations. The RNID is responding to this opportunity by actively seeking contractual arrangements with local authorities, although the question of how a voluntary organization can effectively maintain its traditional role as an independent monitor of provision when it is itself providing services on a commercial basis, has yet to be resolved.

7.10 The National Deaf Children's Society

Harry Cayton* (1990)

The National Deaf Children's Society (NDCS) is the only national charity especially concerned with the needs of deaf children and their families. The Society represents deaf children's interests nationally and locally and supports parents through a large network of self-help groups. It provides advice on welfare, education, health and audiology, publishes information on all aspects of childhood deafness and gives grants for holidays, education, research and equipment for children and families in need.

The Society was founded in 1944 by a small group of parents determined to see an improvement in educational provision and in educational standards for deaf children. The Society has remained essentially a parents' organization acting in the interests of the consumers of the health, social services and educational systems. However, both nationally and locally, professionals, including teachers, doctors, audiologists and social workers, enter into partnerships with parents, grandparents, and deaf people themselves, to promote the interests of deaf children.

The Society is democratically organized. Local groups (known as Regional Associations) are autonomous and elect their own officers and committees. They raise and spend money locally, paying a small annual fee to the national society. Each Regional Association can send a representative to the National Council which meets three times a year. The National Council is the main policy making body of the Society.

The National Society is managed by an elected committee drawn from the members of the society. Elections are held each year and every member has a vote. The National Management Committee comprises mainly parents, who bring their expertise in business, banking, education, administration and commerce, to serve the charity. The senior voluntary members of the Society are the Chairman (supported by a Vice-Chairman) and the Honorary Treasure (supported by a Honorary Deputy Treasurer).

The Management Committee appoints a Director and Staff. In 1989 there were twenty-three full-time staff in five departments divided between Centres in London and Birmingham. The Society's professional staff include qualified social workers, teachers of deaf children, information, library and computer specialists and qualified counsellors. Its five departments cover education, health and social services, information and publications, technology and administration, finance and fund raising.

---

*Director, The National Deaf Children's Society.

The Society's key activities include:

- essential information on all aspects of childhood deafness;
- independent advice on education, including pre-school services, placement in schools and units, Statements and Records of Special Educational Needs, further education and careers;
- an advice, advocacy and counselling service to families of deaf children;
- welfare and holiday grants to families of deaf children;
- independent advice on Attendance Allowance, Severe Disablement Allowance, Income Support and other state benefits;
- a Festival of Performing Arts every year;
- an Annual Scholarship and other bursaries to help train teachers of the deaf, and to help others improve their skills in working with deaf children;
- courses for parents and professionals;
- a wide range of publications, videos and children's books;
- grants for educational and medical research;
- radio hearing aids to deaf children, or a donation of these to schools and individuals;
- advice to families and deaf children on hearing aids and environmental aids;
- working with other national and overseas organizations;
- representing the needs of deaf children and their families to parliament and government departments;
- a network of voluntary Welfare and Education Representatives across the UK;
- helping to run a support group for children with Treacher Collins syndrome, or allied conditions, and their families;
- supporting research into the integration of deaf children in mainstream schools;
- research grants in audiology and education for universities and hospitals.

The National Deaf Children's Society's development plan for the 1990s includes a greater commitment to the involvement of young deaf people in its decision-making processes, and to greater access for minority groups to its services. In a multicultural society, voluntary organizations must ensure that equal opportunities are an essential part of their working methods, not merely an added extra. The Society was the first voluntary organization in the deaf field to introduce equal opportunities and anti-racist training for all staff and to develop an equal opportunities access policy agreed by its National Council. Publications are currently available in six languages, and audio and video information cassettes are being produced. Deaf people are employed by the Society at all levels and serve on all the Society's committees. Sign language interpreters are provided for staff and voluntary members and all staff have an opportunity to learn basic signing skills.

As demands on the Society's services grow, particularly from parents who are dissatisfied with health and education provision in their area, the Society is committing more and more of its resources to improving the effectiveness of local groups. To this end, training for local Welfare Representatives and Education Representatives has been introduced. Qualified representatives will be able to handle a wide range of enquiries in their chosen area and to assist parents with access to local services. The cost of training, support, and the expenses of volunteers, are met by the National Society. It is hoped that by 1994 more than 100 Education and Welfare Representatives will have been trained.

During the first part of the 1990s the Society will be restructuring its services in order to improve access and provide a more national service. A third centre will be opened, concentrating on family support, to complement the National Office in London and the Technology Information Centre in Birmingham. As well as providing a more comprehensive support for families and children with particular problems, the Society plans to improve the range and quality of its already extensive publications list and to provide more regular benefits for ordinary members.

1994 will see the 50th Anniversary of the National Deaf Children's Society; despite changing times in education, the Society remains committed, as its founders were, to *quality* in education and *choice* for parents and children. The NDCS welcomes as members all those who have the interests of deaf children at heart, whether they be natural auralists, supporters of Total Communication or bilingual approaches, or advocates of Cued Speech. Equally, the Society recognizes that integrated education may benefit some children and education in special schools maybe more appropriate for others. What matters is the quality of the education and the opportunity for deaf children to develop their potential.

The Society is not a slave to dogma or ideology but a real society: a community of members whose views are as varied as the needs of the deaf children they seek to help and encourage. In its 50th Anniversary year, the Society hopes to be able to look back on real progress in education, welfare and public and political attitudes towards deaf children, and also forward to greater co-operation, higher standards of achievement, greater choice for parents and a more active role for deaf people in society.

Section 8
Deafness Portrayed: Deaf People in Film and Fiction

Systematic information concerning popular notions of deafness is difficult to come by. We originally hoped that studies of deaf people in film and fiction would provide an insight into public constructions of deafness. It appears, however, that film and fiction, rather than reflecting popular views of the lives and culture of deaf people, appropriate deafness to their own ends and use it as a device within essentially hearing contexts. They almost invariably create a simplistic view of deaf people, who are generally portrayed as either totally good or totally bad, as stupid or as having amazing powers of lipreading. These mythical deaf people generally appear individually so that interaction between deaf people is rarely seen. Schuchman's suggestion that 'the deaf community does not exist in film or television, only deafness and deaf individuals do' may be applied equally to fiction.

The recent introduction into film and television of deaf people using sign language may represent early indications of a changing emphasis and an awareness of deaf people as a linguistic minority rather than as a disability group. There is perhaps some evidence that the simple assimilation of deaf people into hearing cultural productions may be changing as deaf fictional characters become more actively involved in dramatic dialogue.

8.1 Deafness in Fiction

Susan Gregory (1990)

Although a number of deaf characters have appeared in novels and short stories in both classical and popular literature,[1] there has been little fictional writing which has shown an awareness of sign language and Deaf culture[2] which are significant issues for the Deaf community today. The representation of deaf people in literature has been from an essentially hearing viewpoint, and the deaf characters who appear have rarely established themselves as credible people but are usually merely caricatures or useful devices within the story. They are generally portrayed as totally good or, more occasionally, totally bad. Sometimes they are attributed with mystical powers, sometimes they serve as mirrors to reflect aspects of the hearing world while having no identity of their own. Occasionally, the fact that they cannot hear is simply used as a device for furthering the plot.

Studying deaf characters in fiction thus tells us remarkably little about deafness itself, but does tell us something about misconceptions which may influence popular notions of deafness. While it is beyond the scope of one short article to give a comprehensive account of deaf people in literature,[3] it is hoped, by sampling a number of representative stories, to give some indication of how deafness is constructed within fiction.[4]

Where deaf people appear in fiction it seems that it is the deafness rather than the person which is of paramount importance. They are not real people who happen to be deaf, but deaf characters who, on the whole, appear not to be real people. Thus the recourse to stereotypes, and a glance at the titles of many of the novels indicate one of the more popular conventional representations of deafness: *In Silence* (1906), *A Silent Handicap* (1927), *David in Silence* (1965), *The Silent World of Nicholas Quinn* (1977), *The Listening Silence* (1982) and *The Rest is Silence* (1985). Thus, despite evidence that the world of deaf people is not without sound, novelists are keen to perpetuate the myth of a silent world.

A further stereotype endorses the idea that lack of hearing makes deaf people liable to be involved in accidents as a result of not being able to hear the sound of the danger or warnings concerning it. The following are but a few examples: 'The van's exhaust was making a hell of a noise, but without even turning her head the girl stepped out into the road' *(The Listening Silence);* 'She did not hear the car as it approached. When it hit the pram, her screams combined with the screaming of the brakes' *(Kilcaraig);* 'He had not heard the crackling of the flames as they ate their way down the corridor towards his room; he had not heard the shouts, the screams, or the siren of the lone Hastings fire truck as it howled through the night towards the blaze' *(The Acupuncture Murders).*

Thus, when deaf people appear in fiction their deafness often obtrudes to such an extent that it inhibits the development of complex characterizations. The personality of the individual is often irrelevant and the author is concerned merely with what are seen as essential concomitants of deafness: the inability to hear and, perhaps more erroneously, the ability to lipread in what might otherwise be considered impossible situations. These supposed features of deafness are then used as devices to further the plot. In *Gorky Park*, for example, the old woman who is deaf plays the '1812 Overture' and unwittingly covers the sound of the murder. A favourite of detective fiction writers is the lipreading powers attributed to deaf people, and at least two characters, Paulina Paine (in *The Listening Eye*) and Nicholas Quinn (in *The Silent World of Nicholas Quinn*), have been murdered because they lipread information they should not have had. Many would envy the lipreading powers attributed to Paulina Paine who was described as lipreading a long and complicated conversation giving times and places for a robbery. Bernard Guella (1983, see note 4) reports a story by Vivien Bretherton, *Charm*, written in 1926, where a woman who had become deaf testified in a court case, her testimony being based on her ability to lipread a boy's lips while he was three flights directly below her. Nicholas Quinn is more interesting in that a mistake in lipreading is at the crux of the plot: Quinn confuses the lip patterns of 'Doctor Bartlett' for those of 'Donald Martin'. Also in this story, improbable events are combined so that, although Quinn can talk, albeit with difficulty, on the telephone, he is unable to hear the noise of the fire bell. Such inconsistencies are not uncommon.

Inasmuch as deaf people are allowed characters, these are generally limited to demonstrations of goodness, or strength combined with silence in the face of oppression. In Turgenev's story of *Mumu*, the deaf servant Garasim is 'A fine figure of a fellow . . . he had a reputation for being the most punctual and obedient of all the village serfs . . . His perpetual silence lent a solemn dignity to his labours'. The story tells how he rescues a young puppy, Mumu, and cares for it. It becomes his companion, but his mistress orders it to be killed. He obeys the order, but then he leaves her service and walks the long distance back to the village in the country where he was born, and there he lives out his life alone. Riordan, who has published a translation of this story, suggests in his commentary that Turgenev was drawing a parallel with the Russian serfs that could be enslaved but not crushed.

A similar theme of silent strength occurs in the de Maupassant story, *The Deaf Mute*. Gargan, the deaf shepherd, is '. . . an excellent shepherd, devout, upright, knowing how to find all the members of his flock, although nobody had taught him anything'. In the story he kills his wife, but he conveys to the court by mime and gesture his profound anger at finding her with another man, and is acquitted, his master commenting, 'He knows what honour is this man does'. Batson (1980, see note 4) has argued that these stories, typical of the nineteenth century, were part of the moralistic writings of the time, the message being that if 'These brave afflicted souls, as hard a life as they have, still manage to live a moral heroic life, why can't you, who have such a comparatively easy life, also live up to high standards of moral conduct?'.

As indicated above, while the silence, which many authors see as an essential accompaniment to deafness is often viewed as a virtue, it may sometimes be introduced as a device to be used by hearing people. It is as if the deaf person's silence creates a vacuum to be filled by the hearing characters, or by the reader's own projections. McCay Vernon has written '. . . deaf characters in fiction are like rorschach blots, neutral stimuli onto which the author, the reader or other characters in the story can project their own fantasies about life' (reported in Batson, 1980, see note 4). One of the most obvious examples of deafness used to reflect back other characteristics is in *The Heart is a Lonely Hunter* by Carson McCullers, where the central figure John Singer, who is deaf without speech, is the recipient of the confidences of four other lonely people. The writer herself says, 'One of these five persons is a deaf mute, John Singer—and it is around him that the whole book pivots. Because of their loneliness these four people see in the mute a mystic superiority and he becomes in a sense their ideal. Because of Singer's infirmity, his outward character is vague and unlimited. His friends are able to impute to him all the qualities they would wish for him to have. Each of these four people creates his own understanding of the mute from his own desires. Singer can read lips and understand what is said to him. In his eternal silence there is something compelling. Each of these persons makes the mute a repository for his most personal feelings and ideals'. In this article on the outline of 'The Mute', the original title of the book, McCullers describes in detail the development of the characters within the novel. For the four other characters the description is detailed, taking on average two and a half pages. The description for Singer, however, is just one page, and in a revealing comment McCullers herself says, 'He is a flat character in the sense that from the second chapter on throughout the rest of the book his essential self does not change'.[5] Thus the central figure in the story is himself almost without intrinsic content.

Deaf people are rarely portrayed as equals in status to the hearing characters in works of fiction. Equality of status is, however, achieved in an interesting way in *The Listening Silence*. In the early chapters of the book the relationship between the mature Flying Officer, David Turner, and the innocent and immature Sally Barnes, seems doomed to failure. However, when David loses his voice in a flying accident, it is Sally who is the only person with whom he can easily converse without resorting to pencil and paper. Because of her deafness she has developed the ability to lipread. The relationship is thus able to flower. The equality is achieved, not through empathy and understanding, but by the simple expedient of disabling the main character.

Deafness has been employed by novelists in various ways to reveal aspects of the hearing characters and their lives. It has been used to create or magnify positive attributes of the hearing characters who, through association with the perceived virtue of deaf characters, enhance their own moral standing. It is as if disability can be compensated for by more intensified positive attributes, hence the supposed superior hearing of blind people often found in popular lay conceptions of blindness. Deaf people, however, are not accorded a heightened sense of sight, but silence, which is seen as a necessary concomitant of deafness, is considered a virtue with special meaning. In *The Golden Bird*, for example, the deaf girl, by her silent loyalty to the schoolmaster, restores his faith in human nature. 'But for you Sunniva, the schoolmaster would be a poor desolate unkempt creature. You have kept hope alive in me . . . I had no wish to live truly. But the fire was no sooner dead than you rekindled it.'

In both *Hide and Seek* and *Dr Marigold*, the deaf young girls exist as catalysts for the other characters. Through their assumed innocence, they transform the lives of those around them while having no life of their own. In *Dr Marigold*, the deaf Sophy lived to make others happy, by bringing comfort to the life of a man whose own daughter Sophy was beaten to death. In *Hide and Seek*, Madonna, a deaf girl, brings joy to the lives of Mr and Mrs Blythe who have no children of their own. The story is largely the attempt to discover Madonna's origins, while she, through her deafness, remains the mysterious figure around whom the plot unfolds.

Alongside moral superiority is the attribution of mystical powers to certain categories of disabled people. Perhaps the most famous example is the blind oracle of Delphi. Such powers have been granted to deaf people in stories from the earliest novels to the present day. *The History of Duncan Campbell*, by Defoe, is generally agreed to be fiction, though it is probably based on a real character whose life was described by Hawkins in a work on the deaf and dumb published in 1869.[6] The real Duncan Campbell was born in 1680, and renowned for his fortune-telling abilities, though it is, however, not even certain that he was deaf. In the Defoe story, Duncan Campbell was deaf, and famous for his magical powers, and the story includes numerous accounts of his uncanny ability to see into the future and make accurate predictions.

A twentieth-century novel also links mystical forces with deafness. In *Shrine*, by James Herbert, a young deaf girl is born with special innocence. 'She cannot speak, she cannot hear . . . A good child, a curious child. Her disability made her a solitary one. She was frail, yet seemed to carry an inner strength within that small body.' At the beginning of the novel, the child has visions of the lady in shining white who said she was the Immaculate Conception. The girl is able to perform miracles, and the site of her visitation becomes a shrine. By the end, however, she becomes corrupted, and her powers become forces for evil.

Despite, or perhaps because of, the superficial nature of their treatment of deaf characters, some authors attempt to achieve credibility for their portrayal of deafness by providing descriptions of contemporary educational practices with deaf adults and children. For example, in *The History of Duncan Campbell*, the style of writing is suggestive of a factual account and includes an interesting description of contemporaneous educational methods for teaching deaf children, in particular those of the renowned Dr Wallace, who favoured fingerspelling as a route to language. In *Too Much, Too Soon*, Briskin describes in detail a session at the John Tracy clinic, an actual institution in the USA famous for its oralist approach. *A Silent Handicap,* published in 1927, provides a particularly interesting account of the methods of education employed at that time when the transition to oral methods had been made, but teachers remained who were trained in, and sometimes committed to, approaches involving signing. The book includes several discussions of the issues, many of which differ little in form or content from similar debates today.

A Silent Handicap is unusual, not only because it mentions signing, but also it includes more than one deaf character. However, the interactions that occur are between individual deaf children or adults, and hearing people. The perspective remains essentially hearing. In most of the other stories described so far (apart from a section of *The Heart is a Lonely Hunter*) there has been only one deaf character, which has inhibited the development of realistic descriptions of the experience of deafness or valid accounts of the lives of Deaf people. The focus on individual deaf people has promoted themes of isolation and loneliness. It has also served to locate the problem of deafness within the individual. It is then the responsibility of the individual to adapt, and adaptation is usually taken to mean becoming as apparently 'normal' as possible and adopting the values of the hearing world. For example, Sally Barnes is described as '. . . sitting in the first row of class to facilitate her quite remarkable gift of lipreading; accepting the teacher's notes at the end of each session with a dignified nod of thanks' *(The Listening Silence).*

Joanne Greenberg is one of the few novelists to give a compelling account of Deaf people in her novel *In This Sign,* and her short story *And Sarah laughed.* In these she describes the life of a Deaf couple, Janice and Abel Ryder and their hearing daughter, Margaret. By locating the story within the Deaf experience she is able to explore ideas about what it could be like to be Deaf.

However, such stories are rare. Most existing fiction either uses deafness as a device to facilitate an essentially hearing plot, or perpetuates myths about deafness. The deaf person is portrayed mainly as a lonely and isolated person. Because the existence of a Deaf community and of sign language remains hidden, it appears that the only way of life is within the hearing world, and that the Deaf person is viewed only from a hearing perspective. Thus a study of 'Deafness in Fiction' reveals more about the hearing world than it does about Deaf people.

Notes

1   I have been collecting examples of deaf characters in fiction for a number of years, only a few of which are described here. Two collections of writings are particularly useful sources,

Grant, B. (1987) *The Quiet Ear: Deafness in Literature.* London, Andre Deutsch.

Batson, T.W. and Bergman, E. (1976) *The Deaf Experience: An Anthology of Literature by and about the Deaf,* 2nd edn, South Waterford, ME, The Merrian Eddy Co.

I am grateful to all those friends and colleagues, and to the staff of the library of the Royal National Institute for the Deaf, who have drawn to my attention various books with deaf characters. While the classics are usually known, more popular novels are harder to locate and I would be grateful for any further works drawn to my attention.

2   Following other authors (see Padden, this volume) I have followed the convention of using 'deaf' to refer to deafness defined by hearing loss, and 'Deaf' to distinctions based on a cultural notion of deafness. For reasons that become clear in the article, 'Deaf' is rarely used.

3   I have omitted childrens books, and some books published only in the USA, and have concentrated mainly on those where characters are either born deaf, or become deaf in early childhood, rather than adults who gradually lose their hearing as part of the ageing process. I have also omitted those stories, of which there are several, where deafness is feigned.

4   There have been several such previous accounts including the following:

Barnes, F.G. (1915) 'The Deaf in Literature', *The Teacher of the Deaf, 13.*

Batson, T. (1980) 'The Deaf Person in Fiction—From Sainthood to Rorschach Blot', *Bulletin of Interracial books for Children, 11.*

Guella, B. (1983) 'Short Stories with Deaf Fictional Characters', *American Annals of the Deaf.*

Guire, O. (1959) 'Deaf Mutes in Russian Literature', *The Silent Worker,* July 1959.

Guire, O. (1961, 1963) 'Deaf Characters in Literature', *The Silent Worker,* August 1961, July/August 1963.

Guire, O. (1965) 'More Books of Interest to the Deaf', *The Deaf American,* September 1965.

Lindholm, T. (1963) 'A Deaf Character in Charles Dickens's "Master Humphries Clock",' *The Silent Worker,* April 1963.

Panara, R.F. (1972) 'Deaf Characters in Fiction and Drama, *The Deaf American, 24.*

5   See Carson McCullers (1975) *The Mortgaged Heart,* London, Penguin Books. The particular essay to which reference is made, 'The Mute', was first published in 1966.

6   For a fuller account see *The British Deaf News,* February 1905.

Fictional works discussed in the text

Briskin, J. (1985) *Too Much, Too Soon,* London, Corgi Books.

Brown, G.M. (1987) *The Golden Bird,* London, John Murray.

Carothers, A. (1983) *Kilcaraig,* (first published 1982) London, Pan Books.

Coffman, V. (1985) *The Rest is Silence,* London, Judy Piatkus.

Collins, W. (1981) *Hide and Seek*, (first published 1854) London, Constable and Co.

Defoe, D. (1875) 'The Life and Adventures of Duncan Campbell', in *The Works of Daniel Defoe,* (first published 1720) Edinburgh, William P. Nimmo.

Denman, A. (1927) *A Silent Handicap,* London, Edward Arnold.

Dexter, C. (1978) *The Silent World of Nicholas Quinn,* (first published 1977) London, Pan books.

Dickens, C. (1972) *Dr Marigold,* (first published 1865) in Batson, T.W. and Bergman, E. (see note 1 above).

Greenberg, J. (1973) *In This Sign,* (first published 1970) London, Pan Books.

Greenberg, J. (1973) 'And Sarah laughed', in *Rites of Passage,* London, Victor Gollancz.

Herbert, J. (1983) *Shrine,* London, New English Library.

Joseph, M. (1982) *The Listening Silence,* London, Hutchinson.

de Maupassant, G. (1970) 'The Deaf Mute', in *The Complete Short Stories of Guy de Maupassant,* (first published late nineteenth century) London, Macmillan.

McCullers, C. (1981) *The Heart is a Lonely Hunter,* (first published 1943) London, King Penguin.

Reynolds, F. (1906): 'In Silence', discussed in Barnes, F.G., 'The Deaf in Literature', *The Teacher of the Deaf, 13.*

Robinson, V. (1965) *David in Silence,* London, Andre Deutsch.

Smith, M.C. (1981) *Gorky Park,* London, William Collins.

Steward, M.C. (1073) *The Acupuncture Murders,* London, Arthur Barker.

Turgenev, I. (1988) *Mumu,* Bradford, University of Bradford Press. (Original story first published 1852) translated by James Riordan.

Wentworth, P. (1977) *The Listening Eye,* (first published 1957) London, Coronet books.

8.2 Hollywood Speaks: Deafness and the Film Entertainment Industry

John S. Schuchman (1988)

[. . .]

What is the Hollywood image of deafness? In her analysis of the image of women in films, Molly Haskell uses the term 'the big lie' in concluding that the movie industry has served as a popular agent to foster and perpetuate the myth of women as the weaker sex.[1] Is there a comparable 'big lie' in the Hollywood depiction of deaf characters? If so, one must conclude that a collective Hollywood is guilty of the perpetuation of a pathological view of deafness as a disease and of deaf individuals as abnormal. At the same time, it is only fair to observe that the film industry did not invent this perspective.

Film-makers reflect the prevailing American cultural bias toward disability and deafness. There certainly exists a large network, both in the United States and abroad, of educational, rehabilitation and medical professionals who are dedicated to the proposition that deaf people, particularly children, have special needs that require their expertise. Unlike the professional who can take the time to deal with the complexities represented by deafness, movies try to convey their messages as simply as possible and, in doing so, often turn to formulas and stereotypes in their depiction of deafness. It is at this level that films have so much potential for harm. More than any other medium, they have popularized simple-minded views of deafness. This survey of film and television entertainment programmes clearly demonstrates that the deaf community has every right to complain about the practices of Hollywood in the industry's depiction of deafness up to the present.

Often described as the invisible handicap, deafness remains a mystery to most Americans. The motion picture industry has contributed little to a better understanding of the deaf community. Historically, Hollywood's ideal deaf person has been truly invisible—other than the inability to hear, the stereotyped movie ideal invariably speaks clearly and reads lips with unfailing accuracy—both unrealistic exaggerations. Talking motion pictures have continued the negative image of deafness established in silent films. Often, a movie ends with a cure through an experimental drug (*And Now Tomorrow*), an operation (*Flesh and Fury*), or a psychologically traumatic event (*The Story of Esther Costello*). When the character's deafness cannot be cured, the film ends with the character acquiring speech, the symbol of success for the 'dumb' individual (*The Miracle Worker*). In common with the depiction of other disabled figures, the deaf character contemplates suicide (*Sincerely Yours*); and like his or her literary brethren, the deaf character often serves as a symbol for loneliness and alienation (*The Heart Is a Lonely Hunter*). Hollywood has avoided deaf couples or families, and movies very rarely have more than one deaf character. With two exceptions, in 1926 (*You'd Be Surprised*) and most recently in 1986 (*Children of a Lesser God*), actors who could hear always played the role of the deaf persons in theatrically released films. Until 1979, in the movie *Voices*, audiences had not heard real deaf speech from a deaf adult character. Only deaf children, usually portrayed by a class from nearby schools for deaf children, have difficulty with speech.

In Hollywood's view there is little or no humour in deafness. This has been particularly true since the demise of silent motion pictures. Of the more than one hundred movies and television programmes produced since the advent of sound technology, only three associate a deaf character with humour.[2] Westerns and horror films constitute less than a half-dozen films involving deafness; all of the rest are melodramas. In the movie houses of America, deaf people are usually victims, either to be pitied or cured. It is clear that the Hollywood stereotypes of deaf persons as either 'dummies' or 'perfect lipreaders' represent the extremes, which rarely are encountered in the real world.

Deafness is a disability in a society that communicates primarily through sound and speech. Deaf persons have been killed by oncoming automobiles and trains that they could not hear, shot by policemen with whom they could not communicate easily, incarcerated in mental institutions and jailed by professionals who misunderstood and misdiagnosed them and their deafness. They have been denied equal employment opportunities by individuals who equate good speech and English skills with intelligence. It is on this aspect of deafness that Hollywood has focused its camera lens.

There is another view, however. In the past, some deaf people accepted the fact that they would never hear and, as a result, developed cultural reponses to a dominant hearing society that could not and would not assimilate them. At least as early as the antebellum nineteenth century, there emerged a deaf community replete with its own social organization, schools, churches, clubs, self-help societies, newspapers and magazines, and language. In spite of the fact that the American deaf community is considered to be the most independent and progressive such community in the world, and that within the United States the Los Angeles (the spiritual if not geographical centre of Hollywood) deaf community is considered to be one of the most assertive and politically astute groups at the local level, the normal activities of this community are largely unknown to the public, and no movie or television script has dealt with its existence or activities at a substantive level. It is clear that the movie industry has been a primary vehicle for the transmission and perpetuation of an American cultural view that depicts deafness as a pathological condition. The deaf community does not exist in film or television, only deafness and deaf individuals do.

The reason for this is clear. Hollywood cannot or will not deal with the issue of language in the deaf community. Individual deaf characters are excellent victims. Like their blind counterparts, these characters look good; and since film-makers value a pleasing physical appearance, this explains why deafness and blindness predominate among disabled characters in film. It is no accident that in more than 80 years of film there have been no multiply disabled deaf characters depicted, with the exception of deaf-blind portrayals (of course, the deaf-blind characters have met the test of good looks). It is only when two deaf characters appear in a film together that communication difficulties are experienced. Even if they are physically attractive, how will the audience understand them?

As a practical matter, Hollywood treats the deaf community as a linguistic minority; and as such, it has avoided substantive depictions of American Sign Language. At the individual level, Hollywood consistently has its deaf characters speak orally or simply lets the audience guess at the meaning of the deaf character's limited signs. The 1948 film *Johnny Belinda* used a hearing character, the doctor (played by Lew Ayres), to provide contextual clues to the signed dialogue with the deaf character (played by Jane Wyman), but at the time this was an exception to the general film practice. Another 38 years passed before film-makers again used this technique, in *Children of a Lesser God*. Although this is not unlike the situation for Hispanic characters who must speak in accented English, it does explain why there are almost never two deaf characters in the same film. (The two notable exceptions are *The Heart Is a Lonely Hunter* and *Voices*; but in both films, when the two deaf characters communicate in signs, the audience is left to guess at the meaning of the dialogue.) Note that in *Children of a Lesser God*, when James (William Hurt) appears lost and isolated at the party of deaf people, the audience also has no idea what the deaf characters at the party are saying since he is not interpreting their signs.

The obvious solution to this dilemma is the use of captions, but the movie industry consistently has rejected their use since the transition from silent to talking motion pictures in the late twenties. In spite of occasional use of captions for foreign-language dialogue in such films as *The Longest Day* and *Patton*, theatrical films and television have opposed the use of open captions with the rationale that general audiences dislike them. This result has reduced the ability of scriptwriters to get beyond simple-minded dialogue for non-speaking deaf characters and has perpetuated the practice of separate viewing for deaf audiences. In *Johnny Belinda* and *Children of a Lesser God*, the dialogue is complex, but the deaf person is wedded to a hearing person's voice, which reinforces the image of the deaf person as dependent.

This image has not been exclusively negative, however: *Johnny Belinda* did make a difference by demonstrating that deafness could be portrayed substantively and still turn a profit. After the film's success, there was a significant increase in the number of deaf characters in the movies and on television during the 1950s and following decades. Although many of the stereotypes continued unabated, there were films and telvision episodes that provided information to the general public about new developments in medicine, education, hearing-aid technology, and telecommunication devices. In 1968, *The Heart Is a Lonely Hunter* presented an English-literate non-speaking deaf person, and finally, in 1979, the first professional deaf person, a teacher, appeared in *Voices*.

Unfortunately, the only three theatrical films produced in the first half of the eighties that deal with deafness appear to have returned to some of the old formulas. *Eyes of a Stranger* once again shows the cure of a deaf-blind-mute female victim through the device of a traumatic attack by a rapist. And although the screenwriters wrapped *Amy* in a historical guise, that story celebrates the triumph of articulation (lipreading and speech) over dependence on sign language and a parochial deaf community. Finally, the most powerful and potentially independent deaf character to appear in motion pictures, Sarah, in *Children of a Lesser God*, is a cleaning woman who is dependent on a man who earns his living as a speech teacher.

In contrast, television has broken many of the prevalent stereotypes about deafness. A wide range of deaf adult characters have appeared as attorneys, illiterates, dancers, prostitutes, stuntwomen and teachers; and they have been allowed to speak with clear voices or speech-impaired voices, or to remain mute. Although loneliness prevails in the continued predominance of melodramas, deaf couples have appeared in two television movies: *And Your Name Is Jonah* and *Love Is Never Silent*. The most significant and hopeful sign has been the appearance of deaf actors in the roles of deaf characters: since 1968 they have appeared with increasing frequency, capped by the December 1985 Hallmark Hall of Fame presentation of *Love Is Never Silent*, starring deaf actors Phyllis Frelich and Ed Waterstreet and produced by Julianna Fjeld, who is also deaf.

Even though many of the earlier and more pejorative filmic views of deafness will continue to appear on late-night television and on videotape recorders (through rentals), there has been a discernible change in the direction of the depiction of deafness in the eighties, led by television programming.[3] Since much of television continues to be produced in Hollywood, we can only hope that theatrical films will reflect these positive changes within the near future.

Some credit for this recent change in direction for television must be attributed to the presence of deaf persons as actors, technical advisers, and, most recently, as producers. Although most film-makers would not accept the analogy of white actors in blackface, many in the deaf community perceive the continued use of hearing actors in the role of deaf characters as a present-day example of that silent era practice. When Daniel Wilson, the producer of the television programme 'Mom and Dad Can't Hear Me', responded to charges of discrimination by deaf actress Audree Norton, he argued that film-makers should not limit deaf roles to deaf actors. Even though the facts are that less than 10 per cent of the deaf character roles have been played by deaf actors and that virtually all of these have been on television, his argument struck a familiar and responsive chord in Hollywood. While the evidence makes his argument shallow, his rhetoric reflects a basic principle: actors should be free to play any role. Certainly, the testimony of the actors is clear.

Anthony Quinn, referring to his role as Deaf Smith, observed (or at least his publicist did) that 'if every actor could play a deaf-mute once, it would be the best thing that could happen to him. I had to react to everything and everyone around me. It was a terrific experience for an actor'.[4] Alan Arkin recognized that deaf people are as 'multicolored and varied emotionally as they can be', but the 'one thing that the affliction does seem to cause is a great sense of isolation'.[5] In an effort to replicate the experience, Arkin watched television without sound and learned that a deaf lipreader watches the face, not the lips.[6] Jane Wyman worked hard to capture the look of deafness, stuffing her ears with wax and arranging for a young deaf woman to visit her regularly. She strove for a look that tried to anticipate and guess at the meaning of the spoken word.[7]

All of this, of course, misses the point, because these excellent actors focused on the absence of hearing, not of deafness. Although there are actors who are oriented to a visual mode of communication, there have been few of them since the silent era. To use recent examples, the deaf actresses Phyllis Frelich and Marlee Matlin have few peers, among their hearing colleagues, in the use of facial expression and body language, not to mention sign language itself. Their portrayals of the charming deaf prostitute in 'Barney Miller', the deaf mother of a hearing daughter in the television movie *Love Is Never Silent*, and Sarah in *Children of a Lesser God* exemplify the best of a long tradition of deaf actors and expose the shallowness of weak imitations by hearing actors.

Perhaps the silent film actor Lon Chaney understood this better than anyone else. Even with the high-tech gadgetry of modern film-making, few actors have been able to surpass Chaney's ability to master the look of a character. Although he was gifted at make-up artistry, he understood that characterization was more than cosmetics. This son of deaf parents understood, instinctively and experientially, what it meant to be different as well as to look different. Accordingly, he created memorable character-izations that remain classics today. So far, Hollywood has had limited success with the look of deafness.

Although some of the films discussed in this survey demonstrate insights into individual aspects of deafness, none of them deals with deafness in a way that reflects a cultural understanding of deaf people. Until film-makers portray the existence of an active and healthy deaf community, it is improbable that Americans will get beyond the pathologi-cal myths that make daily life difficult for deaf individuals. In this sense, films continue to serve as a major source of public misinformation about deafness and deaf people. The deaf community awaits the next step in the industry's portrayal of deafness.

Earlier, I observed that the deaf community has a right to complain about its treatment by film-makers; at the same time, I have been puzzled by the comparative absence of complaints. A few petitions in 1929 and a boycott 50 years later, in 1979, hardly represents significant protest. Much of this, I believe, can be attributed to our national policy of segregated film and television viewing for deaf audiences. Deafness is a disability of communication. And it is my opinion that the deaf community literally does not appreciate how badly they have fared at the hands of the entertainment industry. For most of the period covered by this survey of film and television, deaf viewers have not been given precise information about the dialogues that accompany the images on the screen. For example, within the past several months, *Beau Bandit* (1930), *Charlie Chan at the Olympics* (1936), *No Road Back* (1957), and *For the First Time* (1959) have appeared on television stations in the Washington, DC, area. Despite the presence of what is considered to be the best-educated deaf community, Washington deaf audiences had no information about the audio content of these films because, like most past and current films, they were not captioned.

Even though most current prime-time network television programmes are captioned for use with television decoders, the overwhelming majority of the films and episodes described in this survey, and in the Filmography, are not captioned. And, as exemplified by the appearance of old films in the Washington, DC, television market, this backlog of films and episode reruns will continue to haunt the deaf community through the depiction of misinformation about deaf people. Simple equity requires that the industry, or the federal government, if need be, correct this communication imbalance with the provision of captioned versions so that the deaf community is fully informed. A society committed to a policy of equal access for all of its citizens can do no less.

Notes

1 Molly Haskell, (1974) *From Reverence to Rape: The Treatment of Women in Movies*, New York, Penguin Books, pp. 1–41.

2 The three are: *Pocketful of Miracles* (United Artists, 1961), *Good Times* (CBS, 1975), and *Barney Miller* (ABC, 1981).

3 Although I do not agree that this has occurred with commercial films about deafness, this positive change has been observed for other disabilities. See Paul K. Longmore, '"Mask": A Revealing Portrayal of the Disabled', *Los Angeles Times Sunday Calendar*, 5 May 1985, pp. 22–3; and Longmore, 'Screening Stereotypes: Images of Disabled People', *Social Policy*, Summer 1985, pp. 36–7.

4 '*Deaf Smith and Johnny Ears:* MGM Pressbook', C–37, Motion Picture, Broadcasting, and Recorded Sound Division, Library of Congress.

5 Alan Arkin to Virginia S. Carr, Personal Correspondence, 22 September 1970, Manuscript Department, Duke University, Durham, NC.

6 Robert E. Miller. Transcript: American Film Institute Screenwriting Workshop, 22 March 1977, Beverly Hills, CA, Center for Advanced Film Studies, 1977, pp. 26–7.

7 Joe Morella and Edward Epstein, *Jane Wyman, A Biography*, New York, Delacorte Press, p. 115.

Source list for articles

Section 1 Deafness: Whose Perspective?

1.1 Learning to be Deaf: Carol Padden and Tom Humphries
From Carol Padden and Tom Humphries (1988) *Deaf in America: Voices From a Culture*, London, Harvard University Press (from Chapter 1).

1.2 Everyone Here Spoke Sign Language: Nora Groce
From Nora Groce (1985) *Everyone Here Spoke Sign Language: Hereditary Deafness on Martha's Vineyard*, London, Harvard University Press (from Chapters 5 and 6).

Section 2 Defining the Deaf Community

2.1 Outsiders in a Hearing World: Paul Higgins
From Paul Higgins (1980) *Outsiders in a Hearing World: A Sociology of Deafness*, London, Sage Publications (from Chapter 2).

2.2 The Role of Sign in the Structure of the Deaf Community: Lilian Lawson
From Lilian Lawson (1981) 'The Role of Sign and the Structure of the Deaf Community', in Bencie woll, Jim Kyle and Margaret Deuchar (eds) *Perspectives in British Sign Language and Deafness*, London, Croom Helm (from Chapter 10).

2.3 The Modern Deaf Community: Paddy Ladd
From Paddy Ladd (1988) 'The Modern Deaf Community', in Dorothy Miles, *British Sign Language*, London, BBC Books (from Chapter 2).

2.4 The Deaf Community and the Culture of Deaf People: Carol Padden
From Carol Padden (1980) 'The Deaf Community and the Culture of Deaf People', in Carol Baker and Robert Battison (eds) *Sign Language and the Deaf Community: Essays in Honour of William Stokoe*, Silver Springs, MD, National Association of the Deaf, USA.

2.5 Is There a Deaf Culture?: David Brien
From David Brien, 'Is There a Deaf Culture Available to the Deaf Young Person?' Paper from the Study Weekend, Loughborough, 1981, National Council of Social Workers with the Deaf.

Section 3 Psychological Perspectives: Understanding Difference or Different Understandings?

3.1 Cognition and Language: Stephen Quigley and Peter Paul
From Stephen Quigley and Peter Paul (1984) *Language and Deafness*, San Diego, College Hill Press and London, Croom Helm (from Chapter 2).

3.2 Looking for Meaning in Sign Language Sentences: Jim Kyle
From Jim Kyle (1983) 'Looking for Meaning in Sign Language Sentences', in Jim Kyle and Bencie Woll (eds) *Language in Sign*, London, Croom Helm (from Part Four).

3.3 Surdophrenia: Terje Basilier
From Terje Basilier (1964) 'Surdophrenia', *Acta Psychiatrica Scandinavica Supplementium*, 40, (1980) pp. 363–372.

3.4 Is There a 'Psychology of the Deaf'?: Harlan Lane
From Harlan Lane (1988) 'Is there a "Psychology of the Deaf?"', in *Exceptional Children*, Vol. 55 No. 1 pp. 7–19, 1988.

Section 4 Audiology and Technology: From Description to Prescription

4.1 Basic Acoustics: Barry McCormick
From Barry McCormick (1988) *Screening for Hearing Impairment in Young Children*, London, Croom Helm (from Chapter 1).

4.2 Assessment of Impaired Hearing: William Noble
From William Noble (1978) *Assessment of Impaired Hearing: A Critique and a New Method*, London, Academic Press (from Chapter 7).

4.3 The Hearing Aid as a System: Ivan Tucker and Michael Nolan
From Ivan Tucker and Michael Nolan (1984) *Educational Audiology*, London, Croom Helm (from Chapter 4).

6.3   Sign Languages of Deaf People and Psycholinguistics: A. van Uden
From A. van Uden (1986) *Sign Language of Deaf People and Psychologuistics: A Critical Evaluation*, Swets, North America Inc. (from Chapters 2 and 3).

6.4   Tell Me Where is Grammar Bred?: 'Critical Evaluation' or Another Chorus of 'Come back to Milano'?: William Stokoe
From William Stokoe (1987) 'Tell Me Where is Grammar Bred? "Critical Evaluation" or Another Chorus of "Come back to Milano"?', *Sign Language Studies, 54*, Spring.

6.5   What Sign Language Research Can Teach Us About Language Acquisition: Virginia Volterra
From Virginia Volterra (1986) 'What Sign Language Research Can Teach Us About Language Acquisition', in Tervoot, B. (ed.) *Signs of Life; Proceedings of the Second European Congress on Sign Language Research*, The Institute of General Linguistics of the University of Amsterdam, publication no. 50.

6.6   A Stimulus to Learning, a Measure of Ability: T. Stewart Simpson
Commissioned article.

6.7   British Sign Language Tutor Training Course: A. Clark Denmark
Commissioned article.

Section 7   Social Welfare: Enabling or Disabling?

7.1   The Development of Local Voluntary Societies for Adult Deaf Persons in England: Kenneth Lysons
From Kenneth Lysons (1979) 'The Development of Local Voluntary Societies for Adult Deaf Persons in England', *British Deaf News*, 38 Victoria Place, Carlisle, UK.

7.2   Deaf People, Ethnic Minorities and Social Policy: George Taylor
From George Taylor (1986) 'Deaf People, Ethnic Minorities and Social Policy', *Journal of the National Council of Social Workers With Deaf People, 2*, no. 2.

7.3   The State, Social Work and Deafness: David Parratt and Brenda Tipping
From David Parratt and Brenda Tipping (1986) 'The State, Social Work and Deafness', *Journal of the National Council of Social Workers With Deaf People, 2*, no. 4.

7.4   Sign Language Interpreting: An Emerging Profession: Liz Scott-Gibson
Commissioned article.

7.5   Social Work and Interpreting: David Moorhead
Commissioned article.

7.6   'We' Are Not Disabled, 'You' Are: Vic Finkelstein
Commissioned article.

7.7   Deaf People and Minority Groups in the UK: Jim Kyle
From Jim Kyle (1986) 'Deaf People and Minority Groups in the UK', in Tervoort, B. (ed.) *Signs of Life; Proceedings of the Second European Congress on Sign Language Research*, The Institute of General Linguistics of the University of Amsterdam, publication no. 50.

7.8   The British Deaf Association: The Voice of the Deaf Community: British Deaf Association
Commissioned article.

7.9   The Development of The Royal National Institute for the Deaf: The Royal National Institute for the Deaf
Commissioned article.

7.10   The National Deaf Children's Society: Harry Cayton
Commissioned article.

Section 8   Deafness Portrayed: Deaf People in Film and Fiction

8.1   Deafness in Fiction: Susan Gregory
Commissioned article.

8.2   Hollywood Speaks: Deafness and the Film Entertainment Industry: John S. Schuchman
From John S. Schuchman (1988) *Hollywood Speaks; Deafness and the Film Industry*, Chicago, University of Illinois Press (from the Conclusion).

Index

(NOTE: The alphabetical arrangement of this index is in word-by-word order. Prepositions etc. at the beginning of subheadings have been ignored in determining the alphabetical order of subheadings. Numbers in italics refer to an article by the person so annotated; the word *passim* means that the subject so annotated is referred to in scattered passages throughout the pages indicated. 'n' means that the reference is in a note on the page mentioned. Emboldened numbers refer to a table or a figure.)